PSYCHOTHERAPY OF ABUSED AND NEGLECTED CHILDREN

Psychotherapy of Abused and Neglected Children

John W. Pearce
Terry D. Pezzot-Pearce

THE GUILFORD PRESS
New York London

© 1997 The Guilford Press
A Division of Guilford Publications, Inc.
72 Spring Street, New York, NY 10012

Printed in the United States of America

This book is printed on acid-free paper.

Last digit is print number: 9   8   7   6   5   4   3   2   1

Library of Congress Cataloging-in-Publication Data

Pearce, John W.
    Psychotherapy of abused and neglected children / by John W. Pearce
and Terry D. Pezzot-Pearce.
        p. cm.
    Includes bibliographical references and index.
    ISBN 1-57230-163-5
    1. Abused children – Rehabilitation. 2. Child psychotherapy.
I. Pezzot-Pearce, Terry D. II. Title
RJ507.A29P43 1997
618.92′ 8582230651 – dc20   96-43650
                                                                     CIP

To Clarissa, Timothy, and Kathleen

Acknowledgments

W E WISH to thank the many people who have helped us while we were writing this book. Dr. Eric Mash of the University of Calgary encouraged us to begin the project and introduced us to The Guilford Press, where Seymour Weingarten, Editor-in-Chief, and Rochelle Serwator were instrumental in the development of the manuscript. They guided two novice authors through the sometimes overwhelming process of writing a book with patience and generous assistance, and their insightful comments and rigorous standards improved the book immeasurably. We also wish to thank Jeannie Tang of The Guilford Press for shepherding the project through the production process. Helen Holmes gave us incisive advice and feedback at a critical juncture in the life of the manuscript.

The staff of the Child Abuse Program at Alberta Children's Hospital provided John with an unending supply of encouragement and friendship. The Program's clinical excellence has stimulated his thinking and practice for many years. John also wishes to thank the former manager of the program, Pat Dougan, and the current manager, Keith Donaghy, for their personal and professional support. Barbara Saies-Jones typed a rambling first draft with her typical efficiency and good humor.

We have disguised the identities of all children and families mentioned in the book; some of the clinical material is a compilation of cases. Although we cannot divulge their identities, it has been a privilege to serve these children and many others over the years. They have taught us much. Our young clients' courage and resiliency in surmounting their histories of abuse and neglect and their will to live happy and productive lives are testaments to the strength of the human spirit.

We have been lucky to have good friends: Doug and Diane Lindbloom, Jane Matheson, David Westelmajer, Karen Walsh, Don Schwartz, Pat Grayton, Elva Jolly, Pat Petrie, and Peter and Vango Smith have always stood by us. Our parents, Claire Pearce and Bob and Vicki Pezzot have, as usual, sustained us with their love and support, as have our sister and brother-in-law, Susan and John Kennedy. Finally, we want to thank our children. Clarissa, Tim, and Kathleen have magnanimously tolerated two parents who, at times, have been preoccupied and distracted. We wish to thank them for their boundless love, and for teaching us everyday what is truly important in our lives.

Foreword

THE URGE to simplify is extremely powerful. Human beings seem to be able to tolerate complexity for only brief periods of time. If one charts the course of scientific thought, particularly our thinking as it pertains to mental health conditions, one can recognize the oscillation from complexity to simplicity. This pattern cycles over and over again.

The simplistic pre-Freudian concept that mentally ill people were possessed was followed by a more complex and humanistic way of thinking, in which the morality of the individual did not enter into the equation. The mental health movement was then followed by the disease model in which gross brain structures were implicated in the emergence of psychiatric conditions. This simplistic notion was then followed by an extremely complex perspective that tried to recognize not only the relationship of a number of environmental factors to emotional disorders, but attempted to explain why it is that some people "weather" these environmental storms whereas others do not.

In the last decade or so we have entered into another period in which simple thinking has taken hold. This is an age represented by a new reductionism. The search for a gene that is responsible for each mental condition is going full bore, and psychopharmacologic treatments are de rigueur. Scientists seem to be unfazed by the fact that single gene theories are outdated or that other research groups cannot identify the same gene–behavior relationship. Treatment intervention studies which point to the efficacy of a combined approach that utilizes cognitive therapy and pharmacotherapy for the treatment of depression get ignored by practitioners who buy into the "chemical imbalance theory."

A recently published meta-analysis of the pharmacotherapy literature on the treatment of children's psychiatric problems points to essentially no consistent treatment effect of pharmacotherapy in the treatment of children's psychiatric problems (Thurber, Ensign, Punnett, & Welter, 1995). However, where I practice, that information certainly has not been incorporated into the clinical management of children. Parents continue to arrive for the first appointment looking for a chemical imbalance, and we, as professionals, continue to provide them with a simple answer. This is usually a chemical that contains a "Z" or "X" in the name. I have an urge to call this new reductionism the Z-factor era.

Given the above context, the authors of this book are ahead of their time in anticipating our field's return to a flirtation with a more complex perspective. As I see it, child neglect lacks panache, physical abuse is passé, emotional abuse is too hard to measure, and sexual abuse is really the only game in town. Witness the plethora of recent books on the treatment of sexually abused children. I say that fully admitting that I am in whole or in part responsible for three of those books.

The authors address the entire scope of parents' cruelty to children. We know that parents can be extremely cruel to children. I say that as both a parent and as a therapist. If we absolve parents of blame, we are assigning blame, in a way, to children, as we sometimes do with victims of crimes. An interesting finding is that victims would prefer to think that they could have done something about the trauma, because then it gives them an answer for how they can make a difference in the future (Briere, 1992). According to attribution theory, external, unpredictable forces create some of the most severe and intractable problems (Lazarus & Folkman, 1984).

Assigning blame to any party is far too simple and reductionistic in its own right. However, caregivers are responsible for the raising of children, and the degree to which we are responsible for a broad range of maltreatment should be acknowledged. In a study that I was involved with (Reams & Friedrich, 1995), we examined the treatment effects of a structured play therapy intervention with physically abused preschoolers. We found that they had routinely experienced at least one other form of maltreatment: physical neglect, emotional neglect, sexual abuse, rejection, or emotional abuse. These types of abuses were not simply additive in their effects. Rather, they had a geometric, even exponential effect on behavioral consequences. For example, the addition of a second maltreatment type did not simply double the score of the child, it raised the behavioral scores by an even bigger factor.

Data from the mother–child project at the Institute of Child Development have also pointed to the multicollinearity of child maltreatment (Egeland, Sroufe, & Erickson, 1983). When one form of maltreatment occurs, the likelihood of a second occurring becomes even greater. The data also show the same relationship of multiple forms of abuse to elevated levels of consequence.

Australian researchers have also noted a large degree of overlap between different types of abuse and neglect. In their study, (Higgins & McCabe, 1996), a disturbing proportion of parents described their own childhood experiences with multiple forms of child maltreatment. In fact, family background factors and family functioning were found to be important factors mediating the adjustment of children independent of maltreatment. The implications of these findings are that the treatment of maltreated children typically must address a number of different consequences, not only of maltreatment, but also of family functioning.

A complex view of maltreatment necessitates a complex perspective on treatment. I strongly recommend adhering to the assessment philosophy espoused by the authors of this volume. They make a very good case for the need to consider all manner of negative factors. The only way to fully comprehend the challenge one is up against is to assess it very carefully.

Repeatedly, the interventions described in this book address not only the parent–child relationship but also examine how the maltreatment experience of the child is mirrored in the relationship between the child and therapist. The authors are very accurate when they state that specific interventions, over and above relationship-correcting experiences, are needed, and the reader will appreciate how these are explicated.

I sincerely hope that the authors presage the return of complexity to our field. Even if it lasts for only a decade before we slide back into triviality and simplicity, we should open ourselves to the complexity of maltreatment and the corresponding complexity of both assessment and treatment.

WILLIAM N. FRIEDRICH, PH.D., A.B.P.P.
Mayo Clinic
Rochester, MN

REFERENCES

Briere, J. (1992). *Child abuse trauma: Theory and treatment of lasting effects.* Newbury Park: Sage.

Egeland, B., Sroufe, L. A., & Erickson, M. (1983). The developmental consequences of different patterns of maltreatment. *International Journal of Child Abuse and Neglect, 7,* 459–469.

Higgins, D. J., & McCabe, M. P. (1996). *Parent perceptions of children's experiences of maltreatment.* Paper presented at the Biannual Conference of the International Society on the Prevention of Child Abuse and Neglect, Dublin, Ireland.

Lazarus, R. S., & Folkman, S. (1984). *Stress, appraisal and coping.* New York: Springer.

Reams, R. A., & Friedrich, W. N. (1994). The efficacy of time-limited play therapy with maltreated preschoolers. *Journal of Clinical Psychology, 50,* 889–899.

Thurber, S., Ensign, J., Punnett, A. F., & Welter, K. (1995). A meta-analysis of antidepressant outcome studies that involved children and adolescents. *Journal of Clinical Psychology, 51,* 340–345.

Contents

ONE

Child Maltreatment and Developmental Outcome

Despite considerable attention to the problem of child maltreatment, thousands of children are abused and neglected every year. Child maltreatment is a serious legal, medical, and psychosocial problem that often has grave consequences for its victims and for society. In a survey in Washington state the mental health status of children aged 3 to 18 years who were recipients of protective services was assessed. Seventy-two percent of these children were statistically indistinguishable from children in the state's most intensive mental health treatment programs (Trupin, Tarico, Low, Jemelka, & McClellan, 1993). Besides the human costs associated with child maltreatment, vast financial resources are spent in providing professional treatment and social service programs.

We will provide a comprehensive description of individual psychotherapy strategies that can be used to assess and treat children who have suffered various types of abuse and neglect. However, we do not want to dismiss the importance or utility of other psychotherapeutic approaches, especially group therapy for victimized youngsters or family therapy. Space limitations preclude a description of these modalities, although we will describe some interventions with the family designed to complement and support individual child psychotherapy.

We would like to state two other limitations to this book. It is intended for clinicians who work with preadolescent school-aged children, although a few of the case examples incorporate material from sessions with young adolescents. Second, empirical evaluation of treatment strategies designed to assist maltreated children has been a neglected area of research; however, some research reports have begun to appear that support the notion that individual therapy (e.g., Lanktree & Briere, 1995) and group therapy (e.g., McGain & McKinzey, 1995) are associated with a reduction in symptomatology in sexually abused children. Finkelhor and Berliner (1995) have prepared a comprehensive review of treatment outcome for sexually abused children. However, there have been virtually no empirical investigations of the effects of psychotherapy on children exposed to other types of maltreatment, and little work has been done to examine the outcome of different therapeutic modalities (individual vs. group vs. family). Furthermore, studies have rarely been done to investigate the efficacy of abuse-specific treatment techniques or strategies, although some research in this area is beginning to be reported (e.g., Stauffer & Deblinger, 1996). Consequently, many of the interventions we describe have not been empirically validated. We hope that sound research will soon become more prevalent to guide our future choice and application of treatment interventions.

The purpose of this first chapter is to provide the reader with a summary of what is currently known about the impact of maltreatment upon children's development. In the next chapter some mechanisms and factors thought to be responsible for the association between maltreatment and its various sequelae are identified and described. A key notion of this conceptual model is that maltreatment is just one of a number of factors that influence children's development and that other variables moderate the impact of abuse and neglect.

First, a word of warning. It would have been easier to write a book without reviewing the impact of maltreatment or generating hypotheses about its effects upon development. Such a volume would have dealt exclusively with therapeutic strategies and techniques and probably would be easier to read. Some readers may find the literature review dry and academic and begin to question its relevance for their daily clinical practice. As clinicians we are often searching for creative interventions, especially when confronted with children and families whose progress in therapy seems almost imperceptible and whose pain is all too apparent. Although in this book we will focus upon practical interventions, we strongly believe that restricting its scope to technique would do us and our clients real disservice. Clinical skills and acumen are refined by understanding and appreciating maltreatment effects and the mechanisms and processes responsible for developmental sequelae. An awareness of the diverse array of outcomes of maltreatment alerts us to the need for comprehensive assessments that evaluate many domains of functioning. A solid understanding of the literature and theory guides clinical decision making and leads to the development of specific interventions in individual cases and eventually, we hope, to rigorous evaluation of treatment techniques. Being a skilled clinician and a good scholar are not antithetical.

Before we review the literature on clinical treatment and techniques, we would like to present a brief overview of child maltreatment with particular focus upon the definitions of the types of maltreatment and information about the scope of the problem.

DEFINITIONS OF CHILD MALTREATMENT: AN OVERVIEW

The term "child maltreatment" is broad and subsumes many different conditions. Garbarino and Gilliam (1980) offer the following general definition of maltreatment: "acts of omission or commission by a parent or guardian that are judged by a mixture of community values and professional expertise to be inappropriate and damaging" (p. 7).

This definition includes acts of both abuse and neglect, as reflected in the term "acts of commission and omission." The combination of "community standards and professional expertise" establishes that standards regarding maltreatment will have a broad base of support, including endorsement by the public. The definition serves as the basis for describing specific subtypes of child maltreatment but also presents a number of difficulties. These difficulties include variability in the standards used to determine when a subtype of maltreatment has occurred and the different purposes various definitions serve (legal, case management, and research). Cicchetti and Olsen (1990) and Wolfe (1988) offer a detailed discussion of these issues.

Physical Abuse

Physical abuse was the first type of maltreatment that attracted professional and public attention. The general definition emphasizes the presence of a nonaccidental injury resulting from acts of commission, such as physical assault, or omission, as exemplified by a caretaker's failure to protect the child. Another basic component of the definition is the presence of consequences (i.e., physical injury) that are, for instance, "substantial and observable" (Province of Alberta, Child Welfare Act, 1984, p. 6). Although many cases of physical abuse are easily identified, others are more equivocal. For instance, the 1984 Child Welfare Act of Alberta says that leaving bruises on a child through the nonaccidental application of force constitutes physical abuse. Leaving welts (elevations on the skin produced by a blow), however, is not defined as physical abuse in that Canadian province. Are the two situations so dissimilar, especially from the child's perspective? Would a caretaker be committing physical abuse if he or she spanked a child on 4 consecutive days and left welts? Do other factors, such as cultural traditions that sanction or condone physical punishment determine whether a particular form of physical discipline is abusive? For instance, several Scandinavian countries have outlawed the use of corporal punishment, even by parents.

Despite these definitional uncertainties, the number of children who are physically abused is alarming. Citing three American studies, Finkelhor and Dziuba-Leatherman (1994) found that the incidence (i.e., new occurrences per year) of physical abuse ranged from 4.9 to 23.5 per 1,000 children. Other studies have shown even higher rates. Gelles and Straus (1990) estimated that 6.9 million American children were assaulted by parents (defined as kicking, biting, punching, choking, beating, and using weapons) at a rate of 110 incidents per 1,000 children during a 12-month period. Despite differences in the definition of physical abuse and sampling methodologies that may account for these discrepancies, the statistics clearly indicate abuse is a significant medical, legal, and psychosocial problem for children. Concern is compounded by estimates that that only one physically abused child in seven is reported to authorities (Schene, 1987).

One of the central points we would like to make is that many children who have experienced one type of abuse have also been subjected to other types of maltreatment. There is significant overlap between physical abuse and psychological maltreatment (Claussen & Crittenden, 1991; Egeland & Sroufe, 1981; Ney, Fung, & Wickett, 1994). Permanent developmental damage is more likely to occur when these kinds of multiple risks are present in the environment (Rutter, 1987; Vissing, Straus, Gelles, & Harrop, 1991).

Sexual Abuse

Schechter and Roberge (as cited in Mrazek, 1981) offer the following definition of sexual abuse: "the involvement of dependent, developmentally immature children and adolescents in sexual activities that they do not fully comprehend, are unable to give consent to, and that violate the social taboos of family roles" (p. 11). The last phrase of this definition seems to imply a genetic relationship between participants, possibly limiting it to incest. Wolfe and Wolfe (1988) have broadened this concept to incorporate "intrafamilial" abuse where the perpetrator is any individual who assumes a parental or caretaking role in the child's life. They also incorporate "extrafamilial" abuse that refers to exploitative sexual contact by an individual who may be familiar or unfamiliar to the child. Finally, other definitions of sexual abuse have encompassed a broad range of sexual activities, including direct sexual contact with a child and exposure of a child to inappropriate sexual activity.

Because of different definitions and sampling methodology, estimates of incidence and prevalence (the latter the total number of cases of sexual abuse existing in a population at a given point in time) vary widely. Finkelhor and his colleagues (Finkelhor, 1979; Finkelhor, Hotaling, Lewis, & Smith, 1989) have found the sexual victimization rate is about 20% to 30% for females and 10% to 15% for males. According to Russell (1983), 16% of the women in this study had at least one experience of intrafamilial sexual abuse before they were 18 years of age, and 12% had been sexually abused before they were 14 years old. The rates of extrafamilial abuse found in this survey were even higher: 31% of the sample reported having had at least one such experience before the age of 18, and 20% reported at least one experience before they turned 14. More recently, Finkelhor and Dziuba-Leatherman (1994) report two studies in which the estimated rate of sexual abuse in children from infancy to 17 years ranged from 2.1 children per 1,000 to 6.3 children per 1,000. As with physical abuse, we may be underestimating the true rate of childhood sexual abuse. For example, Russell (1983) reports that only 2% of the cases of intrafamilial sexual abuse and 6% of the extrafamilial cases had been reported to the authorities.

Psychological Maltreatment

Psychological maltreatment has only recently received attention from professionals and the public. It has been discussed under many labels, including "emotional abuse," "emotional neglect," "psychological abuse," "mental cruelty," and "emotional maltreatment." There has been considerable debate about conceptualizations and definitions of psychological maltreatment. In 1983, the International Conference on Psychological Abuse of Children and Youth proposed the following definition:

> Psychological maltreatment of children and youth consists of acts of omission and commission which are judged by community standards and professional expertise to be psychologically damaging. Such acts are committed by individuals, singly or collectively, who by their characteristics (e.g., age, status, knowledge, organizational form) are in a position of differential power that renders a child vulnerable. Such acts damage immediately or ultimately the behavioral, cognitive, affective, or physical functioning of the child. Examples of psychological maltreatment include acts of rejecting, terrorizing, isolating, exploiting, and mis-socializing. (Hart, Germain, & Brassard, 1983, p. 2)

Hart, Germain, and Brassard (1987) and Garbarino, Guttmann, and Seeley (1986) augmented this definition with the following descriptions of seven forms of psychological maltreatment. Garbarino et al. (1986, p. 8) described the following as "basic threats to human development" and maintained that psychological maltreatment is the core issue in child maltreatment.

1. Rejecting: the adult wishes the child away or refuses to acknowledge the child's worth or the legitimacy of the child's needs.
2. Degrading: the child is labeled as inferior, humiliated, and depreciated, and is deprived of dignity.
3. Terrorizing: the child is verbally assaulted, intimidated, and threatened with psychological or physical harm.

4. Isolating: the child is separated from social contacts or restricted to a limited area without social interaction.
5. Corrupting: the child is encouraged to engage in antisocial activities that in turn may teach and reinforce criminal or socially unacceptable behavior.
6. Exploiting: the child is used for the parents' own advantage or profit.
7. Denying emotional responsiveness: The adult fails to provide responsive caregiving that then impairs the child's emotional development. The core feature of this category is the caregiver's ignoring and neglecting the child (i.e., an act of omission) and is sometimes referred to as "emotional neglect." This term is distinguished from "rejecting" and "degrading," which have an active quality (i.e., an act of commission) and constitute typical forms of emotional abuse.

McGee and Wolfe (1991) maintain that these seven subtypes of psychological maltreatment have a number of limitations, particularly for research purposes. Some subtypes are not discrete, with considerable overlap between categories, and some parent–child interactions such as inconsistent parenting cannot be classified into one of the types. They note that the categories are heterogeneous; some emphasize the negative outcome for the child, while others are defined solely in terms of parental behavior. McGee and Wolfe (1991) define psychological maltreatment as "any communication pattern that could undermine a child's resolution of important developmental tasks" (p. 41) and argue that psychological maltreatment should be defined primarily on the basis of parental behavior, not on the nature of the psychological effects it engenders.

McGee and Wolfe's conceptualization provoked even more debate. For example, Barnett, Manly, and Cicchetti (1991) note that decisions about what constitutes maltreatment cannot be made solely on the basis of research results but must incorporate societal standards of appropriate parental behavior. This absence of a standard definition of psychological maltreatment is not just a matter of academic debate. Studies of the impact of psychological maltreatment using different definitions may well include subjects who have undergone diverse experiences, thereby contributing to mixed or even contradictory results.

Hart and Brassard (1987) suggest that the true extent of psychological maltreatment is difficult to determine, given the absence of operational definitions and standards of severity. However, the incidence of psychological maltreatment in the United States has been conservatively estimated at 200,000 new cases per year (American Humane Association, 1984; National Center on Child Abuse and Neglect, 1981). As we have already stated, most theorists in this area regard psychological maltreatment as inherent in other forms of abuse and neglect. Use of this concept, in turn, would significantly increase the numbers of children experiencing this form of maltreatment.

Physical Neglect

Wolfe (1988) defines neglect as "a chronic pattern of deprivation of necessities that must be remediated in order to prevent sustained and pervasive developmental impairments of the child" (p. 629). These necessities include appropriate food, clothing, and shelter, as well as other aspects of physical care: a safe home environment, adequate supervision of child behavior, and adequate or appropriate use of medical facilities (Wolfe, 1988).

Physical neglect as a type of child maltreatment has received little attention from the public or professionals. However, it is a serious problem, in terms of both its incidence and impact upon children. Daro and McCurdy (1991) report an incidence of 20.2 children per 1,000 or more than 1,200,000 American children. Sedlack (1991) reports a smaller but still alarming incidence of 11.3 children per 1,000, or more than 700,000 children who had been neglected in one year. That child neglect is a significant problem and deserves more attention is borne out by a study conducted by the American Humane Association (1984). Of 484 known child fatalities, 51% died because of neglect, while 40% died of major physical injuries.

THE IMPACT OF MALTREATMENT: A THEORETICAL OVERVIEW

Summarizing and integrating the research findings on the sequelae of child maltreatment have been monumental tasks. We faced a vast amount of research data that sometimes included disparate and conflicting findings. Moreover, the greatest challenge has been to find a conceptual model to help us organize and present this information. We have examined the impact of maltreatment upon the child's journey from infancy to preadolescence within the context of the model proposed by developmental psychopathology. Additionally, we will examine those effects that do not interfere with the child's development but are still associated with considerable pain and suffering.

The basic tenets of developmental psychopathology, especially the transactional model espoused by Cicchetti and Rizley (1981), provide the researcher and clinician with a useful way to understand many effects of maltreatment. One hallmark of this approach is the attempt to integrate knowledge from different disciplines. Among these disciplines are clinical and experimental psychology and psychiatry, sociology, and the biological sciences, including genetics and the neurosciences. Developmental psychopathologists maintain that attempts to understand human development from the perspective of just one discipline do injustice to the complexity of this process. Likewise, exclusive focus upon one factor or variable to explain human behavior (e.g., attributing abusive behavior solely to a parent's own history of maltreatment) is overly simplistic and inaccurate. Considering development across a broad range of functioning and behavioral organization is an approach well suited to the study of the diverse effects of child maltreatment.

According to Cicchetti and Rogosch (1994), developmental psychopathology "adopts an organizational view, conceptualizing development as a series of qualitative reorganizations among and within biologic and behavioral systems as growth of the individual proceeds" (p. 760). These various systems and processes include the biological, behavioral, psychological, as well as broader ones such as the environment, society, and culture. They are in dynamic "transaction" (i.e., interaction) with one another throughout a person's lifespan. This concept of the primacy of interrelations among various systems for human development is antithetical to the notion of a direct, linear (i.e., main-effects) relationship between maltreatment and specific developmental sequelae first used to explain causes of child abuse. Theorists and clinicians regarded one factor (e.g., a parental history of victimization) as the causative variable of abusive behavior (e.g., Steele & Pollock, 1968). There is now general agreement that abusive or neglectful parenting is determined by the interaction of many different variables. Belsky's (1980, 1993) ecological model of child maltreatment is typical of such an approach. He proposes that child maltreatment is more likely to occur when there is a confluence of factors at four different levels: the psychological characteristics of the parents, the family setting and its dynamics, the immediate social network of the family members, and the current state of society as it pertains to maltreatment.

Similarly, child maltreatment can be regarded as one of several variables that may contribute to specific developmental outcomes. Clinicians and researchers must remain cognizant of the complexity of the association between maltreatment and outcome. Given the influence of multiple variables, there are multiple pathways to adaptive and maladaptive developmental outcomes. Likewise, interventions may have to be directed at a number of different targets or variables. A history of maltreatment, although a significant risk factor for many serious emotional, behavioral, and interpersonal problems, does not necessarily condemn an individual to such a fate. In fact, it is upon this basic premise of the possibility of change that this book is based. Figure 1.1 illustrates the linear and transactional models of the impact of maltreatment.

Stage-salient developmental issues must be considered. At each developmental stage, the individual confronts specific developmental tasks that are

LINEAR MODEL

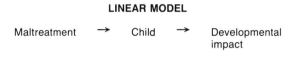

TRANSACTIONAL MODEL

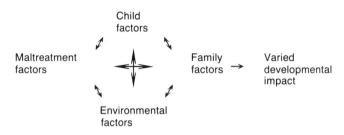

FIGURE 1.1. Models of impact.

central to that age (Cicchetti & Rogosch, 1994). Upon emergence, each remains critical to the child's continual adaptation, although decreasing in salience relative to newly emerging tasks. In optimal development, the child successfully negotiates the progression of stage-salient issues and moves through a course of increasing competence and adaptation. In other words, later competencies build upon earlier competencies. The maltreating environment may have a significant negative impact upon this progression, but numerous other factors can mediate its impact. In Chapter 2 we include a more detailed discussion of these moderator variables.

This notion of maltreatment's impact upon the child's progression through different developmental stages is consistent with one of the two major types of effects arising from child victimization proposed by Finkelhor (1995). *Developmental effects* "refer to deeper and generalized types of impact, more specific to children, that result when a victimization experience and its related trauma interfere with developmental tasks or dysfunctionally distort their course" (Finkelhor, 1995, p. 184). Areas that can be affected include attachment, behavioral and emotional self-regulation, development of the self, cognitive and academic functioning, and peer relations. These developmental outcomes in turn may have a significant effect upon the attainment of future developmental tasks (Finklehor, 1995). In contrast, *localized effects* are "those specific to the trauma experience but without major developmental ramifications . . . these symptoms can be called localized not only in the sense that they are short-term, which they often are (Kendall-Tackett, Williams, & Finkelhor, 1993), but also in the sense that they primarily affect behavior associated with the victimization experience and similar classes of experience" (Finkelhor, 1995, p. 184). Although localized effects can be pervasive and persistent, they do not interfere to a great extent with development. Among localized effects, Finkelhor (1995) includes nightmares and fears of being in the environment where the victimization occurred. Developmental and localized effects are not mutually exclusive. Maltreatment may produce a mixture of both types of effects.

We will now examine the major developmental tasks that children confront as they progress from infancy through preadolescence; we will also examine the potential effects of maltreatment upon their ability to negotiate these tasks and challenges adaptively. We will, as well, review the localized effects that maltreated children evidence. However, before reviewing these findings, we will make some comments about the methodological adequacy of the research.

METHODOLOGICAL CONSIDERATIONS

Clinicians sometimes accept some of the misconceptions that have developed regarding child maltreatment (e.g., "All sexually abused children are 'scarred for life.' ") without any critical thought or reflection. We believe that a knowledge of the empirical research on sequelae of abuse and neglect can provide useful information about the validity of such assumptions and can guide and direct, at least to a certain degree, the design and implementation of assessment and treatment strategies. However, familiarity with the literature is insufficient. As clinicians, we must evaluate it analytically to avoid unwarranted or weakly substantiated conclusions. The following survey provides the clinician with some guidelines to evaluate critically the research discussed below.

Definition of Maltreatment and Subject Selection

The different definitions of abuse and neglect used in various studies limit our ability to make sense of contradictory results. Are the discrepant results attributable to the subjects' having undergone significantly different experiences, or are there other factors that could explain this discrepancy? In a number of studies investigators have grouped together children who have experienced different types of maltreatment, such as physical abuse and neglect. This type of grouping limits conclusions regarding the specific sequelae associated with subtypes of maltreatment. However, making these differentiations may be difficult. Cicchetti and Olsen (1990) have identified several practical limitations of efforts to define specific maltreatment subtypes. The data upon which such classifications are based may be limited, since it is often difficult to obtain highly sensitive and confidential records from the child welfare agencies. These records frequently are not compiled or kept systematically with research considerations in mind. The reliability of maltreating parents' reports may be poor and may fail to include comprehensive or accurate accounts of what happened to the child. Finally, as we have seen, children frequently experience more than one type of abuse or neglect.

Besides giving imprecise definitions, researchers often have failed to define comprehensively what is meant by the term *maltreatment*. Even within a subtype, experiences are not homogeneous. Experiences vary according to the severity, frequency, and chronicity of the abuse or neglect; the identity of the perpetrator; and the child's relationship to that individual. These factors, among others, affect or mediate the association between the act(s) of maltreatment and outcome.

Researchers frequently fail to incorporate other mediating variables (e.g., attributions about the maltreatment, the degree of support afforded the child by parents postdisclosure, and poverty) in their studies. Although more difficult to conceptualize and implement, results of research in which the role of these intervening variables, and especially their interactions, are examined render more accurate depictions of the consequences of maltreatment and the role of these multiple variables. This approach may offer clinical benefits as well. For example, as we shall see later, the impact of childhood sexual abuse is associated with the degree of postdisclosure maternal support. Such research findings alert clinicians to examine this variable with individual clients and intervene accordingly if a lack of support is deleteriously affecting the child's response to victimization.

There are other concerns about subject selection. In studies of maltreated children whose ages cover a wide range and both genders, important distinctions in symptom patterns may be obscured. Sexually abused preschoolers tend to display anxiety, nightmares, symptoms of posttraumatic stress disorder, internalizing and externalizing behaviors, and inappropriate sexual behavior; whereas the most common symptoms of sexually abused adolescents are depression, somatic complaints, illegal acts, running away, and substance abuse (Kendall-Tackett et al., 1993).

Research Design

Results of case studies add little to our knowledge of sequelae because of the absence of comparison data. Small subject numbers also limit the generalizability of findings. In much research, use has been made of retrospective designs in which children are assessed after having been abused or neglected. These designs cannot demonstrate definitive causal relationships between maltreatment and later outcome. For example, some of the "effects" of the maltreatment may in fact be factors that precipitated the abuse (Conaway & Hansen, 1989). Results of prospective, longitudinal studies would help researchers disentangle the maltreatment effects from other factors. These results would allow investigators to establish the equivalency of premorbid functioning prior to the onset of maltreatment, and enable them to better identify relationships between maltreatment and outcome. However, even in such studies we should be careful about assuming a direct, linear connection between the maltreatment (the "cause") and outcome (the "effect"). Longitudinal research in which the focus is upon the processes through which maltreatment, child, family, and societal–environmental factors interact to produce adaptive or maladaptive outcome will, in the long run, be more useful than simplistic research designs in which these multiple variables and their interactions are ignored.

Control Groups

Single-group investigations render no information on how victimized and nonvictimized children differ. A well-designed group comparison can provide information on the behavioral or psychological characteristics of victimized youngsters but not, as we have seen, on the antecedents or consequences of maltreatment. Given the wide range of variables that may mediate the relationship between maltreatment and outcome, controlling them is a daunting and formidable task. Conaway and Hansen (1989) also recommend that control groups of nonmaltreated children who exhibit behavior or psychological problems be incorporated into designs, rather than merely using a comparison of abused or neglected children with nonclinical, nonmaltreated groups. Such an approach would help in determining whether maltreated children demonstrate any unique characteristics or problems.

Outcome Measures

Results of a number of studies must be interpreted cautiously, since the researchers did not employ standardized or psychometrically sound measures. Concerns also emerge about the sensitivity of some instruments that have well-established psychometric properties, such as the Child Behavior Checklist (CBCL) (Achenbach & Edelbrock, 1983), to measure consistently and accurately the trauma of maltreatment (Finkelhor & Berliner, 1995). Although such instruments are useful in screening and providing information about overall functioning, they may not allow for the identification of specific sequelae associated with maltreatment. The failure to use investigators who are blind to group membership also detracts from the validity of the results in some studies.

There is no perfect assessment device or test, and relying solely on one particular instrument or strategy limits the validity of the conclusions. For example, parent ratings of child behavior may be somewhat biased, since abusive and neglectful parents may have unrealistic expectations or distorted perceptions of their children's behavior (Conaway & Hansen, 1989). Assessments in both research and clinical realms should include multiple measures to increase the validity of results. Furthermore, the following review of the impact of maltreatment indicates that many areas of children's functioning can be affected. The aim of future research should be to begin to evaluate a wide range of functioning rather than to examine only one or two domains.

ATTACHMENT
An Overview of Attachment Theory

The establishment of a secure attachment with a primary caregiver is the stage-salient task children confront between the ages of 6 and 12 months (Sroufe, 1979; Sroufe & Rutter, 1984). Although each stage-salient task decreases in importance relative to newly emerging tasks, it does not disappear. Consequently, attachment is not an issue for the first year of life alone. Once an attachment develops, it undergoes transformations and reintegrations, with subsequent developmental accomplishments; it has importance for human development throughout the life span. As we shall demonstrate, abuse and neglect often have a profound impact on the child's ability to form secure attachments to others.

Drawing upon some concepts of ethology, Bowlby (1973, 1980, 1982, 1988a, 1988b) and his colleagues (Ainsworth, 1989; Ainsworth & Bowlby, 1991) propose that attachment behavior keeps the infant close to one or a few principal caregivers through complimentary caregiver and infant behavior. The infant is equipped at birth with species-characteristic behaviors (e.g., crying) that elicit certain behaviors in the caregiver. Caregiving behavior (e.g., feeding the child, protecting the child from harm) that sensitively and appropriately meets the child's needs helps ensure infant survival and that of the species. The caregiver's behavior also generates a feeling of security in the child. At first, the infant's behaviors are not directed at a specific individual. Gradually, the child begins to discriminate among people and establishes an attachment to one or a few select individuals. We refer the interested reader to a volume prepared by Karen (1994), a highly readable and comprehensive account of the emergence and development of attachment theory.

Ainsworth, Blehar, Waters, and Wall (1978) have developed the "strange situation" paradigm to assess the security of mother–infant attachment. In this 20-minute videotaped procedure, the infant is exposed to a series of increasingly stressful events that culminate in being left alone. The infant's reactions to separations, and more specifically to reunions, are believed to measure the degree to which the infant's perceptions and expectations of the mother provide feelings of security and trust. Ainsworth et al. (1978) found that infants with a *secure attachment* (type B) greeted their mothers positively after being separated, actively sought proximity or interaction, and readily accepted comfort if distressed. They directed little, if any, negative behavior toward their mothers. These mothers were responsive, accessible, and sensitive to their infants' needs. Infants who manifested an *avoidant attachment* (type A) showed little stress when separated. Upon reunion, they avoided their mothers by turning and looking away and ignoring them. These infants showed little preference for their mothers over a stranger and evidenced little affective interchange in the preseparation episodes. The mothers were insensitive to their children's needs, avoided physical contact, and were intrusive in interactions with their infants. These interactions were also characterized by instances of covert hostility and rejection. Infants who demonstrated an *ambivalent–resistant attachment* (type C) exhibited a high level of distress upon separation. Upon reunion, they showed angry resistance and appeared ambivalent. They actively sought proximity but angrily pushed away from their mothers. These mothers responded inconsistently and interacted in a very passive, withdrawn manner.

Main and Weston (1982) describe these three attachment patterns as coherent strategies for achieving "felt security" and regulating distress. Sensitive parents react promptly to their infants' arousal states, thereby reducing the infants' distress and allowing them to attend to and explore the environment. As most parents know, it is very difficult for a baby screaming with hunger or fright to settle down and interact with others or explore the environment. Intensely aroused infants are incapable of processing information. The securely attached child readily seeks comfort in the strange situation because of an expectation that the attachment figure will respond sensitively and appropriately. Also, the child can freely explore the environment because of the expectation that the attachment figure is readily available if the child becomes distraught or anxious during these explorations.

The avoidantly attached child expects to be rebuffed, rejected, or subjected to anger and hostility if he or she makes demands in stressful situations; consequently, the child begins to avoid closeness or intimacy with the attachment figure (Crittenden, 1992a; Main, 1981). For these children, closeness, intimacy, and the expression of negative affects are fraught with danger. Some have learned that parents ignore their distress rather than reacting angrily or punitively. Parental neglect of the child who needs soothing or comfort leads to continued intense, emotional arousal, an exceedingly disorganizing effect. To cope, the child excludes feelings and thoughts that would normally arouse the attachment system and begins to suppress or falsify the expression of affects typically used to signal for appropriate parental response (Cassidy & Kobak, 1988; Crittenden, 1992b; Main, 1990). The child dismisses the importance of the attachment relationship and the associated feelings and thoughts. Although this strategy provides relief from intense, emotional arousal, ultimately it may lead to problems in perceiving, interpreting, and displaying feelings. It precludes children from forming close interpersonal relationships that fulfill affectional needs and instead encourages counter expectations that relationships are a source of danger and rejection. Main and Goldwyn (1984) also suggest that children with an avoidant attachment may idealize caregivers. They portray the rejecting, hostile parent as a wonderful caregiver, thereby attenuating the troublesome feelings of anger, sadness, and anxiety associated with an accurate perception of the relationship. McCrone, Egeland, Kalkoske, and Carlson (1994) assert that the avoidant attachment pattern represents a behavioral defense that protects the infant from further trauma and facilitates exploration of the world. As we shall see later, the older child begins to develop "representational" (i.e., mental) defenses for the same purposes.

The child with an ambivalent–resistant attachment attempts to provoke the attachment figure to meet his or her needs via angry and aggressive behavior. Unlike avoidant children, these youngsters learn to overexpress their feelings and needs. The parent tries to modulate the child's distress only after the child's affective arousal has become intense. These children subsequently become "hypervigilant and responsive to signals of maternal unavailability and also to intensify their signals" (Crittenden, 1992b, p. 581). Besides using angry behavior in their attempts to threaten parents into compliance, preschool children use charmingly seductive, disarming behavior that Crittenden (1992b) labels "coercive." Furthermore, with uncertainty about whether the mother will be available, responsive, or helpful, the child becomes dependent and clingy and manifests the kind of anger just described. The child's ability to explore the environment is restricted by this preoccupation with parental unavailability.

This description of attachment patterns as strategies reflects one of Bowlby's (1969, 1973, 1980, 1982; Sroufe & Fleeson, 1986) most important theoretical concepts of attachment theory. The child's *internal working model* of attachment (mental representations of the self and the parent) is inferred from the infant's responses and behavior in the structured separation and reunion episodes of the strange situation. Infants with a secure attachment organization who freely seek comfort, proximity, and contact in the reunion episode and then gradually explore the environment or return to play are inferred to have an expectation that parents can meet needs for reassurance, comfort, and protection. Infants judged to have an avoidant attachment organization actively avoid and ignore the parent in the reunion because of an expectation that their proximity-seeking advances will be rejected or ignored. Their mental representation of the relationship seems to be characterized by danger, rejection, or neglect. Infants classified as having an ambivalent–resistant attachment expect that their parents cannot meet their needs consistently. This expectation is evidenced by the infants' angry yet clingy and dependent behavior in the reunion episode, which seems designed to evoke an appropriate response from their parent.

Main and Solomon (1986, 1990) have reviewed a large number of cases that had not been previously classified or did not fit the criteria of these three patterns. They identified criteria for an additional insecure pattern that they called *disorganized–disoriented attachment* (type D). When confronted with their mother's return, these infants displayed diverse and contradictory behavior patterns (e.g., strong initial proximity seeking followed by strong avoidance; approaching but with head averted), undirected expressions of fear and distress, dazed or disoriented facial expressions, and apprehension. Disorganized–disoriented behaviors do not represent a fourth organized strategy for maintaining access to an attachment figure (Main & Solomon, 1990). These behaviors make sense only if interpreted as reflecting fear and confusion about the caregiver and unresolvable conflict concerning whether or how to maintain access to the attachment figure in times of stress (Goldberg, 1991; Main & Solomon, 1990). Main and Hesse (1990) and Lyons-Ruth, Repacholi, McLeod, and Silva (1991) suggest that this pattern might result, for example, from a relationship in which the child suddenly experiences a previously positive and caring parent as threatening. The maternal behaviors that induce fear in the child are often subtle and contradict other overtly positive aspects of the mother's behavior.

If pervasive enough, this conflict could impede the infant's organization of a consistent attachment-oriented strategy. However, Main and Solomon (1990) propose that this conflict and disorganization might occur in the context of a strategy that was otherwise secure. Likewise, disorganization might exist in relation to the two other coherent strategies, avoidant and ambivalent. Consequently, Main and Solomon (1990) advise investigators to code the best-fitting classification according to the infant's underlying attachment strategy. These best-fitting classifications are usually described as "forced" classifications. Lyons-Ruth et al. (1991) have reviewed the disorganized forms of secure and insecure attachment behavior and their correlates. Disorganized behavior in infants with serious social risks (e.g., infants from low-income backgrounds or who have been maltreated) has been predominantly of the forced–insecure and, especially, forced–avoidant types. Disorganized behavior in infants from low-risk, middle-class backgrounds has been predominantly of the forced–secure type.

The Attachment Organizations of Maltreated Children

As has been suggested in the preceding discussion, quality of attachment depends on the quality of care the infant has received (Sroufe, 1988). In studies following Ainsworth's original investigations (Ainsworth et al., 1978) it was confirmed that mothers of secure infants were rated as more sensitive, responsive, accessible, and cooperative during the infants' first year than mothers of insecure infants (e.g., Belsky, Rovine, & Taylor, 1984). Results of studies in which the attachment patterns of maltreated children were examined consistently show that physically abused and neglected children are less likely to develop secure attachments, with 70% to 100% of maltreated infants exhibiting insecure attachment organizations (e.g., Cicchetti, 1989; Crittenden, 1988). The disorganized–disoriented category also has been found to characterize maltreated infants. For example, Carlson, Barnett, Braunwald, and Cicchetti (1989) found that approximately 80% of maltreated infants could be classified as disorganized–disoriented; compared with less than 20% of a nonmaltreated comparison group.

The Minnesota Mother–Child Interaction Project, a prospective, longitudinal study of the development of a sample of high-risk children, has generated research that merits close attention (Erickson, Egeland, & Pianta, 1989; Egeland, 1991). From the original sample of 267 mothers, four maltreatment groups based upon maternal parenting quality were identified. These mothers were physically abusive, neglectful (defined as a failure to provide adequate physical care), hostile/verbally abusive (defined as harsh criticism and harassment), and psychologically unavailable (defined as passively rejecting the child). The latter two terms may be similar to the respective terms "rejecting" and "denying emotional responsiveness" included in the psychological maltreatment categorization scheme described earlier in this chapter.

In the Minnesota Mother–Child Interaction Project the strange situation paradigm was used to classify the attachment patterns of the children in the project at 12 and 18 months of age. Compared with the control children whose mothers provided adequate care, a larger proportion of the physically abused children were anxiously attached (avoidant and ambivalent-resistant) at age 18 months. Significantly more neglected children than control children were anxiously attached at ages 12 and 18 months. By age 18 months, the number of neglected children classified as anxiously attached had decreased, although it was still significantly greater than the number of control children. There were fewer children who showed an ambivalent-resistant pattern at age 18 months than at age 12 months, especially children who were neglected but not physically abused. The attachment patterns of the verbally abused children were not significantly different from those of the control children at ages 12 and 18 months. However, Erickson et al. (1989) report that several children classified as being securely attached were observed to have a mixture of behaviors that suggested a disorganized–disoriented pattern. At the age of 12 months, 57% of the children in the psychologically unavailable group (children who had been passively neglected but not physically abused) were securely attached, but by the time the children were 18 months old this number had dropped to 14%. The vast majority (86%) of children in this group was classified as avoidant at age 18 months.

Investigations of the attachment classifications of preschoolers (2 to 5 years of age) show that maltreated children continue to exhibit insecure attachments. Cicchetti and Barnett (1991) examined maltreated preschoolers' attachment relationships with their mothers at one or more of three ages: 30 months, 36 months, and 48 months. Children who were physically abused, neglected, emotionally maltreated, and a fourth group judged to have experienced multiple types of maltreatment were evaluated. There were few statistically significant relations among the types of maltreatment and specific classifications of insecure attachment. However, a significantly greater proportion of maltreated youngsters were found to be insecurely attached when compared with nonmaltreated children in each age group. Also, a small number of maltreated children with secure attachments at 30 months were likely to be classified as insecure at later assessments.

The association between maltreatment and insecure attachments has been demonstrated in other studies. van IJzendoorn, Goldberg, Kroonenberg, and Frenkel (1992) conducted a meta-analysis of 34 clinical samples representing 1,624 strange situation classifications. Included in the clinical sample were six studies in which the attachment classifications of maltreated infants were examined using the secure, avoidant, and ambivalent–resistant classification schemes. The maltreatment group showed an overrepresentation of avoidant and ambivalent–resistant classifications. Another analysis was conducted of three studies that also included the disorganized–disoriented category. The maltreatment group contained an overrepresentation of avoidant and disorganized–disoriented classifications.

We were unable to locate any empirical studies regarding the association between childhood sexual abuse and attachment security, although Cole and Putnam (1992) speculate that incest may significantly impair infants' and toddlers' basic trust in their parents. Alexander (1992) maintains that subsequent sexual abuse may erode a previously securely attached child's basic sense of trust. This erosion is consistent with Finkelhor and Browne's (1985) description of "betrayal" as one of four traumagenic (i.e., trauma-producing) dynamics in cases of childhood sexual abuse. The other three are powerlessness, stigmatization, and traumatic sexualization. They describe betrayal as "the dynamic in which children discover that someone on whom they were vitally dependent has caused them harm" (Finkelhor & Browne, 1985, p. 531). Certainly, based on our own clinical observations, many sexually abused children display an impaired sense of trust.

Thus the association between child maltreatment and insecure attachments seems well established. But this does not mean there is no controversy or that attachment theory is free of the methodological problems that have plagued other areas. We must not forget that relationships are complex and include other dimensions besides attachment qualities. In our clinical experience, focusing exclusively upon attachment excludes many important factors (e.g., shared positive emotions, balance of control) that have real significance for our clinical understanding and work with maltreated children and their parents. The focus upon mothers has also limited the conclusions that can be drawn about attachments to fathers and other figures. Moreover, we must be careful to avoid falling into the trap of linear models and asserting that an insecure attachment has "caused" a particular child's maladaptive behavior. Similar to our conceptualization of the impact of maltreatment, an insecure attachment is a risk factor whose role in an individual's development is mediated by many other variables.

Besides the formation of a secure attachment with a primary caregiver, the child must negotiate other stage-salient developmental issues. Child maltreatment may compromise these other aspects of personality organization. We now turn to a brief discussion of the potential impact of maltreatment on other stage-salient tasks the young child must negotiate.

EMOTIONAL AND BEHAVIORAL SELF-REGULATION

An important component of adaptive functioning in childhood and later life is the ability to regulate both emotion and behavior. The successful negotiation of this stage-salient task in toddlerhood and early childhood may well increase chances of competency in later developmentally salient tasks (Shields, Cicchetti, & Ryan, 1994). For example, a child who has previously learned to regulate and modulate feelings may have a greater chance of making and keeping friends. The child is more likely to cope adaptively with classroom demands where children are expected to exert some self-control by sitting quietly and inhibiting the urge to yell out or hit someone.

Maltreated children show numerous difficulties in their emotional and behavioral self-regulation. These problems, ranging from externalizing, acting-out behavior (e.g., aggression) to internalizing behavior (e.g., anxiety, depression), have been comprehensively reviewed in a number of papers (Ammerman, Cassisi, Hersen, & Van Hasselt, 1986; Cicchetti & Olsen, 1990; Cicchetti & Rogosch, 1994; Kolko, 1992; Wolfe, 1988; Wolfe &

Wolfe, 1988). We will review these symptoms, starting with externalizing problems.

Externalizing Problems

Physical Aggression

In the Minnesota Mother–Child Interaction Project it was found that maltreated children as young as 2 years were more angry, noncompliant, and frustrated during an experimental task than were control children (Erickson et al., 1989). Similar difficulties characterized them as preschoolers. They were more hyperactive, distractible, and lacking in self-control, and displayed many negative affects. The findings of Erickson et al. (1989) are not unusual. Physical aggression and antisocial behavior are among the most prevalent sequelae of physical abuse in preschool children (George & Main, 1979; Hoffman-Plotkin & Twentyman, 1984). Physically abused grade-school children have also been found to exhibit a wide array of dysregulated behavior, again characterized by disruptive and aggressive actions (Cicchetti, Lynch, Shonk, & Manley, 1992). Kaufman and Cicchetti (1989) report that day-camp counselors gave children who had been subjected to all three forms of maltreatment (physical abuse, physical neglect, and emotional abuse) the highest ratings on aggressive behavior.

Vissing et al. (1991) have examined the effects of verbal abuse. They found that the rates of physical aggression, delinquency, and interpersonal problems were higher in verbally and physically abused children than in nonmaltreated youngsters. These results are consistent with those obtained by Kaufman and Cicchetti (1989), who found that children subjected to multiple types of maltreatment were regarded as more disruptive by peers. As well, maltreatment may interact with other variables to place a child at risk. Scerbo and Kolko (1995) found that physically abused children aged 7 to 15 years showed heightened physical aggression only if they also exhibited high levels of internalizing problems.

There are, of course, interactions between maltreatment and other variables that influence child outcome. Manly, Cicchetti, and Barnett (1994) have examined the impact of various aspects of maltreatment, such as its frequency, severity, and chronicity, and their relationship to sequelae. Children between the ages of 5 and 11 were assessed on social competence, behavior problems, and peer ratings of cooperation, disruption, and initiation of aggression. The subjects included children subjected to sexual abuse, physical abuse, or physical neglect. Although the maltreated children generally demonstrated poorer adaptation, the severity of the maltreatment, the frequency of child protective services reports, and the interaction between severity and frequency of maltreatment were significant predictors of functioning. The chronicity of the maltreatment also predicted peer ratings of aggression.

Although a discussion of the long-term impact of maltreatment is beyond the scope of this volume, Widom (1989) has examined evidence concerning the relationship between a childhood history of abuse and later involvement as adults, in abusive or aggressive behavior against children. She concluded that although a history of childhood abuse is a risk factor for later aggressive behavior, other variables, such as the provision of psychotherapy, moderate the relationship between it and subsequent violent behavior. This observation is congruent with our experience. We have had numerous discussions with former child clients who have reached adulthood. Although abused as youngsters, they now report that they are nonviolent as adults. This is so even though many still encounter other types of difficulties.

Evidence of behavioral dysregulation has also been found in studies of sexually abused children. For instance, in the Tufts' New England Medical Center investigation (1984) it is reported that 45% to 50% of 7- to 13-year-old sexually abused children showed significantly higher hostility levels on aggression and destructive behavior measures. Using the CBCL, Dubowitz, Black, Harrington, and Verschoore (1993) found that sexually abused children showed significantly more problems with aggression and hyperactivity than did a group of nonabused children. The importance, however, of including appropriate comparison groups was illustrated by the review prepared by Kendall-Tackett et al. (1993). Of the 11 studies in which the frequency of aggression and antisocial behavior problems of sexually abused children were compared with those of nonsexually abused, nonclinical children, results of 10 showed that sexually abused children were significantly more aggressive or antisocial. However, the comparison between sexually abused children and other clinical but nonabused children showed a different pattern. Of the 7 studies in which this design was used, 6 demonstrated that sexually abused children were less aggressive and antisocial than the nonabused, clinical children. The other study revealed no differences.

Sexualized Behaviors

Sexualized behaviors are another type of externalizing problem exhibited more frequently by sexually abused children. Friedrich, Beilke, and Urquiza (1987) report that sexually abused children displayed significantly more sexual problems on the Sex Problems scale of the CBCL than either a nonabused, psychiatric outpatient group or a nonabused, nonclinic group. Friedrich, Beilke, and Urquiza (1988) also demonstrated that sexually abused boys were more sexualized than whose problem was diagnosed as a conduct disorder/oppositional disorder. Subsequently, Friedrich and his colleagues (Friedrich, Grambsch, Broughton, Kuiper, & Beilke, 1991; Friedrich, Grambsch, Damon, et al., 1992) developed a rating scale for parents, the Child Sexual Behavior Inventory (CSBI), to assess children's specific sexual behaviors. They compared 880 nonabused 2- to 12-year-old children to 276 children of the same age with a confirmed history of sexual abuse. They found that 25 of 36 items in the CSBI differentiated the two groups, with the sexually abused children showing higher rates of sexualized behavior.

Cosentino, Meyer-Bahlburg, Alpert, Weinberg, and Gaines (1995) found that 6- to 12-year-old sexually abused girls manifested more sexual behavior problems on the CSBI than did nonabused girls in two comparison groups who did not differ from each other on the CSBI. Sexually abused girls masturbated more openly and excessively, exposed their genitals, indiscriminately hugged and kissed unfamiliar adults and children, and attempted to insert objects into their genitals. Higher scores on the CSBI were associated with sexual abuse perpetrated by fathers or stepfathers and abuse that involved vaginal and/or anal intercourse. The authors also found, using the CSBI, a small group of girls who forced sexual activities on other children. All had experienced sexual abuse perpetrated by a parent for more than 2 years. The victimization by parents had been accompanied by physical force. Four had also been physically abused.

In the preceding studies, the investigators relied upon parental report of children's sexual behavior. Given that a significant proportion of childhood sexualized behavior is probably private and never comes to the attention of parents or other adults, the accuracy of parental reports might be somewhat suspect. In a few studies that have appeared, sexually abused children were directly asked about their sexual behavior. Briere (1996) has developed the Trauma Symptom Checklist for Children (TSCC), a brief child self-report measure that is used to assess a number of dimensions related to trauma, including anxiety, depression, sleep problems, dissociation, and sexual problems. Friedrich and Briere (as cited in Friedrich, 1993) administered the TSCC to 8- to 15-year-old children. All were inpatients and were matched on demographic variables. The mean values for the Sexual Concerns scale differed significantly between the sexually abused children and those without such a history.

In general, the research indicates that sexual behavior is elevated in sexually abused children (for a review, see Friedrich, 1993). The same conclusion was reached by Kendall-Tackett et al. (1993). When compared with other clinic, nonabused children, sexually abused children showed significantly more inappropriate sexual behavior than did the clinical comparison groups (six of eight studies). Sexualized behavior was only one of two symptoms sexually abused children showed more consistently than did nonabused clinical children. Posttraumatic stress disorder was the other. However, sexualized behavior is still not shown by a majority of sexually abused children. Kendall-Tackett et al. (1993) calculate that the percentage of victims manifesting inappropriate sexualized behavior in 13 studies was 28%.

Internalizing Problems

Internalizing problems, including depression, anxiety-related symptoms, and posttraumatic stress disorder, are further manifestations of disturbances in self-regulation and are associated with various types of maltreatment.

Depression

Kazdin, Moser, Colbus, and Bell (1985) examined the relationship between physical abuse and depressive symptoms in 79 child psychiatric inpatients aged 6 to 13 years. Physically abused children, when compared with non-abused psychiatric patient controls, displayed significantly lower self-esteem, more depression, and more negative expectations about their futures on a variety of measures, including the Children's Depression Inventory, the Bellevue Index of Depression, the Hopelessness Scale for Children, and the Self-Esteem Inventory. Abused children with both past and current abuse showed more severe symptoms of depression than did those with either past or current abuse alone. Toth, Manly, and Cicchetti (1992) found that physically abused 7- to 12-year-old children earned significantly higher scores on the Children's Depression Inventory than either neglected or comparison groups. The latter two groups did not differ from each other. However, results of other studies lead to the suggestion that there is an association between neglect and affective disturbances. At 6 years, neglected children in the Minnesota Mother–Child Interaction Project rarely expressed positive affect or a sense of humor (Erickson et al., 1989). Their lack of joy was consistent with the sadness observed in preschool children who were neglected in infancy. Eleven children who had been sexually abused also displayed less positive affect than did controls.

Depressive symptomatology in sexually abused children has been shown in a number of other studies. Kendall-Tackett et al. (1993) calculate that across six studies, 28% of sexually abused children under 18 years of age showed this symptom. Dubowitz et al. (1993); Lanktree, Briere, and Zaidi (1991); Koverola, Pound, Heger, and Lytle (1993); and Wozencraft, Wagner, and Pellegrin (1991) all found higher rates of depression in sexually abused children. They may also be at higher risk for suicide. Lanktree et al. (1991) discovered that sexual abuse victims enrolled in a child psychiatric outpatient program were more likely to have made at least one suicide attempt. They also had made more attempts than had clinic children who had not been sexually abused.

Posttraumatic Stress Disorder

Posttraumatic stress disorder and other symptoms of fear and anxiety have been investigated in maltreated children. Finkelhor (1995) describes many of these problems as examples of localized effects of child victimization. They can cause considerable distress but, unlike developmental effects, do not interfere significantly with the child's progress through developmental stages. Current formulations of posttraumatic stress disorder include a number of elements from Terr's model of childhood trauma (Terr, 1991). Terr (1991) divides childhood trauma into two types. Type I disorders, which follow from unanticipated single events, are characterized by full, detailed memories of the event; "omens" or attempts to develop a reason for the trauma or how it could have been averted; and misperceptions. The last includes mis-identifications, visual hallucinations, and peculiar time distortions after a single, intense, unexpected shock.

Type II disorders follow from long-standing or repeated exposure to extreme external events. One primary characteristic of type II disorders is the child's attempts to preserve and protect the self from painful feelings, memories, and experiences engendered by the trauma. Writers such as Briere (1992) have focused upon the functionality of these "symptoms" and defenses. They regard them as the child's accommodations to early victimization and/or responses to later abuse-related distress. Terr (1991) identifies three major characteristics of type II disorders. First, rage is a common feature. Second, denial and psychic numbing occur as an accommodation to extreme, long-standing, and repeated traumatic situations, including maltreatment. In an extreme form, denial and psychic numbing may be manifested in children who forget whole segments of their childhood. These defensive operations are reflected in a reluctance to talk about themselves, a failure to define or acknowledge feelings, and a hesitancy to say anything about their ordeals. Terr (1991) suggests that the child's relative indifference to pain and lack of empathy for others may be further examples of denial and psyche numbing. Third, children accommodate or cope with this repeated experience through self-hypnosis and dissociation. These devices allow the child to escape mentally and may be reflected in bodily anesthesia, feelings of invisibility, and amnesia for certain childhood periods. In its most extreme form, these behaviors may culminate in multiple personality disorder.

According to the fourth edition of the *Diagnostic and Statistical Manual of Mental Disorders* (DSM-IV), a diagnosis of posttraumatic stress disorder requires the following criteria to be present (American Psychiatric Association, 1994):

> The person experienced, witnessed, or was confronted with an event that involved actual or threatened death or serious injury, or a threat to the physical integrity of the self and others.

The traumatic event is persistently reexperienced through a recurrent and intrusive distressing recollection of the event. In young children, repetitive play may occur in which themes or aspects of the trauma are expressed. The event may also be reexperienced through distressing dreams; a sense of reliving the experience; illusions, hallucinations, and dissociative flashbacks; intense psychological distress through exposure to internal or external cues that symbolize or resemble an aspect of the traumatic event; and physiological reactivity on exposure to internal or external cues.

The individual engages in persistent avoidance of stimuli associated with the trauma and a numbing of general responsiveness, such as efforts to avoid thoughts, feelings, activities, places, or people associated with the trauma.

Persistent symptoms of increased arousal, such as difficulty falling or staying asleep, irritability or outbursts of anger, difficulty concentrating, hypervigilance, or an exaggerated startle reaction. (Adapted from pp. 427–428)

In a number of studies the association between posttraumatic stress disorder and sexual abuse has been examined. Although it is a common reaction, posttraumatic stress disorder is not shown by a majority of sexually abused children. McLeer, Deblinger, Atkins, Foa, and Ralphe (1988) report that 48% or approximately half, of their sample met the criteria for posttraumatic stress disorder contained in the revised third edition of the *Diagnostic and Statistical Manual of Mental Disorders* (DSM-III-R) (American Psychiatric Association, 1987). Merry and Andrews (1994) assessed the psychiatric status of 95 children, aged 4 to 16 years, 12 months after sexual abuse disclosure. Posttraumatic stress disorder accounted for only 18.2% of the diagnoses, whereas anxiety disorders constituted 30.3%. Wolfe, Sas, and Wekerle (1994) compared sexually abused children who fulfilled DSM-III-R criteria for posttraumatic stress disorder with those who did not. The mean age of these children was 12.4 years. For approximately half the sample of 90 children the diagnosis was posttraumatic stress disorder. Children meeting the criteria were more likely to have been abused over longer time periods, whereas nonposttraumatic-stress-disordered children had experienced more isolated abuse episodes. Posttraumatic stress disorder symptoms were related to the presence of violence and to a closer relationship with the perpetrator, which was compounded by feelings of guilt.

Although not extensive, some work has been done on the prevalence of posttraumatic stress disorder in physically abused children. Results vary, and like the sexual abuse findings, demonstrate that while posttraumatic stress disorder is evident in some, it is not shown by a majority of physically abused children. For example, Deblinger, McLeer, Atkins, Ralphe, and Foa (1989) compared the rates of posttraumatic stress disorder in groups of sexually abused, physically abused, and nonabused psychiatrically hospitalized children. The children ranged in age from 3 to 13 years. Overall, 20.7% of the sexually abused children, 6.9% of the physically abused children, and 10.3% of the nonabused children met the DSM-III-R criteria for posttraumatic stress disorder, but the differences across groups were not significant. In a study of 109 children removed from their homes because of serious physical abuse or neglect, Famularo, Fenton, Kinscherff, Ayoub, and Barnum (1994) found that 35.8% of this group met posttraumatic stress disorder criteria. Children who were younger when the maltreatment began were more likely to have met the criteria.

THE DEVELOPMENT OF AN AUTONOMOUS SELF

Development of an autonomous self is another early stage-salient developmental issue confronting the young child. The child's experience of caretaking and subsequent development of attachment patterns have particular relevance for the emergence of the self. The young child who receives good care internalizes these experiences and develops a sense of self as worthy, lovable, and deserving of this care and love (Bowlby, 1973). Caregiving that is sensitive to the child's idiosyncratic needs reinforces a greater awareness of self. Furthermore, the young child who is securely attached to a caregiver can use that person as a secure base from which to explore the environment. This potentiates feelings of autonomy and independence. In turn, these feelings lead to an even greater differentiation of self from others and to enhanced self-esteem and self-confidence.

Internal State Language

Examination of internal state language has been used to investigate the development of an autonomous self in maltreated children. Internal state words "refer primarily to those words that have explicit reference to internal states ('mad,' 'happy') rather than words that have implicit connotations of emotion, motivation, or intention" (Beeghly & Cicchetti, 1994, p. 6). Bretherton and Beeghly (1982) show that by the age of 28 months, most middle-class children master verbal labels for perception (i.e., the five senses), physiological states, goals, intentions, and ability. More than half discuss basic feelings (e.g., anger, sadness), whereas only a few begin to talk about their own thought processes. The use of this internal state language for themselves and others reflects a growing awareness of the self as distinct from others. Internal state language allows young children not only to verbally communicate their feelings but to clarify misunderstandings with others. The ability to talk about internal states promotes behavioral and affective self-regulation in interpersonal situations: rather than hitting another child, a youngster can express anger or frustration through words.

Cicchetti and Beeghly (1987) found that maltreated and nonmaltreated 30-month-old toddlers did not differ significantly in receptive vocabulary but did differ in their internal state language. Maltreated children used proportionately fewer internal state words, showed less differentiation and attributional focus, and were more context bound in the use of internal state language. Maltreated children were less likely to talk about negative affect and feelings (e.g., hate) or about physiological states (e.g., hunger or thirst). Cicchetti and Beeghly (1987) also interviewed the mothers of these children; the content of these interviews confirmed that maltreated children produced far fewer internal state words than did middle-class non-maltreated children of the same age. In contrast, the internal state language of nonmaltreated children from a lower socioeconomic status was very similar to that of middle-class nonmaltreated children. More recently, Beeghly and Cicchetti (1994) again examined the internal state language of 30-month-old maltreated children and a nonmaltreated, demographically matched comparison group. As in their 1987 study, a majority of the children had experienced multiple types of maltreatment: physical abuse, physical neglect, and emotional abuse. The investigators obtained a pattern of results very similar to those in their earlier study and reported that maltreated children with an insecure attachment had the most compromised internal state language.

The tendency of maltreated toddlers to speak less frequently about negative emotions may reflect exposure to mothers who label feelings imprecisely. This difficulty in verbalizing feelings may in turn lead to problems with the subsequent development of emotional control and self-regulation in children. Maltreated children's compromised internal state language may also reflect other aspects of their general child-rearing environment. Dunn, Bretherton, and Munn (1987) and Dunn and Brown (1991) report that children acquire words for feelings and emotions most readily when participating in family discussions about these affective states. However, maltreating families may not participate readily in these discussions about feelings (Burgess & Conger, 1977; Burgess & Conger, 1978).

Development of the Autonomous Self and Self-Esteem

Beeghly and Cicchetti (1994) suggest that children who talk about their internal states, especially their negative feelings, may provoke maternal disapproval and considerable anger, thereby increasing the risk of further maltreatment. Consequently, children avoid these discussions to minimize future abuse and attenuate their anxiety. Crittenden and DiLalla (1988) report a pattern of "compulsive compliance" in insecurely attached/maltreated children who did not openly express negative feelings and passively complied with their mothers. This behavior may be accompanied by ambiguous affect, masked facial expressions, rote verbal responses, and verbal–nonverbal incongruence. Compulsive compliance is consistent with older psychoanalytic notions of the development of the "false self" (Winnicott, 1965). To reduce anticipated conflict with the caregiver, the child may learn to cut off, repress, or falsify the expression of feelings, particularly negative ones. The child then begins to exhibit false positive affects but experiences few feelings of authenticity in regard to the self. This tendency is also similar to the concept of "other-directedness" described by Briere (1989, 1992). The maltreated child or adult is hypervigilant regarding the abuser's emotional demeanor or behavior. Sustained attention may be advantageous, since it allows the individual to either avoid or placate the abuser before maltreatment occurs, but it exacts a significant cost from the developing child. The child is unaware of his or her own needs, feelings, and motivations, and the growth of self is seriously compromised.

Researchers in the Minnesota Mother–Child Interaction Project reported children in the project showed problems with autonomy and self-esteem when they were evaluated at 42 months of age (Erickson et al., 1989). There was considerable similarity among the maltreatment groups in performance on tasks designed to assess reaction to frustration. Physically abused children lacked confident assertiveness, expressed a great deal of negative affect, and showed little creativity. Their self-esteem was low compared with that of nonmaltreated children. Children whose mothers were hostile/verbally abusive also evidenced negative affect and low self-esteem. Neglected children showed poor impulse control, were inflexible and uncreative in their approach to the tasks they were given, and, when first interviewed, showed low self-esteem and greater unhappiness than did other children. These neglected children often withdrew from tasks and were distractible. The children of psychologically unavailable mothers lacked creativity and displayed anger, noncompliance, lack of persistence, and little positive affect.

Early deficits in the development of an autonomous sense of self may be revealed later in low self-esteem. Findings are somewhat mixed, especially for sexually abused children. Tong, Oates, and McDowell (1987) reported that sexually abused girls had significantly lower scores on the Piers–Harris Children's Self-Concept Scale than control girls but there was no difference between sexually abused and control boys on this measure. However, other studies have not found differences in the self-esteem of sexually abused children using self-report measures. Cohen and Mannarino (1988) compared the scores of 6- to 12-year-old sexually abused girls on the Piers–Harris Children's Self-Concept Scale with the scale's normative data. The abused girls did not exhibit significantly low self-esteem by self-report, but parents rated them as having more behavioral problems than girls in a normative sample. Cohen and Mannarino (1988) speculated that sexually abused children may deny feelings of depression and low self-esteem or label them differently from clinical populations. Alternatively, parents of victimized children may have distorted perceptions of their children.

The relationship between maltreatment and self-report of self-esteem is not direct but is mediated by a number of variables. Studies of physically abused, neglected, and sexually abused children suggest that developmental level may significantly mediate the relationship between maltreatment and children's reports. Vondra, Barnett, and Cicchetti (1989) examined the perceived and actual competence of maltreated children; 80% had experienced more than one type of maltreatment, primarily physical abuse, physical neglect, and psychological maltreatment. Only 5% had been sexually abused. Younger children (grades 1 to 3) tended to describe themselves in exaggerated positive terms. They also rated themselves as more competent than they actually were (based on teachers' ratings), especially regarding their physical competence. Older children in grades 4 to 6 described themselves as less competent than their nonmaltreated peers, a finding consistent with their teachers' rating of themselves. Black, Dubowitz, and Harrington (1994) found a similar pattern in a sample of sexually abused children. In their study, preschool children had elevated scores on measures of perceived competence and social acceptance, whereas school-aged children had depressed scores. Vondra et al. (1989) and Black et al. (1994) proposed that perceiving themselves as more competent than they actually were might have been adaptive for younger maltreated children, since it protects them from profound feelings of personal inadequacy. However, by later elementary school, these children could better compare themselves with others, thus undermining their early efforts to preserve positive self-esteem. Furthermore, children may reconceptualize the meaning of their abusive experiences over time, resulting in different patterns of sequelae and adjustment as they grow older. Thus, self-esteem may suffer as they become more cognizant of the implications and meaning of their history of victimization.

Extreme Disturbances in Self-Definition: Dissociation and Multiple Personality Disorder

Maltreatment, especially severe abuse, is associated with extreme disturbances in self-definition and self-regulation, such as dissociative disorders. Dissociation allows the child to cope by escaping mentally from the situation or from thoughts and feelings associated with the experience. As a result, the child does not integrate feelings and perceptions about the traumatizing experience. Lewis and Yeager (1994) defined dissociation as "an automatic, primitive, protective, psychological response to unendurable physical, sexual, or psychological pain. It results in alterations of awareness both at the time of the trauma and subsequent to it" (p. 729).

A considerable body of research has linked dissociative disorders to histories of physical and sexual abuse and trauma in adults (e.g., Chu & Dill,

1990; Sanders & Giolas, 1991) and in children and adolescents (e.g., Putnam, 1991; Vincent & Pickering, 1988). In some investigations a relationship between dissociative disorders and psychological maltreatment in adults was found (Briere & Runtz, 1988; Sanders & Giolas, 1991). Multiple personality disorder, an extreme form of dissociation, is strongly associated with a history of childhood maltreatment. For example, Ross, Anderson, Fleisher, and Norton (1991) reported that of 102 adult patients in whom a diagnosis of multiple personality disorder was diagnosed, 82% had histories of childhood physical abuse, and 90% had sexual abuse histories.

Putnam (1993, 1995) has identified the protective functions afforded by dissociation. Dissociation compartmentalizes and sequesters emotionally painful material out of conscious awareness and protects the child from overwhelming psychological and physical pain. The sense of self is altered so that a traumatic event is experienced as if "it's not really happening to me." In multiple personality disorder, the individual usually switches among a series of alter identities that personify specific capacities, functions, or experiences to protect against overwhelming trauma.

This protective function has been examined in several studies. Stovall and Craig (1990) compared the responses of three groups of 7- to 12-year-old girls on the Thematic Apperception Test (TAT). They found that the mental representations of the physically abused and sexually abused girls did not differ but were significantly different from those of nonabused girls who came from a "distressed home environment." The abused girls were more likely to have negative unconscious perceptions of themselves and others, but their conscious perceptions of others were more positive.

In a more recent study of self-representations of sexually abused adolescent girls admitted to a psychiatric inpatient unit, Calverley, Fischer, and Ayoub (1994) compared the responses of seven sexually abused girls with those of nine nonabused girls on the Self-in-Relationships Interview. This procedure involves creating a graphic self-portrait by arranging self-descriptions on a diagram of concentric circles. The most important characteristics are placed in the center core, less important ones in the middle circle, and the least important in the outer circle. Compared with nonabused counterparts, victimized girls placed negative characteristics as central to their core self and produced an unusually large number of negatives. Second, the sexually abused girls showed a complex form of dissociation not evident in the nonabused group. In this "polarized affective splitting," three of the seven sexually abused girls generated diametrically opposed descriptions of the "real me." For example, one 17-year-old girl who had been sexually abused by an adult male neighbor from the age of 6 to 12 described the "real me" as "good," "bad," "happy," "lonely," and "dead" (Calverley et al., 1994, p. 208). Furthermore, none of these girls recognized any contradictions in their self-descriptions, asserting that these descriptions were compatible and similar. Although the sample size was small and limited to hospitalized female patients, results of this study suggest that sexually abused youngsters may develop an exaggerated sense of their own badness. Similar to the younger children in Stovall and Craig's (1990) study, these girls seemed to sequester the trauma of the abuse by constructing segregated and polarized views of the self in order to cope with these episodes of victimization.

LANGUAGE DEVELOPMENT

Between the ages of 24 and 36 months, the use of language emerges and becomes more differentiated. The available research suggests that maltreatment poses a substantial risk to the development of language competency in children.

Receptive and Expressive Language

As we have already seen, maltreated children use less internal state language than nonmaltreated children. Studies have been done to examine other aspects of language development in toddlers. Gersten, Coster, Schneider-Rosen, Carlson, and Cicchetti (1986) found that attachment security was significantly related to the language performance in both maltreated and nonmaltreated 2-year-old children. Securely attached children displayed a more elaborate vocabulary and used syntactically more complex language than did toddlers with an insecure attachment.

Believing that the adverse effects of maltreatment might only become apparent when children are older, Coster, Gersten, Beeghly, and Cicchetti (1989) examined differences in two groups of children: 31-month-old maltreated and nonmaltreated toddlers. Although there were no differences in receptive language between the groups, maltreated toddlers had less well-developed expressive language. They used syntactically less complex language, scored lower on measures of expressive vocabulary, and showed deficits in their discourse abilities, for example, using fewer descriptive phrases and sentences. The maltreated children also talked less about their own activities. They made fewer requests for information and fewer references to persons or events outside the immediate context.

An association between expressive-language deficits and physical aggression was demonstrated by Burke, Crenshaw, Greene, Schlosser, and Strocchia-Rivera (1989). Expressive language deficits were significantly more prevalent in physically aggressive, physically abused children than in physically abused children who were not physically aggressive. Although expressive language abilities differed, these groups did not show any significant difference in general verbal ability.

Studies have demonstrated the deleterious effect neglect has on language development (e.g., Fox, Long, & Langlois, 1988; Pezzot, 1978). Katz (1992) found that in a review of studies conducted from 1975 to 1992, both physically abused and neglected children evidenced language delays and disorders, but those of neglected children were more severe.

Play and Symbolic–Representational Development

Children's play can also reflect their symbolic and representational development. Play becomes more social and cognitively more symbolic over the preschool years, as evidenced by increasing dramatic play and games with rules. Alessandri (1991) compared the play behavior of 4- to 5-year-old maltreated children with that of nonmaltreated children of the same social economic status. The maltreated group included children who had been physically abused, sexually abused, emotionally mistreated, and neglected. Of the 15 children in this group, 10 had experienced more than one type of maltreatment. Maltreated children engaged in less play overall and more simple and repetitive play than did nonmaltreated children. The former displayed a routine, stereotyped use of play materials, more frequently touched toys but did not directly manipulate them, and engaged in more pounding activities. Nonmaltreated children showed more frequent constructive play (learning to use materials, creating something), in which the play was sequentially organized and purposeful. Alessandri (1991) speculates that the more restricted and less elaborated play of maltreated children might be related to their insecure attachments, which undermine their use of the attachment relationship as a secure base from which to explore the environment, thereby contributing to developmental delays in their play. In a subsequent study, Alessandri (1992) found some indirect support for the presence of significant problems in the mother–child relationship. Maltreating mothers were more negative, less involved with their children, and used fewer physical and verbal strategies to direct their children's attention.

COGNITIVE DEVELOPMENT
AND ADAPTATION TO SCHOOL

In general, the literature indicates that maltreatment poses a risk to the child's cognitive development and adaptation to school. In early work, the cognitive functioning of physically abused children, especially its association with neurological damage, was examined. Martin, Beezley, Conway, and Kempe (1974) found that 40% of the physically abused children they studied were functioning within the range of mental retardation. The authors link these deficits to the neurological impairments sustained due to physical assaults by parents.

Intellectual and Academic Performance

In more recent work, cognitive functioning unrelated to neurological damage has been examined. This research in which a variety of measures are used, has been accompanied by an increase in methodological rigor (e.g., the inclusion of appropriate control groups). In most of the studies of physically abused and neglected children, researchers report significant differences in IQ scores between maltreated children and controls (e.g., Barahal, Waterman, & Martin, 1981; Pezzot, 1978).

In other studies, the differences between maltreated children and controls in variables such as reading ability and academic outcomes have been studied. Again, the general finding is that maltreatment poses a risk to success in these areas. For example, Salzinger, Kaplan, Pelcovitz, Samit, and Krieger (1984) evaluated the academic performance of a mixed group of physically abused, sexually abused, emotionally abused, and neglected children. On tests of standard achievement in English and mathematics, significantly more maltreated children than children in the control group were performing at 2 or more years below grade level.

Fortunately, in some research an attempt has been made to examine differences in intellectual and academic functioning of children subjected to different subtypes of maltreatment. In the Minnesota Mother–Child Interaction Project, the Vocabulary, Comprehension, Animal House, and Block Design subtests from the Wechsler Preschool and Primary Scale of Intelligence (WPPSI) were administered when the children were 6 years old (Erickson et al., 1989). The physically abused children earned lower scores on the Block Design, Vocabulary, and Comprehension subtests individually, and on a total of the four subtests as well, than did the control group. The scores of these physically abused children, however, did not differ significantly from those of other maltreatment groups. Using the Devereux School Behavior Rating Scale, teachers rated physically abused children as extremely high in classroom disturbance and low in comprehension. Of the 16 physically abused children, 44% had been referred for special help when they were in kindergarten, compared with 21% of the control children.

On the WPPSI, 6-year-old physically neglected children earned much lower scores on the Comprehension, Vocabulary, and Animal House subtests, as well as on the total for the four subtests. Their scores were significantly lower than those of the psychologically unavailable, sexually abused, and control groups. Teachers rated neglected children as having much more difficulty comprehending day-to-day school work than controls did, and as extremely inattentive, uninvolved, and lacking creative initiative. The neglected children were aggressive and unpopular with their peers. In general, these children evidenced a marked deficit in cognitive functioning and serious problems in the classroom. Of the 17 children, 11 had been referred for special help when they were in kindergarten. By grade 2, all the neglected children were in special education programs (Egeland, 1991).

At 2 years of age, children of the psychologically unavailable mothers showed a marked decline in functioning during their preschool years. By the time they were 6 years of age, their differences on formal measures of intelligence relative to those of control children were not as great. On the WPPSI, the former group earned lower scores on the Block Design subtest and tended to earn lower overall scores on the total of the four subtests. They continued to show significant problems with learning and problem solving, and they manifested difficulties relative to peers and teachers. Their teachers rated them as aggressive, unpopular, overactive, and lower in social competence than control children. Six of the 16 children had been referred for help when they were in kindergarten.

In the group studied by Erickson et al. (1989), 11 children at the 6-year evaluation period were found to have been sexually abused. These children earned lower scores than the control group only on the Block Design subtest of the WPPSI. They were rated much higher on the Need for Closeness Scale than the children in the control group and in all other maltreatment groups. They also showed poor comprehension of day-to-day school tasks and were rated as causing more disturbance in the classroom and being less involved and more likely to make irrelevant responses in class than the control group. Most notable were their anxious, inattentive behavior and their strong need for closeness with, and dependency on, adult help and approval. Five of the 11 sexually abused children had been referred for special intervention when they were in kindergarten.

Investigations of the intellectual functioning of older children support the notion that maltreatment poses a risk to cognitive development. In a well-controlled study, Kurtz, Gaudin, Wodarski, and Howing (1993) evaluated the school functioning of 22 physically abused and 47 neglected children, as well as 70 children with no maltreatment history, all between 8 and 16 years of age. When the effects of socioeconomic status were covaried out, it was clear that the physically abused children displayed serious academic and socioemotional problems. They performed poorly on standardized tests of language and mathematical skills, received low performance assessments by parents, and were more likely than nonmaltreated peers to have repeated one or more grades. The neglected children scored far below the control group on standardized tests of language, reading, and mathematics. In contrast to the physically abused children, the neglected children did not display significant behavior problems in the classroom and did not differ from controls on any of the socioemotional measures over time. Kurtz et al. (1993) speculate that the characteristics of the physically abused children, such as anger, distractibility, anxiety, and a lack of self-control, seriously compromised their learning ability. Neglectful parenting, which may include a lack of encouragement for learning, little language stimulation, and unresponsiveness to the child's achievements, undermines school success and poses a direct threat to the intellectual development of the neglected child.

Eckenrode, Laird, and Doris (1993) found that neglected children had the lowest test scores but that sexually abused children did not differ from control children in their scores on academic measures. Besides having academic problems, maltreated children exhibited social and behavioral problems in the classroom. Maltreated children, especially those who had been physically abused, were more likely than nonmaltreated children to be referred to the principal for discipline problems and had significantly more suspensions in junior and senior high school. School suspension rates did not differ among sexually abused, neglected, and nonmaltreated students.

Using a secondary data analysis of the Eckenrode et al. (1993) data, Kendall-Tackett and Eckenrode (1996) examined the effect of neglect, alone and in combination with either physical or sexual abuse, on the academic achievement and school disciplinary problems of elementary, junior high, and high school students. While Kendall-Tackett and Eckenrode (1996) confirmed the deleterious effect of neglect on academic achievement reported by Kurtz et al. (1993), their data indicate that neglect may also be associated with behavior problems in the classroom. Neglect alone was equally as detrimental to grades and number of suspensions as neglect in combination with physical or sexual abuse. The combination of neglect and abuse had a particularly strong effect on the number of disciplinary referrals and grade repetitions, with abused and neglected junior high schol students having the highest number of grade repetitions. The academic performance of all subjects dropped in junior high; neglect and neglect in combination with abuse exacerbated this decline.

In regard to sexually abused children, Einbender and Friedrich (1989) found that 6- to 14-year-old sexually abused girls had lower scores on the Wide Range Achievement Test than did girls in a control group. Trickett, McBride-Chang, and Putnam (1994) compared the classroom academic performance and behavior of 6- to 16-year-old sexually abused girls with those of a nonabused comparison group. Sexual abuse was related to lower classroom ratings of social competence, lower competent-learner ratings, and lower academic performance. Sexually abused girls scored lower on a test of cognitive ability (Peabody Picture Vocabulary Test). These girls showed higher levels of anxious depression, bizarre destructiveness, and dissociative hyperactivity, which in turn were predictive of academic performance, than nonabused girls. Thus the relationship between sexual abuse and academic functioning is complex and probably mediated by a number of socioemotional variables.

Nonorganic Failure-to-Thrive
and Psychosocial Dwarfism

The insidious effects of neglect, especially emotional neglect, are revealed in other studies. Spitz (1945, 1946) reported an infant mortality rate of over 33% in a sample of 91 institutionalized orphans, despite adequate physical care. The syndrome of nonorganic failure-to-thrive, in which children fail to grow and are apathetic and lethargic, has been described as a consequence of emotional neglect (Bullard, Glaser, Hagarty, & Pivchik, 1967; Garbarino et al., 1986). Besides showing compromised physical health and emotional and behavioral problems, many of these children evidence academic and intellectual delays. Oates, Peacock, and Forrest (1985) assessed 14 children who had admitted to a hospital 12½ years earlier and whose condition, in each case, was diagnosed as failure-to-thrive. Their mean age was 13.4 years. Compared with a group of children matched for age, sex, social class, and ethnic group, the children with previous failure-to-thrive syndrome had significantly lower Verbal IQ values on the Wechsler Intelligence Scale for Children–Revised (WISC-R) than did the control group. Eight were more than 3 years behind their chronological age in reading ability, while only one control group member showed such a delay. Children who had suffered from failure-to-thrive also scored significantly lower on a verbal language development scale. In other follow-up studies, children with nonorganic failure-to-thrive syndrome have shown deficits in intellectual and academic functioning (e.g., Elmer, Gregg, & Ellison, 1969; Glasser, Heagarty, Bullard, & Rivchik, 1968; Hufton & Oates, 1977). Polansky, Chalmers, Buttenwieser, and Williams (1981) also described the hostile, defiant behavior of young adolescents whose condition had been diagnosed as failure-to-thrive when they were infants.

Other syndromes have been linked to severe neglect during childhood. In 1967, Powell and his colleagues (Powell, Brasel, & Blizzard, 1967; Powell, Brasel, Raiti, & Blizzard, 1967) published evidence linking abuse and neglect to psychosocial dwarfism, a syndrome characterized by short stature, intellectual deficits, and behavior problems. Money (1977) and Money, Annecillo, and Kelly (1983) have reported intellectual delays in such children. The IQ level rises in those rescued from their abusive or neglectful environment. Increases in IQ are correlated with increases in height (Money et al., 1983). Using multiple regression analysis, Money and Annecillo (1976) found that the length of time spent away from the abusive or neglectful environment was the primary variable associated with an increase in IQ scores. A return to the maltreating environment was associated with a decrease in IQ that paralleled a deceleration of the rate of statural growth and puberty onset. Gardner (1972) suggests that the recovery of these children, including their intellectual functioning, may not be complete and that they may continue to evidence deficits in personality structure and intellect.

PEER RELATIONS

Establishing peer relations during the preschool and school-age years is an important stage-salient developmental issue. The successful negotiation of this issue depends, in part, upon the successful resolution of earlier stage-salient issues. These issues include the establishment of a secure attachment relationship with the primary caregiver and the attainment of effective emotional and behavioral self-regulatory processes. Failure to establish adaptive relationships with peers and others may interfere significantly with a child's ability to negotiate developmental tasks successfully in later life, leading to continued incompetence and maladaptation. Poor interpersonal relationships are not only strongly associated with concurrent psychiatric disorders in children, they have predictive validity for future interpersonal difficulties as well (e.g., Garmezy & Streitman, 1974).

Although maltreatment poses a significant risk to the establishment and maintenance of adaptive peer relations, there is considerable diversity in research findings. Furthermore, much of the work has focused upon physically abused and neglected children. We know much less about children exposed to other forms of maltreatment. Conaway and Hansen (1989), Mueller and Silverman (1989), and Youngblade and Belsky (1990) have prepared comprehensive reviews of the association between maltreatment and peer relations in children. We will only briefly describe some of the major findings included in these reviews.

Physical Aggression in Social Interactions

Hoffman-Plotkin and Twentyman (1984) report that physically abused 3- to 6-year-old children exhibited more aggressive behavior than did neglected and nonmaltreated children. In studies of older maltreated children, a heightened level of physical aggression in their interactions with peers was also seen (e.g., Dodge, Bates, & Pettit, 1990). However, the relationship between maltreatment and physical aggression directed at peers may be more complicated than results of these studies suggest. Howes (1984) demonstrated the importance of context in determining whether a maltreated child will behave aggressively. When interacting with a familiar peer, maltreated and comparison children behaved similarly. In some dimensions, the maltreated children were more socially competent than comparison children. However, this similarity disappeared when interactions with unfamiliar peers were compared. In a free-play situation, comparison children tended to ignore unfamiliar children, whereas maltreated children tended to become involved in physically aggressive interactions with them. Howes and Espinosa (1985) reported similar findings. This difficulty in relating to unfamiliar peers might compromise the ability of maltreated children to establish new peer friendships (Cicchetti & Toth, 1995). Howes and Eldredge (1985) found that maltreated children tended to respond aggressively to peer aggression, while nonmaltreated children responded with either distress or resistance. Furthermore, physically abused children responded aggressively to a peer's emotional distress, while nonmaltreated children responded with prosocial behavior.

Withdrawal and Avoidance in Social Interactions

Heightened aggressiveness in peer interactions is not the only reaction physically abused children display. George and Main (1979) found, for instance, that physically abused infants and toddlers avoided interacting with adult caregivers and other children. They tended to respond indirectly to a friendly approach, perhaps walking to the adult from the side or behind. Sometimes they turned around and walked backwards to the adult. Straker and Jacobson (1989) found that physically abused children engaged in less social interaction in free-play situations than did control children, but the former did not show significantly more hostility or aggression. In later studies (e.g., Dodge, Pettit, & Bates, 1994; Kaufman & Cicchetti, 1989) maltreated children were also evaluated as being more withdrawn in social interactions. Based on their results in other studies (Hoffman-Plotkin & Twentyman, 1984; Howes & Espinosa, 1985), researchers have suggested that social withdrawal and avoidance may also be more prevalent in neglected children.

The overlap among the characteristics of maltreated children's peer relations is illustrated in the Minnesota Mother–Child Interaction Project (Erickson et al., 1989). By 6 years of age, physically abused, neglected children and children of psychologically unavailable mothers all ranked lower in social competence than those in the control group and were regarded as unpopular and aggressive. The neglected children were also described as withdrawn.

Generally, however, few studies have been done of the peer relations of sexually abused children. Manly et al. (1994) assessed the social competence of abused children between the ages of 5 and 11 years. Children in the sexual-abuse group were rated as more socially competent than the physically abused and physically neglected children. As well, the sexual-abuse group did not differ in social competence from the nonmaltreated group. Manly et al. (1994) postulated that some of these children were truly asymptomatic or that interpersonal difficulties may become more pronounced only in later developmental periods such as the emergence of opposite-sex relationships in adolescence. Conflicting results were obtained by Hibbard and Hartman (1992) who administered the Child Behavior Checklist to male and female alleged sexual-abuse victims aged 4 to 8 years. The authors reported that the subscale profiles all tended in the direction consistent with withdrawal and impairments in social interaction. The sexually abused children who first joined the Minnesota Mother–Child Interaction Project at age 6 years were described as socially withdrawn and unpopular, and their dependency upon adults was striking. Clearly, this area requires further investigation before any definitive conclusions can be drawn.

In studies of the peer relations of maltreated children the focus has been on other variables as well as the degree of aggression or withdrawal. In general, results of these studies reveal that maltreated children are less popular and more likely to be negative when interacting with peers (Dodge et al., 1994; Haskett & Kistner, 1991; Kaufman & Cicchetti, 1989). We have found, in our clinical experience, that peer relationships are identified as a common problem in referrals for therapy. For abused and neglected school-aged children, difficulties with their peers clearly set them apart from their age mates.

SUMMARY

Maltreated children are at significant risk for the development of a number of problems, including insecure attachments, poor emotional and behavioral self-regulatory skills, and a compromised sense of self. Maltreatment has been associated with lowered cognitive functioning, poorer adaptation to school, deficiencies in language, and poor peer relationships. According to the literature, despite being at increased risk for psychological and behavioral problems, maltreated children do not demonstrate a uniform response or reaction to abuse or neglect. Furthermore, there is considerable overlap in the characteristics of children exposed to different subtypes of maltreatment, and some children subjected to abuse or neglect experience only transient effects whereas others display no symptoms. The outcomes of maltreatment do not fall neatly into one diagnostic category and do not comprise a homogeneous syndrome that can be called "the maltreated child."

This diversity of outcome argues against the notion of a simple or direct connection or pathway between maltreatment and sequelae. The transactional model briefly described in this chapter offers a tentative way of conceptualizing the impact of maltreatment upon children. Abuse and neglect, although significant risk factors for many serious problems, interact with other variables, which in turn mediate the impact of maltreatment upon the developing child. In the next chapter we identify and describe the mechanisms and factors that may contribute to this complex relationship.

The somewhat mixed and conflicting results and our consequent inability to draw clear and unequivocal conclusions may also be partially attributable to methodological inadequacies in the research. Problems with subject selection and definitions of child maltreatment, research design, control groups, and the choice of outcome measures have characterized the literature. Remedying the methodological flaws can only contribute to a more thorough and comprehensive understanding of the relationship between various types of maltreatment and outcome and of the possible mechanisms and factors involved. Moreover, researchers must begin to conceptualize the impact of maltreatment as a multidimensional and transactional phenomenon under which numerous variables are subsumed. While less complex conceptualizations are simpler to understand, we must move beyond them to attain a fuller and richer understanding of the lives and experiences of maltreated children. This increased knowledge will enhance our clinical work with these children and their families.

TWO

Mechanisms of Impact

W E NOW TURN to a description of some mechanisms that may mediate between maltreatment and some of the more common symptoms described in Chapter 1. Although this discussion of these mechanisms and processes is somewhat hypothetical and more research is needed to corroborate these tentative and incomplete ideas, hopefully it will assist clinicians' attempts to understand the impact of maltreatment upon their young clients and suggest useful intervention strategies.

ATTACHMENT THEORY AND INTERNAL WORKING MODELS: GENERAL CONSIDERATIONS

We believe that Bowlby's (1969, 1973, 1980, 1982) concept of the "internal working model" is central to an understanding of the association between maltreatment and developmental outcome and has special relevance for clinicians who work with maltreated youngsters.

Although we briefly mentioned the concept of internal working models in Chapter 1, we will expand upon this fundamental notion here before we discuss the way they may mediate the relationship between maltreatment and outcome. Through actual interactions and interchanges with the primary caregiver, the child begins to acquire mental representations, or internal working models, of this parent–child relationship. The internal working model has two primary components. The first comprises children's information about, expectations of, and affects about other people (whether these individuals will be responsive, trustworthy, accessible, and caring or, on the contrary, unresponsive, untrustworthy, inaccessible, and uncaring). Children's corresponding representations of themselves and their own role in these relationships (whether they are worthy and capable of obtaining the other's care or whether they are unworthy and incapable of obtaining adequate care) make up the second component. According to this concept, early relationship experiences become internalized as mental representations and create anticipatory images that shape attitudes and reactions to, and perceptions of, individuals encountered in the future (Flaherty & Richman, 1986). In this model, the individual is provided with a basic context for subsequent transactions with the environment, especially social relationships (Sroufe, 1988). For instance, if a child experiences and mentally represents caregivers as available, nurturing, and trustworthy, this information contributes to the child's more general model of others as available and trustworthy. Furthermore, the self will be regarded as competent and effective in relationship to these other individuals, and worthy of being treated in a sensitive and caring manner. Conversely, if children's experiences of their relationships with caregivers have been characterized by unavailability, uncertainty, and insensitivity, they may develop negative expectations of other relationships. They may begin to regard themselves as unworthy and incapable of obtaining adequate care from parental figures. For example, children abused for many years and from an early age may expect similar treatment in new relationships.

A question arises regarding how these internal working models are constructed. Bretherton (1985, 1987, 1990) proposes that general patterns are first abstracted from and organized according to the actions and outcomes involved in day-to-day infant–parent interactions, such as how the caregiver responds to the infant's distress. This concept is similar to that of "procedural memory," in which information regarding recurrent patterns of sensory stimuli and behavioral responses are encoded (Crittenden, 1992b). The central point is that this memory system relies upon behavioral evidence. Nelson and Gruendal (1981) call these abstractions "generalized event representations" and describe them as the basic building blocks of mental representations. As children mature, their semantic memory develops. This memory system "encodes verbal representations of experience. As children begin the transition to preoperational intelligence (Piaget, 1952), they are able to process information, that is, to think, without immediately experiencing the phenomena of interest. Instead, words substitute for the sensory-action patterns that characterized procedural schemata" (Crittenden, 1992b, p. 577). As they grow, children begin to develop verbal representations of themselves, other individuals and their experiences. Crittenden (1992b) maintains that parents' verbal responses to children and their experience have a substantial influence on the content of semantic memory, such as telling a child that he or she is a "bad kid" and deserves to be beaten. Episodic memory is presumed to develop after procedural and semantic memory. These unique memories are encoded by multiple means—verbal, visual and auditory—and are "recalled as sequentially ordered episodes with characters, movement, sounds, smells, etc. Especially important is recall of the feelings experienced" (Crittenden, 1992b, p. 578). Thus information about attachment may be encoded in different memory systems, represented by multiple working models. We would like to emphasize that the actual construction and mechanisms of internal working models are still a matter of debate. The preceding discussion is tentative and speculative (see Erickson, Korfmacher, & Egeland, 1992, for a cogent and succinct review of these issues).

As well as consisting of expectations about the self and others derived from experience, the internal working model includes the unconscious rules for processing attachment-related information and memories. It affects how the individual perceives, remembers, interprets, and reacts to these experiences (Bretherton, 1985; Solomon, George, & De Jong, 1995; Zeanah & Zeanah, 1989). Given different internal working models, one child may interpret another's refusal to play as a devastating rejection and evidence of personal unworthiness. Another child with a more positive internal working model may perceive and interpret such a refusal as a minor slight. The internal working model of the first child might have developed in association with a chronic history of parental physical abuse and has now been generalized to relationships with others, including peers. The subsequent behavior of these two children may well be different (sulking or an angry outburst by the former versus readily approaching another potential playmate by the latter).

The child is hardly a passive recipient of experience. Rather, he or she is an active constructor of reality who both creates experiences and differentially attends to diverse information in the social world. There is empirical support for this concept. Dodge and Richard (1985) demonstrate that aggressive, school-aged boys are biased in their interpretations of peers. Such boys perceive malicious intent and hostility when no such motives are present. In turn, this perception may result in a heightened tendency to relate aggressively to peers. Unfortunately, this interpersonal style may elicit rejection and, possibly, even aggressive responses from other children, thereby confirming the expectation of unsatisfying and hostile reactions from others. In their study, Rieder and Cicchetti (1989) also found that maltreated children were more hypervigilant to aggressive stimuli than were nonmaltreated children. The introduction of aggressive distractions into a practiced task disrupted performance of the former more than it did for the nonmaltreated children. Also, maltreated children recalled a greater number of distracting aggressive stimuli than did nonmaltreated youngsters. Thus internal working models can affect the range of what can be perceived, how perceptions can be interpreted, and how the person behaves in accordance with these models. A clinical example illustrates this important concept:

Gary was taken into the care of child welfare authorities at 6 years of age because of severe physical abuse, neglect, and psychological maltreatment. A woman to whom his mother had entrusted his care when he was much younger repeatedly subjected him to this abuse and neglect. He was placed in foster care and began attending grade 1 at a large elementary school when the new school year began. At recess, Gary began to experience intense anxiety. He told his therapist that he was distressed with the behavior of some children in the playground. When some ran toward him yelling, he automatically interpreted these advances as threats. According to Gary, "They were screaming at me and chasing me, and they was gonna hurt me!" Discussions with teachers on supervisory duty revealed that the children in question were running while playing an enthusiastic game of tag; and some had happened to run in Gary's general direction. He had not only misinterpreted their behavior (i.e., that they were running toward him to assault him) but had not even perceived the smiles or laughter of his peers.

Given the years that Gary had been terrorized by his female caregiver, his internal working model of others was not open to this discrepant information about how people would treat him; it limited his perception to that which fit his existing model. Additionally, Gary's internal model influenced how he interpreted this experience. Rather than changing the model to fit his experience (accommodation), Gary changed his experience on the playground to fit his model (assimilation). According to Crittenden (1992b), "Representational models can, thus, become a double-edged sword. They both speed the process through which infants respond adaptively to their environments and also skew the processing of future experience to fit existing models of experience" (p. 578).

A basic assumption of attachment theory is that the child's initial relationship with the caregiver, usually the mother, in all probability affects and predicts later relationships. Attachment theorists contend that there is continuity in development when interpersonal and other environmental experiences maintain developmental trajectories already established. This continuity occurs when the individual's experiences are consistent with his or her internal working model of the self and others. Discontinuity occurs when the individual's experiences run counter to this internal working model (Bowlby, 1988b). As we shall see later, a central therapeutic task with many maltreated children is to generate this sense of discontinuity to modify these maladaptive internal working models of the self and others.

Although these internal models are open to change (as suggested by the term "working"), Bowlby (1980) and Bretherton (1987) postulate that models become so ingrained or overlearned they begin operating outside awareness. On the one hand this is advantageous, since it economizes effort and makes people efficient processors in different situations. Returning to our example of maltreated children who perceive malicious intent in their peers: such children may well be efficient processors of information, since interpersonal behaviors are subjected to the same interpretation repeatedly. These children need not engage in the kinds of mental efforts associated with a more critical analysis of others' motivations. McCrone et al. (1994) also postulate that individuals adhere rigidly to these maladaptive assumptions and beliefs, even in the face of discrepant information, because they are stable and protect the child from the surprise and disorganization that a reworking of these models would entail. However, once automated, these internal working models become difficult to change. Models not open to new and discrepant experiences or information pose a real risk to the individual. The child never learns to question the validity of the assumptions and expectations of the internal working model, and it remains intact. In other words, stable organization is counterbalanced by oversimplification and possible distortion (Bretherton, 1987). Sroufe (1988) suggests that, given the increasing firmness of these internal working models, changing the environment may modify but not completely erase the individual's models of relationships.

The development of defense mechanisms in middle childhood occupies a central position in psychoanalytic and psychodynamic theory. Defense mechanisms protect the child from internal pain and conflict (Freud, 1966). McCrone et al. (1994) integrated this traditional notion with the idea of multiple working models. They claim that young, maltreated children cannot integrate discrepant and incompatible information from different models. For example, a child who has been beaten from infancy or toddlerhood may have developed painful and unpleasant procedural memories and a subsequent model of parents as dangerous and rejecting figures. However, parents perhaps told the child they were carrying out beatings because they loved and cared for the child; that is, "It's for your own good." Such statements may have generated a semantic memory far more tolerable to the child. Acknowledging that the beatings reflect parental lack of regard, or even hate, for the child is so painful and threatening that the child retains them at a less conscious level. Other models, such as semantic ones ("My parents really do love me, and that's why they are punishing me like this"), mask the unpleasant procedurally based model. Using another model thereby affords the child some relief from the distressing affects associated with this particular internal working model; in an extreme form the child may idealize the parents. This defensive strategy, although adaptive in the short term, leaves children with little awareness of their sadness, anger, and anxiety. This is one example of defensive exclusion, the process that prevents individuals from consciously experiencing their own feelings, noticing what is going on in their lives, or signaling a need for help.

Incompatible information from different models is kept apart by defenses such as projection, displacement, splitting, preoccupation, and introjection as well as exclusion (McCrone et al., 1994). However, the models and feelings that are excluded from consciousness still exert a potent and sometimes malevolent influence upon the child's adaptation to the world. For instance, McCrone et al. (1994) compared maltreated children's responses on a projective storytelling task with those of nonmaltreated children. Maltreated children's stories revealed that these children had a significantly greater tendency to attend selectively to, and elaborate upon, the negative aspects–especially aggression–of interpersonal relationships. This finding is consistent with the hypersensitivity of maltreated children to aggressive stimuli reported by Rieder and Cicchetti (1989). Our earlier description of Gary's responses to social stimuli is also consistent with this notion that maltreated children have internal working models operating outside awareness yet influencing responses to interpersonal situations.

ATTACHMENT THEORY, INTERNAL WORKING MODELS, AND SEQUELAE OF MALTREATMENT

As we have just described, internal working models generate expectations and rules about processing information related to relationships and attachment. Basing their work upon this core concept of attachment theory, Dodge, Bates, and Pettit (1990) hypothesize that "maltreated children are likely to develop biased and deficient patterns of processing social information, including a failure to attend to relevant cues, a bias to attribute hostile intentions to others, and a lack of competent behavioral strategies to solve interpersonal problems" (p. 1682). Results of their prospective study of 309 children support the existence of such patterns, which, in turn, are predictors of later aggressive behavior development. Thus maltreated children, many with insecure attachments and a consequent lack of basic trust in the world and other people, may perceive and interpret social information and behavior as evidence of hostile intent or threat. In turn, they may react in an aggressive, externalizing manner.

Mueller and Silverman (1989) believe that the maltreated child's reliance upon identification with the aggressor may play a significant role in this process. Expecting more maltreatment, the child may transform into the aggressor not only to fend off the expected assault but to compensate for concomitant feelings of helplessness, inadequacy, and vulnerability. A maltreated child may react aggressively and provocatively to provoke a similar response from the abusive adult. By successfully eliciting this response the maltreated child gains a sense of control and predictability over events (i.e., aggressive interchanges) that are believed to be inevitable. In a much earlier paper, Littner (1960) used psychoanalytic concepts to make the same point: abused children tend to provoke abusive reactions from caregivers, including foster parents, as a way to gain control and mastery over a frightening and unpredictable world.

Mueller and Silverman (1989) have identified another function of aggressive behavior in maltreated children. Drawing upon Bowlby's (1973, 1980) idea that adults sometimes have multiple internal working models of the self and others, they suggest the same may be true of maltreated children. These children might construct a conscious image of caretakers as available and caring and of the self as adequate and worthy. More painful models of the self and others are defensively dissociated or split off to avoid the pain and overwhelming feelings of threat associated with such negative representational models. However, these dissociative models are thought to be able to influence behavior, although they may operate outside conscious awareness. This process may help to explain the reported finding that abused children frequently strike out at a peer who is exhibiting emotional distress (Howes & Espinosa, 1985; Main & George, 1985; Troy & Sroufe, 1987). A peer's distress may elicit mental images and memories of instances when the maltreated child was similarly distressed and attachment figures had rejected the youngster or had not met his or her needs. As these memories and images may be intolerable, the child might strike out at the peer who exhibits this distress to terminate it and thereby avoid personal feelings of anxiety and pain.

The internal working models of maltreated children may mediate their adaptation in other ways. Given their negative expectations of relationships, they may relate to others with a corresponding lack of enthusiasm, confidence, and overall positive affective stance (e.g., Howes & Espinosa, 1985). Friendlier and more cooperative children are more highly regarded by their peers, whereas aggressive children tend to be rejected by others (Asher & Coie, 1990; Denham, McKinley, Couchoud, & Holt, 1990). The absence of a positive affective stance in maltreated children may impede them in establishing and maintaining positive peer relationships and may lead to further incidents of rejection. Such incidents would then reinforce their internal working models of others as unreliable, unresponsive figures who reject them and of themselves as unworthy of friendship.

Our review has provided indications that maltreated children are more likely than nonmaltreated children to engage in more disruptive, withdrawn, and aggressive behaviors and less prosocial behavior. These behaviors, reflecting problems in self-regulation, may well impair the maltreated child's ability to interact positively and proactively with others. As happens with the successful resolution of other stage-salient developmental issues, many factors contribute to competence in behavioral and emotional self-regulation. These factors include the child's level of physiological arousal and his or her capacity to articulate verbally internal affective states (Buchsbaum, Toth, Clyman, Cicchetti, & Emde, 1992). Qualities of the attachment relationship may have significance for the attainment of behavioral and affective self-regulation in the young child. One principal task of parents when their children are infants is to help the infants to modulate their physiological arousal. Buchsbaum et al. (1992) describe some of the processes responsible for this development; for example, parents respond to particular affective displays by the child and discourage others. Parents also begin to teach the child alternate ways of expressing feelings. As we have seen, the parent's use of language – for instance, in articulating a perception of the child's internal states and corresponding needs – facilitates the child's own use of internal state language. Rather than acting out feelings such as anger in impulsive, destructive ways, the child slowly begins to learn to talk about them. Parents who pay little or no attention to their child's feelings or who cannot perceive these feelings accurately encounter grave difficulty in soothing the child. The parents will have difficulty in talking about these emotions in a way that helps the child acquire and refine the special vocabulary of internal states. These characteristics of parenting are, of course, consistent with those that promote a secure attachment.

The importance of the child–parent relationship for a child's development of emotional and behavioral self-regulation was demonstrated by Gaensbauer and his colleagues (Gaensbauer & Sands, 1979: Gaensbauer, Mrazek, & Harmon, 1981). They showed that communication between abused and neglected infants and their mothers was developmentally and affectively retarded, depressed, ambivalent/affectively labile, and angry. Many features of these mother–child interactional patterns contributed to the infants' poor regulation of their own emotional arousal. As a result, the children exhibited negativity, withdrawal, inconsistency, unpredictability, shallowness, and a lack of pleasure. Given their involvement in these kinds of interactional patterns with their mothers, it is not surprising these maltreated infants displayed early problems in their own emotional self-regulation. They displayed excessive levels of negative affects, especially fear, or blunted patterns of emotional expression. Gaensbauer and Hiatt (1984) identified the differential effects of various maltreatment types on patterns of emotional expression. Physically abused infants evidenced high levels of negative affect and little positive affect, while emotionally neglected infants displayed blunted affect.

The importance of the attachment relationship for the development of emotional and behavioral self-regulation continues as children grow older. A "goal-corrected partnership" in which the child increasingly takes the attachment figure's own motivations and plans into account is a major result of a child's establishment of a secure relationship with a primary caregiver (Bowlby, 1969). In this phase, which usually begins some time after the third birthday, verbal interchanges between child and parent are a principal means for the two parties to communicate their respective needs and successfully negotiate a plan that takes these needs into account. Several factors account for this developmental advance. A secure attachment between the child and parent, characterized by parental sensitivity to the child's feelings and internal states, may play a significant role in the parent's ability and willingness to engage in these discussions with the child. Furthermore, the parent's ability to meet the child's needs models a particular style of interaction for the young child; that is, the child incorporates this same kind of sensitivity and an appreciation of the parent's and others' needs and perspectives into his or her interpersonal style. Consequently, the child's burgeoning language skills and developing ability to see the world through the perspective of another individual result in more effective communication between the child and parent. Rather than acting out these feelings and behavior in maladaptive ways, the child can engage in dialogue; the two can then negotiate conflicts and disagreements successfully. These parental qualities that promote secure attachment (accessibility, warmth, and contingent responsiveness) may afford the young child an initial model of reciprocity and sharing. This model can then be applied to other relationships, in turn contributing significantly to rewarding adaptive interchanges with others. On the other hand, the maltreated child who has not experienced a reciprocal relationship may encounter real difficulty in relating empathically to other individuals.

There may be other ways that internal working models mediate a child's response to maltreatment. A key concept of attachment theory is that of the "secure base." Bowlby (1988b) maintains that a basic component of human nature is the urge to explore the environment, which is antithetical to attachment behavior. However, if the child feels secure in the relationship with a caretaker, this person can be used as a secure base from which to explore the world and become acquainted with it. Essentially, the child develops a mental representation of the caretaker as reliable and responsive, someone who will take care of the child if difficulties are encountered while exploring the world.

Experience with the physical and social environment is critical to an infant's and young child's cognitive, language, and social development. Studies by Aber and his colleagues (Aber & Allen, 1987; Aber, Allen, Carlson, & Cicchetti, 1989) have shown that maltreated preschoolers and school-aged children (physical neglect, emotional maltreatment, and physical abuse) exhibit increased dependency upon others and decreased "effectance motivation"; that is, the child's motivation to deal competently with the environment for the intrinsic pleasure of mastery (Aber et al., 1989). High effectance motivation, low dependency, and high cognitive maturity comprise the "secure readiness factor" (Aber et al., 1989). Low secure readiness-to-learn is manifested by maltreated infants and toddlers. They have difficulty in balancing feeling comfortable with adults while exploring new aspects of the environment, and this difficulty may be accompanied by cognitive deficits. Maltreated children also may not feel comfortable enough to engage in new social relationships, which may well compromise the development of their social skills.

An impaired ability to explore the environment is by no means the only factor associated with the academic and cognitive difficulties of maltreated children. Other features of the caretaking environment in which the abuse or neglect occurs play a contributory role. One that must be considered is inadequate cognitive stimulation. For example, Vondra, Barnett, and Cicchetti (1990) demonstrated that the receptive language abilities of physically abused/neglected preschoolers were related to the quality of the home environment, especially the physical condition of the home and the availability of toys. We have already reviewed the detrimental effects of a neglectful environment, including little stimulation, lack of encouragement for learning, and an unresponsive attitude to the child's intellectual efforts or achievements.

One central component of an internal working model comprises the perceptions and representations of the self and the self in relation to significant others. Negative self-esteem and self-evaluation are consistent with the experiences of a child who has received inadequate care. A child may begin to regard himself or herself as ineffectual or powerless either in eliciting adequate caretaking from others or in terminating maltreatment. This latter concept is analogous to Finkelhor and Browne's (1985) concept of powerlessness, one of the four major traumagenic dynamics of child sexual abuse. They defined powerlessness as "the process in which the child's will, desires, and sense of efficacy are continually contravened" (Finkelhor & Browne, 1985, p. 532). Although Finkelhor and Browne (1985) developed the model of traumagenic dynamics to explain the impact of childhood sexual abuse, the model has applicability to other types of abuse. Youngsters who have been physically abused or psychologically maltreated may experience a sense of powerlessness because of their inability to avoid or stop the physical and emotional invasion of their bodies and internal lives. Children feel a similar sense of inadequacy and a lack of control over their worlds when they cannot effect changes in the neglectful and inattentive child-rearing practices of their parents. Children's feelings of powerlessness may be exacerbated by the perpetrator's coercion and manipulation or by the ineffective responses (e.g., denial, lack of protective action) of parents or caregivers. Larger social systems (e.g., child welfare programs, the judicial system) may respond to children's disclosures in ways that diminish the child's self-efficacy, for example, by requiring children to undergo multiple investigative interviews or court appearances.

Finkelhor and Browne (1985) also describe the dynamic of stigmatization: "The negative connotations—e.g., badness, shame, and guilt—that are communicated to the child around the experiences and that then become incorporated into the child's self-image" (p. 532). Again, this description is similar to the concept of the negative internal working model of the self. That many children who have been subjected to abuse or neglect should exhibit negative self-esteem makes intuitive sense: the maltreatment conveys a powerful message to the child (e.g.,"You are not worthy of being treated well," "If you were a better child, we would treat you better"). These attitudes may be reinforced by the negative response (such as shock, revulsion or blame) of caregivers or other significant people to the child's victimization.

We have examined the concept of defense mechanisms from the perspective of internal working models and attachment theory. Incompatible information from different models is kept apart by defenses such as projection, displacement, splitting, and dissociation. Although these defenses arise to help the child cope with the painful and overwhelming affects and cognitions arising from traumatic experiences, they lead to an unintegrated sense of self. The growth of an autonomous self may also be stunted by the phenomenon of "other-directedness": to monitor the abuse or rejection they believe is inevitable in interpersonal relationships, maltreated individuals become hypervigilant and focus upon the other person's emotional state to the exclusion of their own (Briere, 1992).

We believe that attachment theory, particularly in its emphasis upon internal working models, offers much toward an understanding of the association between maltreatment and developmental outcome. There is a potential danger here, however. The theory's extensive empirical base and growing popularization in the media may lead some overzealous proponents to rely upon it exclusively to explain every human problem or suffering. This would be a grave mistake. A secure attachment in infancy and toddlerhood does not necessarily ensure later competence. Conversely, although an insecure early attachment is a significant risk factor for the development of a later psychopathologic condition, a poor outcome is not inevitable. There are many pathways between maltreatment and later adaptation. We would be remiss if we failed to describe other factors, processes, and mechanisms that may contribute to the emergence of maladaptive behavior and psychopathologic conditions. It is to these conceptualizations that we now turn.

CONDITIONING THEORIES

Mowrer (1960) proposed a two-factor (classical and instrumental conditioning) learning theory to explain the development of anxiety and avoidance. Berliner and Wheeler (1987) and Deblinger, McLeer, Atkins, Ralphe, and

Foa (1987) applied this theory to sexually abused children; one might well argue that the basic principles can also be applied to other maltreated children who experience significant levels of fear. In this paradigm, a previously neutral stimulus becomes associated with an unconditioned stimulus that innately evokes discomfort or fear. Applying this paradigm to maltreatment, the abuse or maltreatment is the unconditioned stimulus that evokes fear, whereas other aspects of the situation (e.g., perpetrator, environmental context) represent the neutral stimulus. The neutral stimulus then acquires aversive properties such that its presence elicits anxiety. It now becomes a conditioned stimulus for fear responses (see Figure 2.1).

In a case of child sexual abuse, the fears the child experienced as a direct consequence of the sexual abuse would be associated with the perpetrator or other stimuli. The child would then experience feelings of fear and anxiety in the presence of these stimuli, particularly in situations most similar to those in which the abuse occurred (e.g., being alone with the perpetrator or being in a room where the abuse occurred). Over time the child's fear could, through generalization, produce anxiety in the presence of persons (e.g., other males) or other stimuli (e.g., physical surroundings, sights, sounds, smells) similar to those associated with the abuse. Through higher order conditioning, these more recently conditioned cues for anxiety could themselves become paired with other previously neutral stimuli, producing still more cues for anxiety and leading to feelings of pervasive anxiety.

The second factor of Mowrer's (1960) theory postulates that avoidance or escape responses, which decrease or end the discomfort that arises in the presence of the conditioned stimuli, are reinforced when this discomfort or anxiety decreases. Wachtel (1973) argues that defenses such as repression can be understood as a learned process of avoiding thoughts and events associated with anxiety. By not thinking of the abuse, the abused person minimizes his or her own discomfort, and these avoidant behaviors or thoughts are reinforced as the individual learns to redirect attention from the cues or signals associated with fear. In effect, repression is conceptualized in terms of avoidance learning. This defensive maneuver has some harmful consequences. If a child's avoidance of thoughts or discussions about the abuse is reinforced, the child never learns at what point, if any, fears are no longer justified or adaptive. By not examining or talking about the maltreatment, the child minimizes discomfort but also eliminates the possibility of exposure to the cues and affects of his or her fears. Therefore, the anxiety is not extinguished. Furthermore, the child is unable to examine other central issues critically, such as whether the maltreatment was deserved. Thus the seemingly protective reaction on the part of parents of telling children "to forget about what happened" is not beneficial.

There has been considerable debate about this model's appropriateness for the emergence of posttraumatic stress disorder. Foa, Steketee, and Roth-

DEVELOPMENT OF SYMPTOMS (Classical Conditioning Paradigm)

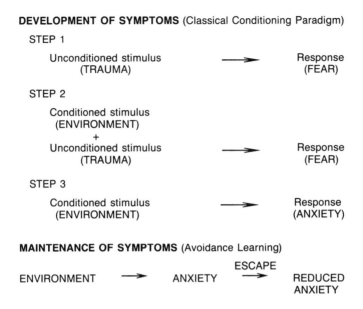

MAINTENANCE OF SYMPTOMS (Avoidance Learning)

ENVIRONMENT ⟶ ANXIETY → ESCAPE → REDUCED ANXIETY

FIGURE 2.1. Development and maintenance of symptoms.

baum (1989) suggest that the case for using Mowrer's theory to explain posttraumatic stress disorder is compelling. It accounts for the addition of fear to trauma-related cues that previously were neutral. The theory also explains why individuals with posttraumatic stress disorder avoid nondangerous situations and why such avoidance persists despite its disruption of daily functioning. Foa et al. (1989) also raise some objections. They note that Mowrer's two-stage theory does not explain other posttraumatic stress disorder symptoms and ignores the etiological significance of the meaning ascribed to the aversive event. For example, the event may destroy or compromise formerly held basic concepts of safety and inviolability: one's world becomes less predictable and controllable. Citing evidence that perceived threat better predicts posttraumatic stress disorder than does actual threat, Foa et al. (1989) argue that any model of the development of posttraumatic stress disorder must incorporate the significance of the meaning of the event for the individual.

LEARNED HELPLESSNESS, ATTRIBUTION THEORY, AND PHENOMENOLOGY

The focus of both learned helplessness and attribution theory has been upon the subjective or phenomenological meaning of the traumatic event for the victim. Learned helplessness also has been used to explain the depressive symptomatology and negative self-esteem of maltreatment victims, particularly those who were sexually abused. According to this paradigm, individuals learn that their responses in traumatic incidents involving personal danger will be ineffective (Petersen & Seligman, 1983). This conclusion is, in turn, generalized across situations and time to generate expectations of future inadequacy. The theory incorporates causal attributions to explain the loss of self-esteem that accompanies these feelings of helplessness and inadequacy. These attributions contain three dimensions: the source (internal/external), the generality over time (stable/unstable), and the generality across situations (global/specific). In this theory, it is posited that victims who attribute the abuse to themselves (an internal attribution) are more likely to develop a negative self-esteem and self-concept. Wolfe et al. (1994) report that sexually abused children who met the DSM-III-R criteria for posttraumatic stress disorder were more likely to report feelings of guilt than those who did not. Mannarino, Cohen, and Berman (1994) have also found that sexually abused 7- to 12-year-old girls reported a heightened sense of self-blame for negative events compared with nonabused controls. Personal attributions for negative events were significantly related to children's self-reports of lowered self-esteem and feelings of depression and anxiety.

When examining this issue of internal attributions, it is important to make the distinction between "characterological self-blame" (attributing the cause of the maltreatment to some uncontrollable aspect of themselves; e.g., "I'm a bad boy and I deserve to be hit") and "behavioral self-blame" (attributing the cause of the maltreatment to specific behavioral responses or a failure to react; e.g., "I kept going over to his house where he abused me") (Janoff-Bulman, 1979). As we shall see in subsequent chapters, such distinctions may have important implications for clinical work. Clinicians have a strong tradition of telling their child clients that they were not to blame for the sexual abuse. Others (e.g., Lamb, 1986) have claimed that such broad statements diminish a child's sense of efficacy: acknowledging behavioral self-blame may confer a sense of mastery upon the child and may serve to identify different behavioral strategies the child can use in the future (e.g., "I'll stay away from his house from now on") to prevent further revictimization.

Feelings of depression and helplessness may be associated with the child's belief that she or he will remain vulnerable to abuse in the future ("stable attributions"). Wolfe, Gentile, and Wolfe (1989) found that higher levels of negative affect and feelings of betrayal, stigmatization, and intrusive thoughts, as well as of lowered social competence, were related to stable negative attributions about the sexual abuse (i.e., that sexual abuse would happen again). They also examined the role of global attributions and found that sexually abused children tended to report a belief that adults are likely to exploit children and that sexual abuse is pervasive. Wolfe et al. (1989) predicted that these beliefs that the world was dangerous and that many people exploit children would be related to negative affect, but the direction of the correlations was opposite to that predicted. They speculated that such beliefs may be comforting to children, since they suggest the children are not alone in their experiences.

In both Foa et al.'s (1989) reformulation of Mowrer's theory and the learned helplessness model considerable emphasis is placed upon the meaning of the abusive event for the child. These models take a "phenomenological" approach. Briere (1992) states that "phenomenology refers to the survivor's personal experiences and perceptions as an important criterion for therapeutic reactions, rather than sole reliance on theoretical notions that may or may not fit the survivor's experience" (p. 84). Most concepts of trauma have incorporated this phenomenological perspective. As Lewandowski and Baranoski (1994) note, the definition of a trauma as a sudden, untoward event depends on one's perspective. For example, in cases of physical trauma like motor vehicle accidents, adults tend to define these events as the disruption of social order. They mark the end of the event by the return of order, i.e., the arrival of help. Children may have a different conception of what is traumatic in a similar event. Children may identify rescue after the trauma as a further source of hurt and fear. Their course while they are in the hospital, replete as it is with painful medical procedures and separation from parents, may continue to be interpreted as traumatic.

We can apply the same concepts to maltreated children. The meaning (i.e., different types of attributions) the child imputes to the maltreatment plays an important role in subsequent adaptation to this trauma. For example, in a recent meta-analytic review it was empirically demonstrated that interpersonal violence (childhood sexual and physical abuse, rape, criminal assault, and domestic violence) has deleterious effects on the psychological functioning of children and adults (Weaver & Clum, 1995). In this review, it was found that "subjective factors" (general appraisal of the incident, self-blame, and perceived life threat) contributed twice as much to the magnitude of psychological distress as did "objective factors" (e.g., physical injury, force, and use of a weapon). Although we will return to this point in our discussions of assessment and therapy, it is important that adults not impose, onto a particular child, their own definition or interpretation of what might have been traumatic or aversive about the maltreatment. A central task of assessment and therapy is the attempt to understand the meaning of the maltreatment for each child client. Furthermore, a child's perception or interpretation of the meaning of maltreatment may change as a function of progress through different developmental stages. The following clinical example illustrates this point well.

Eight-year-old Chris had been sexually abused by his father and his father's female partner. The central theme of therapy at this time was Chris's feelings of powerlessness and vulnerability, reactions that seemed to reflect the physical coercion and threats he received (e.g., statements that he would be killed if he did not participate in the activity or if he ever disclosed it). After a year of therapy, Chris's nightmares, somatic complaints, and intrusive thoughts and images of the abuse had disappeared, and therapy was terminated with the consent of Chris and his mother.

At his request, Chris's mother again contacted the therapist when Chris was 12 years of age. The interviews at the time of the second referral revealed that Chris, who had begun puberty, was now worried about the implications of the actual sexual activity for his own emerging sexual identity. In particular, Chris was distraught in that he had been sexually abused by a male and had shown some physiological responses, such as sustaining an erection, during this activity. Initiation of a short course of therapy resulted in a significant reduction in his anxiety and a return to a more adaptive level of functioning.

Chris's experience illustrates the notion that maltreatment may have different meanings for a child at different developmental stages. When he was 8, sexuality was not a primary focus, but it emerged as one when Chris began puberty. It was only then that he recognized the significance of this aspect of his victimization. The recognition that one has been victimized may, in part, depend upon concepts that are only acquired at a later stage of development. This issue became even more salient for Chris when he began junior high school. He was exposed to more frequent and usually negative discussions of homosexuality, which exacerbated his sense of stigmatization.

The meaning a child ascribes to a particular episode of maltreatment or abuse may be influenced by the child's more general set of attributions about himself or herself and the world. Returning to the concept of internal working models, a child maltreated for a prolonged period, typically beginning in infancy and toddlerhood, may have already formed an expectation of himself or herself as undeserving of care and of being responsible for this poor parenting. Consequently, another episode of maltreatment, although somewhat different from previous maltreatment, may be interpreted similarly; that is, the child deserved the abuse, it was the child's fault, and it was yet another example of other people's unreliability and untrustworthiness.

OTHER MECHANISMS

Other mechanisms or processes contribute to the maltreated child's maladjustment. Belsky (1980) identifies broader societal values according to which the use of physical aggression is condoned, particularly by males, which may reinforce this interpersonal style. The modeling of physical aggression or sexual behavior as a coercive exchange in interpersonal relationships may have considerable impact upon children. In turn, they may engage in similar behavior with others. Besides the influence of modeling, physical and sexual aggression provide some powerful reinforcers for maltreated children. For instance, a child may use physical aggression against peers, which may result in their compliance with the child's demands. Coercive sexual behavior directed toward others may compensate for low self-esteem and feelings of vulnerability and inadequacy. For a child who has experienced both physical and sexual aggression, identifying with the aggressor may be an underlying mechanism that serves to maintain that behavior in the child. The child feels stronger and in control when behaving aggressively, thereby countering feelings of powerlessness and inadequacy. Finkelhor and Browne (1985) describe another traumagenic dynamic, "traumatic sexualization," as "a process in which a child's sexuality (including both sexual feelings and sexual attitudes) is shaped in a developmentally inappropriate and interpersonally dysfunctional fashion as a result of the sexual abuse" (p. 531). For example, the perpetrator rewards the child for sexual behavior through the exchange of affection, attention, privileges, or gifts. Consequently, the child learns to use sexual behavior to manipulate others to satisfy a variety of needs. Briere (1992) and Wolfe and Wolfe (1988) suggest that the sexually abused child may use sexualized behavior to manipulate others or to obtain favors from other people. Finkelhor and Browne (1985) also argue that the child's genitals are fetishized during episodes of sexual abuse. Sexual behavior becomes physiologically arousing for the child, increasing the later likelihood of the child engaging in sexual behavior. Of course, the maladaptive patterns of abused and neglected children may reflect in part the influence of other family variables, such as inconsistent parenting or high rates of coercive exchanges between parent and child.

In summary, there are many different mechanisms and processes that may contribute to the association between maltreatment and developmental outcome. Different mechanisms may be operating in different children and in any one child, there may be multiple mechanisms or processes underlying his or her response to the maltreatment. We will now describe some major factors thought to moderate maltreatment's impact.

MODERATOR VARIABLES

The notion that every child does not succumb to dire circumstances seems well supported in the literature. Studies of these "resilient" children have shown that one third of children in a sample who experienced perinatal stress, poverty, parental psychopathology, and family disruption developed into competent and well-adjusted young adults (Werner, 1989). Rutter (1985) estimates that half of the children exposed to severe stress and adversity do not develop symptoms of psychopathology. Similarly, there are maltreated children who do not show evidence of major dysfunction. Estimates of the rates of asymptomatic sexually abused children in four studies range from 21% to 49% (Caffaro-Rouget, Lang, & van Santen, 1989 [49%]; Conte & Schuerman, 1987 [21%]; Mannarino & Cohen, 1986 [31%]; Tong et al., 1987 [36%]).

These figures, however, do not indicate that all these children will necessarily continue to do well in later life. This is why we prefer the term "resiliency" to "invulnerability." As Rutter (1993) points out, "invulnerability" seems to imply an absolute resistance to damage. Although abatement of symptoms has been shown in at least seven longitudinal studies of sexually abused children, with one half to two thirds of all children becoming less symptomatic (for a review see Kendall-Tackett et al. 1993), in other studies it has been demonstrated that a sizable proportion (10% to 24%) of children get worse (Bentovim, van Elberg, & Boston, 1988 [10%]; Gomes-Schwartz, Horowitz, Cardarelli, & Sauzier, 1990 [24%]; Hewitt & Friedrich, 1991 [18%]; Runyan, Everson, Edelsohn, Hunter, & Coulter, 1988, [14%]). Some children whose condition subsequently deteriorated were asymptomatic at the time of the initial assessment (Gomes-Schwartz et al., 1990).

A central focus in the study of resiliency has been the attempt to identify these moderator variables. Baron and Kenny (1986) define a moderator variable as a qualitative or quantitative variable that "affects the direction and/or strength of the relation between an independent or predictor variable and a dependent or criterion variable" (p. 1174). Cicchetti and Rizley (1981) and Cicchetti and Rogosch (1994) classify moderator variables into two broad categories: "potentiating factors," which increase the probability of negative developmental outcomes, and "compensatory factors," which decrease the risk of negative outcome. Within each of these broad classifications, Cicchetti and Olsen (1990) distinguish between "transient" factors, which are temporary and fluctuating influences; and "trait" factors, which represent more enduring conditions or characteristics.

Moderator variables have been classified into three broad sets of factors: (1) Individual factors: those variables pertaining specifically to the child; (2) family factors: those variables pertaining to the families of these children; and (3) environmental factors: those variables in the broader environmental and cultural milieu (Malinosky-Rummell & Hansen, 1993). Malinosky-Rummell and Hansen (1993) add another, fourth, variable, "maltreatment characteristics" (variables associated with the abusive incident), which must be considered in any model of the effects of maltreatment upon developmental outcome.

We will briefly review the importance of some of these factors. However, the reader must be aware of two caveats relating to this discussion. First, although the relevance of some variables for maltreated children's developmental outcomes has received empirical support, there are others that have not yet been investigated empirically. Second, the reader is cautioned against thinking of these variables in categorical ways. As Rutter (1993) points out, the same variable may be a risk factor in one situation and a protective factor in another.

Table 2.1 depicts a summary of some variables found, or thought to be associated, with the developmental outcome of maltreated children. Alternatively, we would like to highlight some factors that may have particular salience for clinicians.

Maltreatment Factors

Kendall-Tackett et al. (1993) reviewed the influence of these factors on the outcomes of sexually abused children that had been documented in 25 studies. Their review shows that sexual abuse that included a high frequency of sexual contact; long duration; the use of force; oral; anal, or vaginal penetration; and a close relationship between child and perpetrator was associated with more symptoms. Factors such as frequency, duration, and the relationship between the child and the perpetrator have not been sufficiently explored in the literature pertaining to physically abused children, although results of a few studies have been reported. However, as discussed in Chapter 1, the severity of abuse, the frequency of child protective services reports, and the interaction between frequency and severity were significant predictors of outcome in youngsters subjected to different types of maltreatment, including physical abuse and neglect (Manly et al., 1994). The clinician who evaluates the condition of a physically abused child must remain aware that frequency and severity may moderate the association between maltreatment and developmental outcomes. Similarly, we know little about the actual significance of these factors for the impact of other forms of maltreatment, such as neglect and psychological unavailability.

Individual Factors

The child's developmental status influences the impact of maltreatment in a variety of ways. Children's interpretation and understanding of their maltreatment play a significant role in their adjustment to victimization. Maltreatment may have different meanings and significance for children at different developmental stages. Some very young children may not even recognize they have been abused (e.g., sexual abuse). They become cognizant of the significance of what happened to them only as they become

TABLE 2.1. Known or Suspected Moderator Variables for Developmental Outcome of Maltreated Children

1. Maltreatment factors
   Frequency
   Duration
   Relationship betwen child and perpetrator
   Penetration (in child sexual abuse)/Severity of the maltreatment
   Use of force
   Occurrence of other forms of maltreatment

2. Individual factors
   Child's age and stage of development
   Sex of the child
   Temperament and other biological factors
   Premaltreatment adjustment
      Intelligence and cognitive skills
      Internal versus external locus of control
      Coping strategies (e.g., active vs. passive stance)
      Self-esteem
   Child's perception of, and attribution regarding, the maltreatment

3. Family factors
   Family's support of the child postmaltreatment
      Acknowledgment of the maltreatment
      Belief in the child/feelings and attitudes toward the child
      Provision of adequate parenting postmaltreatment
      Ability to protect child from further maltreatment

   Family functioning and parenting premaltreatment
      Adequacy and health of marital relationship (e.g., communication, support, spousal abuse, discord, problem solving)
      Individual functioning of parents (e.g., psychiatric illness, substance abuse, maternal depression)
      Poverty; stability of residence, income; social network and supports
      Single parent
      Discipline/parenting effectiveness and appropriateness
      Accurate perception of child's needs and capacity to respond to them
      Impulse control

4. Environmental factors
   Cultural–societal toleration of maltreatment
   Community's reaction to the child and family
   Supportive social relationship for child and family
   Provision of appropriate services for child and family (including continuing protection of the child)
   Criminal justice involvement

older and, for instance, more aware of the social prohibitions and sanctions attached to this behavior (Finkelhor, 1995).

A child's cognitive development may affect his or her responses to the abuse or neglect in other ways. Children's thinking becomes "decentered" as they enter the concrete operational stage of thought. They recognize that other people may have both positive and negative traits and that they (the children) may experience simultaneously positive and negative feelings toward others (Harter, 1977). The attainment of this developmental stage may contribute to a child's feeling of ambivalence toward the perpetrator, leading to even greater confusion and conflicted feelings.

Shirk (1988) proposes that a child's developmental stage will affect the types of symptoms evidenced by maltreated children. For example, sexually maltreated adolescents may be more likely to engage in running away, substance abuse, or suicidal behavior when distressed, since these behaviors are within the adolescents' repertoire. Younger children are much less likely to show these patterns and more likely to display behavior more common to their age group (e.g., disruptive behavior or sexualized behavior).

The child's temperament and medical status are moderator variables often neglected by clinicians who evaluate maltreatment impact. For instance, a 5-year-old with a difficult temperament may react differently to abuse or neglect than a same-aged child who has a placid, regular temperament. The former might become distressed, not only by the maltreatment but by subsequent changes in family routine or structure, such as placement in foster care. Grizenko and Pawliuk (1994) note that generally an easy temperament serves as a compensatory factor. Besides eliciting more positive responses from their caregivers and being better equipped to cope with changing environmental circumstances, children with easy temperaments appear to have higher intelligence and more advanced problem-solving skills, cognitive–integrative abilities, social skills, and coping strategies (Mantzicopoulos & Morrison, 1994; Werner, 1993).

Medical, biological, or physical conditions that predate abuse—for example, sensory deficits such as blindness or hearing impairments—may influence a child's adjustment to maltreatment. A number of the children whose conditions we have assessed and whom we have treated had primary attention deficit disorders that had had significant effects upon their social, behavioral, and academic functioning. Of course, some problems may result from the maltreatment and in turn influence the child's subsequent adaptation to the trauma. In a fascinating series of papers, Lewis and her colleagues (Lewis et al., 1988, 1991; Lewis, Lovely, Yeager, & Della Femina, 1989; Lewis, 1992) report that a constellation of neurological–neuropsychiatric vulnerabilities and a violent, abusive upbringing are closely associated with physical aggression. Lewis et al. (1989) describe elements of a transactional model in accounting for this association. For example, family violence serves as a model of aggressive behavior and elicits intense feelings of rage. As well, it may create those very neurological vulnerabilities that make it difficult for children to resist these models and control their anger. Lewis et al. (1989) also suggest that neuropsychiatrically impaired children, by virtue of their impulsivity, irritability, and hyperactivity, may be at higher risk for being abused.

Precrisis adjustment is another factor that must be evaluated. Rutter (1993) reports that above-average IQ and positive experiences at school are compensatory factors. Success in these areas generates and strengthens feelings of self-esteem and self-efficacy that attenuate the impact of adverse events. Masten, Best, and Garmezy (1990) and Werner (1993) broaden these areas to include athletic, mechanical, or artistic pursuits as well as academic ones. Consequently, a child with strengths in these areas may be more able to withstand the negative impact of being abused or neglected.

Family Factors

Good and stable care increases a child's chances of establishing a secure attachment with parents, which in turn may serve as a significant compensatory factor for those children who are subsequently maltreated. Children who have an internal working model characterized by a basic trust of people may not be seriously compromised by the offender's actions, especially if the abuse is time limited and committed by someone without a particularly close relationship to the child. These children regard the maltreatment as unfortunate incidents that speak more to the untrustworthiness or even dangerousness of the specific offender than evidence of the ubiquitous badness of people. Consequently, the capacity of such children to form healthy and intimate relationships with others may not be deleteriously affected, although they may display some localized effects such as anxiety-related symptoms. This intact trust in others may increase the chance that they will reach out for help and support concerning issues related to the assaults, thereby increasing the probability of a good outcome. Furthermore, children with a secure attachment may not suffer the same threat to their self-esteem as would youngsters who had always felt unworthy, inadequate, and deserving of maltreatment. Secure attachments also influence language development and the inclination and ability to learn. As we have seen, these capabilities enable children to express feelings in healthy and adaptive ways and provide further confirmation of their personal strengths, capabilities, and effectiveness.

Other aspects of parenting and family support can moderate the impact of maltreatment. Family support is an important moderator of the effects of child sexual abuse. There seem to be no studies in which the specific influence of such support on the outcome of other types of maltreatment has been investigated. However, support from the family seems critical for children's adjustment to almost any kind of trauma. There may be many mechanisms that account for this association. Via the phenomenon of "social referencing," young children take their cues from their caretakers regarding how to respond to situations of potential or actual threat (Lewandowski & Baranoski, 1994). Parents may transmit their own anxiety about the maltreatment, thus escalating the child's apprehension and distress. Maltreated children whose parents disbelieve their accounts or blame them for the abuse may feel even greater stigmatization, which would contribute to a poorer outcome (Finkelhor & Browne, 1985). As well, children's adjustment is significantly dependent upon the actual parenting they receive, especially when they display behavioral or emotional problems associated with maltreatment. Parents who cannot apply firm and consistent limits to their children's behavior and who cannot maintain a regular and consistent routine for their offspring may inadvertently contribute to their children's maladjustment. The deterioration in parenting may occur after the child discloses the maltreatment, or the child might have been subjected to inadequate parenting prior to or concurrent with abuse and neglect episodes. Many variables affect parenting, including the parents' own victimization history, psychiatric illness, and broader factors such as poverty and social isolation. Chapter 3 is devoted to discussion of the assessment of these family factors that may critically influence a child's adjustment to maltreatment. In Chapter 6 some interventions are described that are designed to increase the support parents or caregivers are able to offer their victimized children.

Environmental Factors

Mental health professionals have tended to ignore environmental variables, despite their importance for a child's and the family's adjustment. Broad social factors such as poverty pose significant risk to developmental outcome in general (Duncan, Brooks-Gunn, & Klebanov, 1994; Lipman, Offord, & Boyle, 1994). More specific factors, such as a negative reaction to the child's disclosure of maltreatment by the larger community (e.g., peers and neighbors), exacerbate a sense of stigmatization. A criminal justice system that is unresponsive and insensitive to the idiosyncratic needs of child witnesses may compound feelings of powerlessness and stigmatization. Kendall-Tackett et al. (1993) reviewed studies pertaining to sexually abused children's court involvement and found the children's adjustment deteriorated when cases were not resolved quickly or when they were compelled to testify on multiple occasions. Children who were frightened of the accused also fared poorly. Although in these cases these particular conditions functioned as potentiating factors, the same variable (i.e., testifying at court) might function as a compensatory factor under somewhat different circumstances. For example, Runyan et al. (1988) reports that children who testified in juvenile court proceedings recovered more quickly when cases were resolved with a conviction or a plea bargain.

The influence of other social relationships as a compensatory factor for maltreated children should not be discounted. Egeland, Jacobvitz, and Sroufe (1988) demonstrate that high-risk mothers pose less risk to their children if they have been able to form a supportive relationship with another adult, such as a spouse, or if they have participated in psychotherapy.

We will now turn our attention to a discussion of clinical work with maltreated children. We will attempt to translate these broad theoretical and conceptual notions into viable and, we hope, useful clinical strategies and interventions. Given our strong belief in the importance of the family context for the child's adaptation to maltreatment, we next discuss the significance of a comprehensive family assessment.

THREE

Family Assessment

THE PRIMARY FOCUS of this book is the assessment and treatment of the individual maltreated child. Consistent with the transactional model of development described in the preceding chapters, however, this does not mean the child should be assessed or treated in isolation from those other variables or factors that are critical in an individual's adaptation to maltreatment. The family has special relevance for a comprehensive understanding of the child's response to maltreatment. In this chapter we provide an overview of family assessment, and in Chapter 6 we discuss interventions with caregivers and families that support and maximize individual psychotherapy with the child.

Before dealing directly with the topic of family assessment, we would offer some preliminary comments about our ideas regarding clinical assessment in general that have guided our thinking and practice.

CLINICAL ASSESSMENT: UNDERLYING ASSUMPTIONS

Clinical Assessment Is the Foundation for Therapy

We are traditionalists. We believe strongly that treatment of a child or family should not be undertaken until the clinician has a good understanding of the problems and of the factors that have contributed to their emergence. Treatment should not begin until the clinician has formulated a set of treatment recommendations that has been accepted by the parents or caregivers.

A guiding ethical principle of all mental health professions is that of informed consent. We believe that the guardians of maltreated children must have as full an understanding as possible of the professional's opinion about the problem and of the basis for the treatment recommendations. It is only when these conditions have been met that informed consent for treatment can be given. How can clients provide informed consent if they do not understand the reasons for a particular treatment modality?

As well as being founded upon ethical practice, this stance, we believe, is consistent with the transactional model of development. Sometimes we are overwhelmed with the pain and suffering of a child or family when we first meet them. We feel compelled to "do something" immediately to make things better. However, interventions based upon little or minimal assessment data may be ineffectual, since they would be undertaken with no consideration of the potentially diverse and numerous factors that influence the child's or the family's life. For example, encouraging an open discussion in the family about a child's sexual abuse may be met with resistance by parents who have their own victimization history or cultural values that prohibit such conversations. Such intervention, like this with no prior knowledge of this aspect of parental history and its ramifications, may well lead to ineffective treatment, thereby increasing the frustration and distress of both therapist and clients. We have seen numerous examples in which therapists have not conducted comprehensive assessments. They then intervened in ways that caused significant damage to their clients, such as insisting that the clients provide a full and detailed account of their history of victimization. These approaches were used with no appreciation of the clients' brittle and fragile defensive structures or knowledge of their history of psychiatric admissions associated with therapy, whose goal is to uncover unconscious conflicts and motivations. Conversely, the lack of a comprehensive assessment may result in the therapist's failure to capitalize upon the strengths of a particular child or family.

The child's progress throughout the course of therapy should be assessed at regular intervals. Such assessments range from brief, weekly contacts with the child's parents or caregivers that provide material for informal reports about the child's functioning to one or more readministration of formal assessment instruments. The latter is especially important for long-term therapy, in which there is greater difficulty in keeping the treatment goals in clear focus. Therapists conducting long-term treatment are well advised to review their clients' progress formally at regular intervals and to consider not only readministering evaluative measures that can help determine what progress has been made in reaching goals but also making any necessary modifications in the treatment plan.

Assessments Must Be Comprehensive

Given the wide diversity of outcomes arising from maltreatment, the large number of potential moderating variables that affect a child's response, and the complexity of the interactions among these variables, it should be obvious that the needs of maltreated children and their families vary considerably. Although some common themes have to be addressed with many maltreated children, the clinician must first conduct a comprehensive assessment to identify the child's response to the abuse or neglect. Then the clinician must formulate a specific treatment plan to meet the child's and family's unique needs.

Comprehensiveness includes three dimensions. First, assessments must be ecological. Children do not develop in vacuums but in families that, in turn, fit into a larger societal and cultural context. Clinical assessments of maltreated children require an understanding of the historical and current influence of parents or caregivers. As well, there must be an appreciation of larger societal forces (e.g., poverty) and their impact upon parents and families, and upon children's responses to the maltreatment.

Second, comprehensive assessments must focus upon a broad domain of child behavior. In the preceding review it was shown not only that there is great variability in children's responses to maltreatment but that many areas of functioning can be affected. Therefore, the clinician should be prepared to evaluate numerous and diverse facets of a child's behavior and functioning. Besides being problem areas requiring intervention, these domains of functioning may be moderators of the child's response to maltreatment. We have already seen that good academic achievement and intelligence may function as compensatory factors for some children who have undergone dire experiences. Similarly, many different aspects of family functioning may be affected by the maltreatment. A child's victimization may elicit great emotional distress in a parent and may also result in situational changes (e.g., losing the income of the offending parent who must leave the home). These changes play important roles in helping or hindering the child's attempts to cope with the maltreatment. Such changes may be legitimate targets of intervention, as are problems that predated the maltreatment, such as an attention deficit disorder.

Third, comprehensive assessments of the child and family must use multimethods and be based in multisettings. Relying on any one evaluation format or modality is foolish. No one assessment strategy or test is infallible or renders all the information needed about a child or family. In this chapter and the next, we argue for adopting a multimethod approach that incorporates data from different assessment methods and that places the highest confidence in those findings that recur across different methods. As well, the clinician must attempt to gather information about the child and the family's functioning in multiple settings. Functioning may vary across different environments, which may have significant implications for intervention. For example, the clinician may discover that the child functions well at school. This may point to strengths that can be capitalized upon in treatment. Likewise, the family may show difficulties only in certain environmental contexts, such as when they are being confronted by authority figures.

There Is a Distinction between Clinical Assessments and Forensic/Legal Assessments

Clinical assessments should be conducted only after child protective services or police have completed their investigations. Although there is a certain amount of overlap, the purposes of these two types of assessments differ. The purpose of a forensic/legal assessment is to determine whether the child was maltreated and, if so, to ascertain the identity of the perpetrator. Other issues include establishing the specific details of the maltreatment (e.g., what was done to the child, when, and where) and of other aspects of the abuse (e.g., presence of threats or coercion). Conducting these assessments requires specific training and skills. Leading or suggestive questioning is strictly contraindicated, since it may contaminate evidence and jeopardize the chances of successful court prosecution. In a clinical assessment, suggestive or leading questions are sometimes used in an attempt to confirm or refute working hypotheses about the maltreatment's impact upon the child and to obtain further information. Clinicians should not undertake forensic/legal investigations unless they have been properly trained. The chance of evidence contamination, which might result in harm to either the child or the accused, is too great.

The questions to be addressed in a clinical assessment are different from those in a forensic/legal evaluation and include the following (Broder & Hood, 1983, p. 130):

1. What is the nature of the problem?
2. Is it a problem that requires action?
3. What are the factors causing and maintaining the problem?
4. What action, if any, is needed and by which members of the family system?
5. Who can best carry out the intervention?
6. What is the prognosis for change?

Clinical Assessments Should Have a Therapeutic Component

Although clinical assessments should not be construed as formal treatment, they can still have a therapeutic component. Assessment is the first step in establishing a collaborative alliance with parents or caregivers. Their observations, feelings, and perceptions are legitimized, and they are assured that their concerns are respected by the clinician. They are acknowledged as the most important influences in the child's life, which indeed they are, and are assured that their role in any subsequent treatment is critical to its success. Although this part of the assessment does not constitute treatment per se, it creates a therapeutic atmosphere in which the parents/caregivers receive intelligent caring, listening, and empathy. In Chapter 4 we discuss the therapeutic components of the assessment process for maltreated children.

Assessments Must Be Culturally Sensitive

The assessment and intervention techniques we describe below are based upon a consideration of relevant theory and empirical findings. They also reflect our own cultural heritage. The emphasis we place upon the verbalization of feelings and beliefs associated with victimization is congruent with the notion held by most white, middle-class North Americans that it is "good" to talk about affective and personal issues. However, therapists must guard against applying this assumption indiscriminately in working with clients from different cultural backgrounds. For example, some cultures may not condone explicit discussions of sexuality between children and people outside the family, or with adults of the same sex (Bowman, 1989). For example, Arce (1982) states that Puerto Ricans as a group encounter difficulty in dealing with anger and aggressive feelings and that the direct expression of such affect is followed by intense guilt feelings. Although these descriptions of cultural norms and traditions are useful guides for interactions, therapists must avoid stereotyping all members of a cultural group the same way. There is enough diversity even in homogeneous groups to make it necessary to assess the specific relevance and importance of cultural traditions for an individual child and family. The therapist cannot assume that every member of a particular group will ascribe the same importance to its traditions and teachings. It may well be that some of the techniques and strategies we describe in this book are inappropriate for children from various cultural backgrounds. Therapists must evaluate their utility and appropriateness for children from diverse backgrounds, modify them if necessary, and even discard those that will not be helpful. Obvious examples include the judicious choice of formal psychological assessment instruments (some of which may not have been normed for the particular ethnic or racial group to which the child belongs), the specific meaning of body language, eye contact, loudness and manner of speech, tone of voice, and the importance of timing and appropriateness of talking about culturally acceptable topics (Canino, 1988; Gutierrez, 1989).

Children and their parents are the best sources of information about their cultural traditions and what constitutes appropriate interventions. In our experience, a sincere interest in the family's culture and a willingness to learn about its traditions convey a genuine respect that is usually associated with a useful exchange of information. Many families are willing to share knowledge of their culture with a therapist who asks for their help and guidance. A failure to inquire about specific cultural traditions and the family's adherence to them often leads to treatment recommendations that are mismatched to the family's and the child's context. Therapists can prepare themselves for meeting a child and family from a different cultural background by reading relevant material or talking with other individuals from the same cultural group. By doing so, they can devise some preliminary guidelines and begin to formulate tentative hypotheses regarding the relevance of cultural variables for the sequelae of the maltreatment and for possible treatment approaches. However, as useful as these general guidelines might be, therapists must inquire about the specific meaning and relevance of cultural traditions for a given child and family and then make appropriate adjustments in the assessment or intervention strategies as required.

ASSESSMENT OF PARENTAL
AND FAMILY FUNCTIONING

Reasons for Assessing Parental and Family Functioning

One obvious difference between child and adult therapy is that children usually must be brought to therapy by adults, especially if they are young. If parents or caregivers are hesitant about, or opposed to, therapy for the child, they often will not bring him or her for sessions. If they do bring the child, they may still undermine or sabotage the therapist's efforts. Although we discuss working with parents in much more detail in Chapter 6, we would like to note here that involving parents or caregivers in the beginning of the assessment phase conveys a strong signal to them that their information and participation are important. It is the beginning of the development of a collaborative alliance between therapist and parent or caregiver, a relationship that may be especially significant for those adults who have played a direct role in the maltreatment of their child. Their involvement may afford them some relief from guilt and anxiety as they collaborate to help their child. Even something as simple as providing a developmental history may ease their feelings. We also believe that successfully engaging caregivers in the assessment process conveys a positive message to the child: despite their past parenting difficulties, parents are willing to make the effort to become involved on their child's behalf. Of course, some parents are not able or willing to follow through with either the assessment or the subsequent therapy. The child may realistically regard failure as yet another example of the parent's inadequacy.

A sizable proportion of the maltreated children whom clinicians see do not live with their parents but reside in foster homes or group homes. We believe it is just as important to involve these caregivers in the assessment and therapeutic phases, although the level of involvement may differ. Unfortunately, some mental health professionals regard foster parents merely as individuals who clothe, feed, and house the child and transport the child to and from therapy sessions. This condescending attitude is often associated with a failure to obtain the often insightful and valuable knowledge foster parents have of the children in their care. The clinician sees the child for only 1 to 2 hours per week, whereas the foster parent lives with the child and is, in many ways, the real expert. Similarly, foster parents may be enlisted as significant collaborators and allies in treatment. Failure to engage them in the therapeutic process usually ensures that therapeutic gains are not maximized and even raises the possibility that therapy will flounder or be terminated prematurely. The same basic principle applies to relationships with group-home staff. They, too, are an invaluable source of information about the child's functioning and, like foster parents, must be included as collaborative partners in subsequent treatment.

Besides establishing a collaborative alliance with parents and caregivers, involving these individuals facilitates a much more comprehensive understanding of the maltreated child. Parent/caregiver involvement gives the clinician an appreciation of those potentiating and compensatory factors within the family that have contributed or are presently contributing to the child's level of adaptation. Identifying these factors is not just an intellectual exercise: knowledge of them may suggest possible intervention targets. For example, inconsistent parenting that exacerbates the child's aggressive response to maltreatment will have to be addressed, as would any other potentiating factor, such as blaming the child for the assaults. Information concerning the history of these factors may have relevance for treatment planning. Factors that have been long-term problems and predate the onset of maltreatment may require a different therapeutic approach than others that are more reflective of a family's situational reaction to maltreatment. Returning to our example of inconsistent parenting, a therapist may have to use certain interventions with parents who have always had problems with setting limits. Chronic difficulties, especially those that have continued despite previous, different interventions, may necessitate intensive interventions such as in-home teaching of parenting skills. Blindly recommending a short-term parenting group for a chronically troubled, multiproblem family may lead to further failure and frustration for these parents, and it will do little to help their child. In contrast, a family with numerous strengths and resources, including good parenting skills, may not require the same intensity of treatment or level of commitment of professional resources. These parents may respond rapidly to an approach that validates their distress but also encourages them to place firm and consistent limits upon their child's acting-out behavior.

A knowledge of parental and family functioning helps the clinician develop other aspects of a child's treatment plan, including basic decisions about whether the child should be treated individually and when treatment should begin. Knowledge of past and current family functioning is a critical component in this decision-making process. For example, play therapy, which teaches children more effective ways to articulate feelings such as sadness or anger, may anger parents unused to such openness. They may not be able to tolerate overt emotional displays, thereby increasing the risk that they will physically abuse the child. Instituting such a therapeutic program without information about the parent's or caregiver's ability to accept and manage these changes may place the child in significant danger. As past behavior is often the best predictor of future behavior, the therapist must carefully evaluate the parent's previous responses to expressions of strong feelings by the child and the kinds of coping mechanisms they used. The clinician should consider this historical perspective while evaluating their current ability to accept and support their child's affective expression.

Components of "Family Support"

What are some strengths that generally seem to aid a child's recovery from episodes of maltreatment? It is an important issue to address in this chapter, since clinicians first must be aware of the possible range of compensatory factors before they can identify these factors in any particular family. Again, we turn to the literature for some guidance.

That family support, particularly maternal support, plays a key role in the treatment outcome of the sexually abused child seems well substantiated in the literature (e.g., Conte & Berliner, 1988; Everson, Hunter, Runyon, Edelsohn, & Coulter, 1989; Johnstone & Kenkel, 1991; Kendall-Tackett et al., 1993). Unfortunately, there seem to be no studies in which the influence of family suppport on other maltreatment types has been investigated empirically, although family support seems critical for children's coping with almost any kind of trauma (Lewandoski & Baranoski, 1994). But what does the term *support* mean? It is a broad term that might subsume many different components. Everson et al. (1989) developed the Parental Reaction to Incest Disclosure Scale (PRIDS) by which parental support is measured in three areas: emotional support (e.g., commitment to the child versus abandoning the child psychologically), believing the child (e.g., making clear public statements of their belief versus totally denying the abuse occurred), and action toward the perpetrator (e.g., actively demonstrating disapproval of the perpetrator's abusive behavior by effecting a separation or cooperating with the criminal prosecution versus choosing the perpetrator over the child). Consistent with other investigators, Everson et al. (1989) find a significant relationship between low maternal support on this scale and psychological disturbance among children. In a more recent study, Leifer,

Shapiro, and Kassem (1993) describe three components of maternal support: overt protective actions, such as taking the daughter to the hospital or calling the police; belief in the daughter's account without disputing its truthfulness; and not blaming the daughter for being abused. The authors reported that 49% of the mothers provided an adequate response to their daughters' disclosures of sexual abuse as assessed by these three components. Those children whose mothers provided little support demonstrated poor functioning. Compromised support was associated with maternal substance abuse, which in turn was correlated with mothers' histories of childhood sexual abuse.

Table 3.1 represents an attempt to summarize some of the key variables subsumed by the term "family support." The table does not provide an exhaustive list; there may be other supportive attitudes or behaviors by caregivers and parents. Although they are based upon the child sexual abuse literature, we argue that some of these variables may be relevant for children maltreated in other ways. The child who has been physically abused, neglected, or psychologically maltreated would probably benefit from the same kind of emotional support, belief of the nonoffending parent in his or her allegations, and protection from the abusive or neglectful individual as would sexually abused children. Furthermore, this table may serve as a rough guide for clinicians who are attempting to help parents and caregivers develop ways of supporting their children postdisclosure.

Getting Started:
Who Should Attend the Initial Interview?

Even before meeting the child and family, the clinician faces several decisions. One of the first is whom to invite to the initial interview. Some clinicians interview the entire family first and then interview parents or caregivers separately. Others prefer to see parents by themselves first. We do not believe clinicians must adhere to rigid rules about this issue. However, there are several considerations to keep in mind. Children probably should not be present when parents are asked about their own history, which may include the possibility that the parents themselves were somehow victimized. Similarly, in-depth discussions about the parents' reactions to the child's maltreatment may provoke strong and intense feelings in the parents. Children exposed to this level of parental distress in the assessment phase may experience an exacerbation of their own anxiety. For instance, children may become even more concerned about their own well-being upon learning that the parent is so upset about what happened. They may begin to feel they have been irreparably damaged, or they may stop talking so as to alleviate their parents' pain and suffering. Consequently, we believe that at some point in the assessment phase parents or caregivers need the oppor-

TABLE 3.1. Components of Family Support (Postdisclosure)

1. Emotional support
   For example: committed to the child, has not abandoned the child psychologically, does not blame the child, ascribes responsibility to the perpetrator

2. Belief of child
   For example: believes in the child's account and does not dispute its truthfulness

3. Instrumental support
   For example: ensures the child receives appropriate medical/psychosocial interventions, protects the child from further abuse (e.g., prohibits the child from being alone with the perpetrator again)

4. Actions toward the perpetrator
   For example: notifies the police and/or protective services and cooperates with subsequent investigations, makes the perpetrator leave the home, chooses the child over the perpetrator

Note. Adapted from Everson et al. (1989) and Leifer et al. (1993).

tunity to talk privately with the therapist about these very personal and sensitive issues. Generally, we prefer to conduct several interviews with parents or caregivers by themselves. These interviews provide an opportunity to focus our attention upon the caregivers' concerns and to start establishing a collaborative alliance with them. Having children present during the initial interviews may deflect the therapist's attention onto the child, which in turn, may elicit feelings of jealousy or frustration in those adults who have significant unmet emotional needs.

On the other hand, some may argue that excluding children, even in this very early stage, results in a less than comprehensive perspective on family interactional patterns. Therapists may be interested in observing the reaction of children to their parents' distress about the victimization. Do the children, for instance, stop talking about what happened to them? Do they become upset themselves? Do they attempt to nurture and engage in caretaking behavior with the distressed parent?

Clarifying the Purpose of the Assessment with the Parents

Before being questioned about relevant issues, parents or caregivers deserve an explanation about the purposes of the assessment process. The therapist should briefly review the referral process that resulted in the parents' attendance at the first appointment. They can then be asked for their understanding of the assessment's purposes, and the clinician can clarify any misunderstandings. Many parents are already defensive about their role in the child's difficulties and have not had positive past relationships with professionals. They may believe the clinician will be determining their fitness as parents or conducting a forensic/legal investigation of the child's allegations of maltreatment. A thorough discussion of the assessment's purpose helps eliminate the confusion or conflict that usually ensues when the therapist and parents have divergent ideas about the evaluation. The therapist should make it clear that the purpose of the assessment is to evaluate the impact of the maltreatment on the child and to formulate some appropriate recommendations regarding intervention. The therapist's failure to clarify these issues may compound the parents' anxiety. This united approach also conveys a stronger message to the child about the importance of participating and cooperating in the evaluative process. Children already exposed to inconsistency between their parents will not benefit from a similar relationship between their parents and a clinician.

Discussing the assessment process also alleviates parental anxiety and makes parents feel part of the whole endeavor. The therapist can explain the purpose of the first session, which includes obtaining the parents' account of the child's difficulties, providing a tentative plan for subsequent sessions, and then addressing any parental concerns or questions. As mental health professionals, we often assume that our clients know what will happen in a typical assessment. We also tend to assume that they are comfortable with what may actually be an alien process for many individuals. It is important to emphasize that the therapist is most interested in the parental account of what happened to the child and its effects upon the child's functioning. By stressing that the parents have a wealth of information to offer, the therapist often alleviates some of their guilt and reinforces the collaborative alliance.

Because of the child's distress and their own difficulties in managing it, parents or other caregivers, including foster parents, often ask for advice during the first session. Also, after only one or two assessment sessions they may expect an opinion about their child's difficulties and what can be done. To promote realistic expectations about the limits of advice that can be given in the assessment process, it is helpful to broach this subject in the first session even if the parents do not request immediate advice or assistance. The clinician may empathize with the parents' desire for solutions to alleviate their child's distress. However, the therapist should inform the parents that he or she prefers to wait until the assessment is over, so that treatment recommendations can be based upon as comprehensive a picture of the child and family as possible. In addition, parents or caregivers should be encouraged to tell the clinician of any significant developments in the child's presentation or behavior during the assessment that might merit quick attention. Clearly, any child who becomes acutely suicidal or a danger to others during the assessment will need immediate crisis evaluation and intervention.

Finally, parents and caregivers should be alerted to the limits of confidentiality. These limits include the obligation to report any incidents of abuse or neglect to child protective services. The policy of the agency or clinician regarding the release of information to other individuals should also be reviewed at this time.

History of Presenting Problems

Once the parents or caregivers are oriented to the assessment purpose and process and have reached a consensus with the clinician about the goals and overall plan of this exercise, the clinician can start focusing upon relevant content. Although the clinician will want to assess the child's perception of the presenting problems directly, obtaining this information from parents or caregivers is critical. This is especially so for younger children who may not be able to give a detailed account. This preliminary information enables the clinician to begin forming some tentative hypotheses about the child's response to the maltreatment and serves to highlight those areas that would require particular attention when assessing the child's condition.

Asking parents for their account of the child's presenting problems serves as a relatively benign opportunity for them to become comfortable with the evaluative process and the clinician. Immediately inquiring about some of the more sensitive areas, such as their personal response to the maltreatment or aspects of their own history, may prove to be too threatening for some parents and may diminish the chance of establishing a strong collaborative alliance with them.

Table 3.2 illustrates a fairly standard outline of the information regarding presenting problems that the clinician may want to gather from parents.

It is often useful for the clinician to ask the parents for concrete and specific examples of the child's problems and their manifestations in all

TABLE 3.2. History of Presenting Problems

1. Behavioral description of the problem
2. Onset
3. Where in the child's environment are the problems manifested?
4. How frequently do the problems occur?
5. What precipitates the problems?
6. What makes the problems better or worse?
7. How do the problems create difficulties, and for whom?
8. Child's and family's feelings about the problems, and their explanations of the causes.
9. What attempts have been made to help (duration of efforts, consistency of efforts, outcome, feelings about past efforts)?
10. What are the goals in seeking help now?

of the child's environments. These environments include home, school, the neighborhood among friends, and other situations such as recreational activities. Parents may describe difficulties that predated the abuse or neglect. Rather than dismissing these difficulties, the clinician must inquire about them in the same detailed fashion used for symptoms that are more closely associated with the maltreatment. Although some of these symptoms may not be directly related to the abuse, they may serve as important moderator variables and may require therapeutic intervention.

Besides furnishing detailed information about the child's functioning, history taking affords the clinician the opportunity to form some initial impressions of the caregivers on several different dimensions. First, the clinician may begin to see signs of parental psychopathology in the parent or parents while they are describing the child's behavior. Symptoms of major psychiatric disturbances such as depression or psychosis in the parents may be quite apparent. However, applying a psychiatric diagnosis such as a major depressive disorder to an individual based solely upon impressions derived from an account of the child's problems is not warranted. With this caveat in mind, these parental behaviors or characteristics may serve as indicators for a more in-depth inquiry into the parents' own mental health issues later in the assessment.

Second, parental accounts of the child's difficulties may convey useful information about their feelings toward that child. Do they talk about the child's difficulties in a very hostile, angry tone of voice? Do they seem to have little, if any, understanding of why the child may be reacting in a particular way to the maltreatment? Do they describe the problem behavior as a manifestation of a "bad" child, or do they see the behavior as symptomatic of the child's distress and a reflection of his or her attempts to cope with overwhelming experiences? The clinician may begin to wonder whether the emotions associated with this account are merely situational reactions to the child's negative behavior, a reflection of the parent's own issues about maltreatment and victimization, or indicators of chronic and ongoing problems in the relationship between parents and child. Also, the parents' presentation in this phase of the assessment may generate tentative hypotheses that warrant exploration in subsequent sessions.

Third, if the child has more than one parent or caregiver and both are present at the initial interview, the clinician should observe how they relate to each other. Do they present a fairly consistent picture of the child, or do they have divergent perspectives? If they do have differing perspectives, are they aware of these differences? If they are, how do they reconcile them? Do they undermine each other in the interview, and does one member of the dyad fight for control? Do their divergent perceptions of the child extend to inconsistency in the way they actually manage some of the child's behavior? If the whole family is present, the clinician must be alert to these and other interactional patterns that may have relevance for the child's functioning and recovery from the maltreatment. We discuss family functioning at a later point in this chapter.

Clinicians should supplement informal parental reports of the child's behavior with more standardized measures. The CBCL (Achenbach & Edelbrock, 1983) and the Eyberg Child Behavior Inventory (ECBI) (Eyberg & Ross, 1978) are both parent-completed checklists of child behavior (see Wolfe, 1988, for a good review of these and other instruments). These instruments can used for other purposes besides generating profiles of different behavioral dimensions compared with age-based and sex-based normative data. The clinician may request each caretaker to complete these instruments independently to determine the degree of consistency between their respective perspectives of the child's behavior. Consistent with one of our basic notions of assessing children's behavior in multisettings, it is often useful to ask foster parents, school teachers, or others who have significant involvement with the child to complete one of these instruments. The teacher may complete the Teacher Report Form (TRF) of the CBCL which provides normative comparisons between the child and other youngsters in the school setting. In Chapter 1 we reviewed the CSBI, a comprehensive, parent-completed report of children's sexual behavior. In Chapter 4 we discuss the process of gathering information from collateral sources in more detail.

Developmental History of the Child

We believe strongly that obtaining a detailed developmental history of the child is an important endeavor. Such a history furnishes critical information regarding the child's previous ability to negotiate the stage-salient developmental issues described in Chapter 1, as well as the influence maltreatment might have had upon the child's developmental course. A developmental history may highlight potentiating or compensatory factors that perhaps moderated the association between the maltreatment and the developmental outcome. For instance, is this child now seen to have developmental delays that are a result of the mother's difficult pregnancy or delivery, or the child's prematurity? The clinician can then begin to speculate and eventually gather data about the effects of these delays upon the child's subsequent adaptation to maltreatment. Have speech and language delays had a significant effect upon the child's ability to articulate feelings about the maltreatment verbally? Are these delays a factor that has contributed to the child's aggressive, externalizing style? Is this a child who has always evidenced a difficult temperament and has never adjusted well or easily to change? Has this difficult temperament had a negative influence on his or her response to the disruption of being removed from the parental home and placed in a foster home? Table 3.3 presents an outline of the typical developmental history.

TABLE 3.3. Developmental History of the Child

1. Pregnancy and delivery
   a. Was the pregnancy planned?
   b. Was this the mother's first pregnancy?
   c. Parents' feelings about the pregnancy?
   d. Did the mother have medical care and consultation during the pregnancy?
   e. Health of the mother during the pregnancy
      (1) Weight gain
      (2) Medications taken, including substance abuse
      (3) Medical concerns and treatments
   f. Was the child born preterm or postterm?
   g. Labor
      (1) Were both parents present?
      (2) Duration
      (3) Medications administered
      (4) Special procedures used
      (5) Was the baby healthy at birth?
      (6) Baby's weight
      (7) Was the baby held and fed immediately?
      (8) Did the baby require time in the intensive care nursery?
      (9) How long did the mother and child stay in the hospital?
      (10) How and when was the name selected?

2. Neonatal period and infancy
   a. Constitution and temperamental syle (e.g., activity level, reaction to stimuli, general responsiveness, reactions to change and transitions)
   b. Growth patterns
   c. Establishment of eating, sleeping, toilet routines

3. Developmental milestones
   a. Parents' general memory regarding whether concerns were apparent
   b. Specifics regarding approximate age at first smile, sitting, walking, first words, good communication understandable by others outside the family, day and night toilet training achieved, sexual maturity and puberty

4. Quality of early relationships and attachment history[a]
   a. Who was the child's primary caregiver during early years, and did the child show protest behavior at separation from this person? What age was the child?
   b. Did the child show affection spontaneously? Would the child initiate a hug, kiss, or touch?
   c. Did the child seek affection in an indiscriminate manner? Did the child show selective preference for adults?
   d. Was the child clingy? Did the child allow the adult to have body space? Did the child seem to get enough gratification from the adult to permit separation even briefly?
   e. Did the child have difficulty tolerating emotional intimacy, seeking instead objects as an expression of caretaking? Was it more important to this child that he/she had an object given to him or her than an emotional response from the caretaker?
   f. Did the child show empathy? Was he/she responsive to the emotions of others?

(continued)

TABLE 3.3. *cont.*

5. Stresses
   a. Physical illnesses/injuries (acute and/or chronic)
   b. Emotional (e.g., separation/divorce of parents, death of significant family members or pets, family moves)
   c. History of maltreatment
      (1) Type of maltreatment
      (2) Age at onset
      (3) Duration
      (4) Perpetrator(s)
      (5) Child's reaction (behavioral, emotional, physical) to the maltreatment
      (6) Response of the environment to the maltreatment (e.g., parents/caregivers, siblings, wider community [including teachers, legal/justice system])
      (7) Previous or concurrent treatment or other services to the child and family and their outcomes

6. Other placements
   a. Number of placements and duration; type of placement
   b. Reason(s) for each placement (e.g., maltreatment, breakdown in placement because of the child's behavior)
   c. Feelings and attitudes of previous caretakers toward the child
   d. Child's behavior in each placement (e.g., any significant difficulties: if so, obtain as full a description as possible)
   e. Were alternate child-care arrangements used when parents worked? Who were the caregivers, and what was the child's response to them?

7. Response to discipline

8. School history
   a. Emotional reaction
   b. Progress at school
   c. Behavior with teachers and classmates
   d. Special class placements or other educational and psychological assistance

9. Hobbies, interests, sports, chores

10. Peer relationships
    a. Number of friendships
    b. Nature and intensity of friendships (e.g., has the child been detached or overly dependent upon peers? Did the child have to take all the initiative to establish and maintain peer relationships, or did other children take the initiative?)
    c. Problem areas in relationships with peers (e.g., fighting, withdrawal)
    d. Issues and attitudes about sexuality (e.g., sexual maturity, identification as a male or a female, sexual interest—age at first interest; dating habits, attitudes, and feelings about sexual behavior)

11. History of any other previous problems
    a. Nature of the problem
    b. Onset; frequency; duration
    c. Treatment or other services; outcome

*[a]*Adapted from Carson and Goodfield (1988, pp. 118–119).

The clinician may interview parents to obtain a history or request they complete one of the commonly used developmental history forms, the Aggregate Neurobehavioral Student Health and Educational Review (ANSER) (Levine, 1985), then review it and follow up with any supplemental questions. A review of other collateral documentation (e.g., obstetrical records) sometimes yields valuable information that enriches the clinician's understanding of a child.

The parents' or caregivers' report of the developmental history may reflect their own problem areas or strengths. Does the parent have difficulty in remembering details of the child's history? Is this problem a manifestation of a lack of interest in the child; a reflection of the parent's own difficulties, such as significant substance abuse during the period for which he or she cannot remember information; or symptoms of a mental health problem in the parent?

Inquiry about the Child's History of Maltreatment and Parental/Caregiver Reactions

At this point, the clinician may want to gather more information about the child's maltreatment and the parents' or caregivers' feelings or reactions to these episodes of victimization. The therapist may already have some detailed information from the referral source about what happened to the child. It is usually a good idea to corroborate this account with the parent. When discussing the history of presenting problems or the developmental history of the child, the parent may have brought up the subject of the episodes of maltreatment. The clinician can then request more details about what actually happened. Typical content should include the type of abuse, age of the child at its onset, its duration, the identity of the perpetrator and his or her relationship to the child, the use of physical or psychological coercion or threats, the frequency of the episodes, and the presence of any medical symptomatology. Additionally, the clinician should inquire about how the abuse or neglect was discovered or disclosed, the response of protective or legal/justice systems, and the child's response to the maltreatment (if not already fully explored when a history of the presenting problems was taken). Again, we refer the reader to Table 2.1 in Chapter 2 for an outline of the maltreatment characteristics that deserve careful inquiry.

Parents usually begin to express their own feelings and concerns about what happened as they talk about their child's maltreatment. These reactions and feelings can influence the support they provide to children who have been sexually abused or exposed to other forms of maltreatment. Regehr (1990) provides a useful way to organize the different types of parental responses to extrafamilial child sexual assaults that can be applied to other forms of maltreatment.

Parental Feelings about the Self

Some parents or caregivers may feel extremely guilty about their child's victimization. This is especially so if they have a history of maltreatment themselves and had promised themselves they would never allow anything like that to happen to their own children. They may feel inadequate as parents and are embarrassed to disclose their children's experiences, since they expect criticism from others (Regehr, 1990). Unfortunately, such guilt feelings may contribute to a deterioration in their parenting skills. We have seen some parents who allowed their children to engage in out-of-control or excessive behavior postdisclosure because of their excessive sympathy for the child. Parents' failure to set firm limits may reflect an attempt to alleviate a sense of guilt for what the child has experienced but is rarely helpful for the child. In other cases, parents may become overprotective and severely restrict the child's activities to ensure the abuse never happens again. This strategy may convey the implicit notion that the child is powerless and unable to protect himself or herself from future dangers. His or her role as victim is thereby intensified for the child. Restricting the child's normal activities may impede his or her recovery by limiting the child's opportunities to be successful and interact in healthy ways with peers. Both parental responses may result in an even lower sense of self-esteem for the child and reduce the support the child could have received from friends.

Parents or caregivers with their own maltreatment history may have particular difficulty in managing their reactions to their child's victimization. Such a history in families of abused or neglected children is not uncommon. Goodwin, McCarthy, and Divasto (1981) report that 24% of mothers of physically abused and/or sexually abused children had a prior incest history, compared with 3% of mothers of nonabused children. Leifer et al. (1993) found that 53% of mothers of 68 sexually abused girls aged 5 to 16 had their own history of sexual abuse and that 52% had poor relationships with their own parents.

The notion that a prior history of maltreatment, at least of child sexual abuse, may have significant effects upon later parenting has been reported in several studies. For example, Cole, Woolger, Power, and Smith (1992) found that adult female incest survivors reported significantly less confidence and a diminished sense of control as parents than other mothers. These mothers also reported they were less consistent and organized and made fewer demands on their children. These characteristics impeded the emergence of their children's autonomy, thereby subverting their desire for their children to become autonomous as quickly as possible. The association between a parental victimization history and the subsequent deterioration in parenting and level of support has not been empirically examined for other forms of maltreatment or for fathers. However, the data described above are consistent with our own clinical observations and experiences not only of sexually abused children and their parents, but of families that have experienced other forms of maltreatment.

In general, a child's victimization experiences may elicit parents' feelings, such as sadness, anger, or anxiety, about their own history of maltreatment. These feelings may be overwhelming for parents, especially if they have been repressed and avoided for many years. To cope with this intense pain and distress, parents engage in a number of defensive maneuvers that in turn may have deleterious effects upon their parenting. They may deny the child's emotional reaction or the child's experience to avoid their own pain, which leaves children questioning the validity of the maltreatment and the legitimacy of their feelings. Parents may deal with their own or their children's emotional reactions to the victimization in an intellectualized manner. This approach again leaves children feeling unsupported and unable to articulate or express strong emotions. On the other hand, parents may become excessively preoccupied with issues related to their own victimization, leaving them little time or energy to devote to their children. Consequently, children may feel unsupported and abandoned or may be exposed to inadequate parenting practices such as poor supervision or inconsistent limit-setting.

Given the potential impact of parents' victimization history upon their coping mechanisms and responses to their child's maltreatment, it is crucial to inquire about this variable. Clinicians should preface direct questioning about this issue by noting that a substantial number of parents have such a history and add that it often has important implications for parental reactions to their children. If the child lives with a mother and a father, the clinician should ask both parents about this matter. The following clinical example clearly demonstrates the importance of this inquiry.

A family of three children was referred for an assessment. The children had been deserted by their mother, Joan, several years prior and raised by George, the father of one of the children. The children had been placed in the care of child welfare services because they had experienced significant sexual abuse, physical abuse, and neglect. Shortly after the children had been removed from the home, Joan returned to regain custody of the children. The clinician was asked to evaluate Joan's potential for parenting and supporting the children. Joan herself had been deserted by her father and removed from her mother's care. In foster care, she was physically and sexually abused. She was subsequently placed in other facilities as an adolescent, where she was further maltreated, fleeing when she was 16 years of age. She then became pregnant, had a baby, and entered a relationship with George. Here she continued to be passive and was further maltreated. She fled and left her children behind even though she thought they might also be abused by George. Joan entered another relationship in which she continued to be physically, sexually, and emotionally assaulted. Joan's reactions to her own maltreatment were muted, and she demonstrated little overt distress and no empathy about her childrens' experiences. She clearly was not dealing with her own issues and could not protect herself, let alone begin to support, nurture, and provide safety for her children.

The clinician should attempt to gather enough information to form some tentative impressions about the significance of a parental victimization history for the child's response to maltreatment. We must caution the clinician to be prudent when conducting this inquiry, since it can sometimes provoke intense feelings in the parent or caregiver. The inquiry should not go so far that the parent's defensive structure is stripped away and the parent's functioning deteriorates, functioning that includes parenting and the ability to manage the child's emotional distress and behavioral disturbance. This caveat is especially important if there are no services in place to provide immediate and ongoing assistance to the adult. Although the choice of strategies is partially a matter of clinical experience and judgment, certain approaches may prove useful to contain these strong parental feelings. Although information about the type of parental maltreatment is useful (e.g., did the parent and child experience the same type of abuse?), asking the parent for specific details of his or her abuse may be too provocative. The clinician may want to ask about the identity of the parent's perpetrator to determine if it is similar to the child's (e.g., a paternal figure), whether the parent ever disclosed the maltreatment and if others knew about it, and the response of his or her own parents or caregivers. It may be profitable to ask the parent about their perceptions of how they coped with their own maltreatment, how it has affected their feelings and responses to their child's victimization, and what they need now regarding their own history to help themselves and their offspring. Although such questions may be safer areas of inquiry than asking for a full and detailed account of the parental maltreatment episodes, they may still be provocative, and the clinician must proceed cautiously.

Empathizing with and normalizing parents' distress may attenuate the sense of isolation and stigmatization that may accompany their disclosure of maltreatment. Clinicians should also commend parents for their strength in acknowledging their own history and should reinforce the notion that in doing so, these parents have taken a significant step in helping their child. One component of the treatment plan might be a recommendation for such parents to participate in therapy so as to be effective in addressing those historical issues that are significant obstacles in their attempts to cope adaptively with the child's history of maltreatment. The importance of acknowledging and processing this history for subsequent parenting is demonstrated by Egeland and colleagues (1988) and Main and Goldwyn (1984). Both teams found that parents who had recalled and discussed their own histories of abuse and neglect were less likely to maltreat their own children.

Other caregivers, such as foster parents, may also exhibit intense reactions and feelings regarding maltreated children, particularly if the caregiver was abused as a child and still harbors many unresolved feelings. On occasion, caregivers sometimes come into the work of providing care for maltreated children, seemingly to help themselves resolve personal issues or to make it better for another child than it was for them. Inquiry may be a more sensitive matter, especially as foster parents are part of the treatment team and occupy paraprofessional status. It may be more appropriate for the social worker supervising the foster home to initially address these issues, and then refer the foster parent for appropriate counseling.

Feelings toward the Child

Although parents may believe their child's account of the maltreatment, some are angry at a child who did not stop or prevent the abuse or who did not disclose it sooner. Our clinical experience suggests that this attitude may be particularly prevalent in the reactions of fathers to their abused sons, especially those boys who have been sexually assaulted. These fathers may be anxious about the boy's masculinity or even fearful that the boy consented to the sexual activity. They may have numerous concerns about the boy's sexual identity or preference. Other parents, especially those whose children have been sexually abused, may regard them as "spoiled goods" or see them as so damaged that any chance of recovery is slim. These reactions compound the child's sense of stigmatization and helplessness. Others may outright disbelieve their child's allegations and accuse the youngster of fabrication. They may blame the child for the perpetrator being charged, convicted, or incarcerated, or for the resulting family disruption if the perpetrator is a family member. At its most extreme, this attitude is exemplified by the parent who chooses to support the alleged perpetrator rather than the child, insisting the child leave the home rather than the offender. These sentiments can engender or compound the child's internal attributions of self-blame and feelings of betrayal and stigmatization.

Feelings toward the Offender

Anger is, of course, a normal and expected reaction in any parent whose child has been maltreated. However, this anger may become so extreme that the parent begins to voice a desire to hurt or even kill the offender. Such statements are not helpful for those children who have been abused or neglected by somebody they know well and for whom they hold many positive feelings, including love. Many victimized children are ambivalent about their perpetrator and do not want to see the individual harmed. Parental threats to harm or kill the perpetrator escalate the child's anxiety, especially when he or she is aware that such actions might result in that parent's incarceration or punishment. The child would then be deprived of parental availability and support at just that time when they are most needed. Furthermore, extreme displays of parental anger at the perpetrator may lead the child to believe that his or her positive feelings are in some way deviant. This reaction is highly likely if the parent has been unable to empathize with the child's positive feelings toward the abuser or condemns the child for harboring them. Other parents may feel extremely guilty about pressing charges and are overly concerned about the welfare of the offender or his or her family (Regehr, 1990). They may begin to question the validity of the child's disclosure, thereby making them less supportive of the child. The situation can be magnified if others pressure the parent to consider the offender's welfare. This situation most often occurs when the offender is a family member and other members of the family ally themselves with the perpetrator.

Feelings toward the System

Regehr (1990) reports that parental distress over a child's victimization may be heightened by fears and anxiety associated with the investigation and judicial proceedings. Parents may be apprehensive about the impact of their child testifying in court and may feel they have little control over the whole investigatory and judicial process. Some feel their own parenting capabilities are being questioned by representatives of these various systems, adding to their distress. This reaction may be especially true in families where parents have been responsible for the child's maltreatment and have had extensive involvement with child protective or legal/justice systems. Such parents sometimes feel great antipathy toward these systems and their representatives. These feelings may be communicated directly to the child, who in turn begins to regard contact with staff of these agencies with similar suspicion and hostility. This attitude may be generalized to mental health professionals, and may prove to be an obstacle in establishing a therapeutic alliance between the child and clinician.

Parents' Behavioral Responses to the Maltreatment

Besides inquiring about their affective and cognitive reactions to the child's maltreatment, the clinician must ask about the parent's or caregiver's behavioral responses to the maltreatment. As indicated in Table 3.1, the clinician should ask about the parent's immediate instrumental responses to the maltreatment. Such questions may include whether the parent brought the child for a medical examination, contacted the appropriate legal or child protective services, or took immediate steps to ensure the child's protection from the alleged perpetrator. When the history of the presenting problems was being discussed, the clinician may have inquired about the parent's behavioral responses to the child's initial displays of symptomatology. If this area was not explored at that time, the clinician should now ask for a description of the specific strategies the parent used and is now using to manage the child's behavior. For instance, if the child had displayed many anxiety-related symptoms, such as nightmares, how had the parent dealt with these symptoms? Were the parent's actions effective? What was the child's response? If nightmares are still a problem, had there been any change in the parent's strategies? If so, what has the effect been? Similarly, the clinician will want to know about the parent's response to any aggressive or sexualized behavior the child might have manifested. A parent's inappropriate or ineffective strategies may well exacerbate the child's symptomatology, whereas other practices may prove to be extremely helpful for the child's adaptation to the maltreatment.

Parental and Family History

A knowledge of the parents' and family histories provides an essential context that helps the clinician more fully appreciate the nature and development of the child's difficulties and strengths. Table 3.4 presents a summary of the information the clinician may find relevant. This summary is based upon the work of others (Broder & Hood, 1983; Wolfe, 1988; Wolfe & Wolfe, 1988), which the reader may consult for a more detailed discussion.

We have seen that a parent's own maltreatment history may significantly affect the parent's feelings about and responses to, the child's victimization. Many other characteristics of a parent's history may affect that parent's current ability to support the child. Do present difficulties in talking with the child about the maltreatment reflect longstanding problems in communication and the sharing of feelings that had their origins in the parent's own family? Has the parent always had difficulty making friends or is his or her current social isolation more a situational reaction? Have chronic problems with educational attainment or employment resulted in present poverty? The parent's psychiatric history may be especially helpful in understanding current difficulties coping with the child's victimization. Inquiries in this area may reveal that the parent or caregiver had chronic mental health difficulties that predated the child's maltreatment. The distress of a different parent who does not have this kind of psychiatric history might reflect more of a situational reaction to the child's maltreatment.

TABLE 3.4. Parental and Family History

---

1. Parental history
   a. Quality of relationship with parents/significant caregivers; relationship with siblings
   b. Description of family life during childhood: management of conflict and discipline; patterns of communication, including sharing of affection and feelings
   c. History of maltreatment in childhood and adolescence
   d. Quality of relationships with peers during childhood and adolescence
   e. Educational history
   f. Employment history
   g. Parental and family history of psychiatric/psychological problems, including efforts to seek assistance and outcome of professional involvement
   h. Problems with the law
   i. Other previous relevant life events (e.g., deaths, significant illnesses, financial problems)

2. Marital and family history
   a. Description of previous relationships or marriages, including any problems (e.g., spousal violence); reasons for termination of these relationships/marriages; problems regarding divorce or custody/access
   b. Current relationship/marriage—how the couple met and what attracted them to each other
   c. Length, stability, and quality of the relationship
   d. Presence of any previous problems in the relationship or family (e.g., spousal violence, substance abuse); lack of support regarding family responsibilities

3. Parenting history
   a. Planning for children (e.g., planned vs. unplanned pregnancies); pregnancies; births; adoptions; abortions or miscarriages
   b. Reactions to pregnancies; effect of pregnancies and arrival of children
   c. Brief description of physical, emotional, and behavioral problems of all children; previous attempts to seek help and outcome of these problems
   d. History of parenting difficulties; reasons; previous attempts to seek assistance and outcome of these difficulties
   e. History of maltreatment in the family; type of maltreatment, identity of perpetrator, time of onset, duration, and frequency; emotional and behavioral response of family members and involvement of other systems/agencies (e.g., child protective services, police)
   f. Placements of children (type of placement, reasons, reactions of parents and children)

The history of the parent's significant relationships, including marriage, must also be examined. A longstanding history of parental relationship problems, including spousal violence or a series of many relationships, each having ended abruptly, may bode poorly for a maltreated child's subsequent adjustment. For instance, for a long time a parent might have been so preoccupied with these dysfunctional relationships that his or her attention had been deflected from the child even before the maltreatment began. Furthermore, the child may continue to be exposed to significant conflict or even violence at home. Such a situation would only exacerbate the child's anxiety or distress associated with the maltreatment.

The actual parenting given the child has an enormous influence upon his or her current adjustment. Again, the historical parenting pattern in the family may be a rich source of data. Had this child been exposed to inadequate or ineffectual parenting even before the onset of the maltreatment? Is the maltreatment just one instance of broad and generalized parenting deficits, or has the parent never evidenced any previous difficulties in this area? Are the current problems more a reaction to the child's distress, or are they a reflection of the parent's personal issues about the maltreatment? Despite the time and effort needed to gather the information in Table 3.4, we believe that the clinician will find it well worth doing so. This information will help the clinician form a more complete description of the maltreated child and how he or she fits into this broader family environment.

The main method of obtaining this information is through interviews with the parents. The clinician should reiterate the rationale for these very personal questions. Parental reports may be supplemented by examining documentation from other agencies, such as child welfare reports or records of past involvement with helping agencies, including past therapy records.

Current Parental and Family Functioning

The main purpose of examining current parental and family functioning is to identify parental and family characteristics that are presently serving as potentiating or compensatory factors for the maltreated child. Table 3.5 gives a summary of the major variables in this area, which range from the individual, intrapsychic to broader areas such as financial status.

A positive emotional attachment between the child and parent may serve as a compensatory factor for the maltreated youngster. As we have seen, a secure attachment may contribute to a solid sense of self-esteem and self-efficacy, which in turn may lead the maltreated child to feel less traumatized. A child with a secure attachment to a parent feels and believes that the parent will be psychologically available. The youngster may more readily seek out support and comfort from the parent after disclosure of the maltreatment, resulting in less distress and the emergence of fewer symptoms. The parent who has formed this kind of relationship with his or her child may be more likely to protect that child from further abuse, and be consistently psychologically available. Such a parent probably will not resent the time, effort, and energy required to help the child recover. Specific ways to evaluate attachment will be reviewed in Chapter 4.

The clinician must ask parents whether they have any current psychiatric

TABLE 3.5. Current Parental and Family Functioning

---

1. Parental functioning
   a. Presence of any identifiable psychiatric/psychological problems; substance abuse; health problems; current involvement in any treatment for these problems
   b. Quality of current relationships, including marital relationship; presence of problems (e.g., spousal violence, serious discord); efforts to seek assistance and current involvement
   c. Degree and quality of other social supports
   d. Current employment and financial status; stability and adequacy of living arrangements

2. Parenting ability
   a. A positive emotional attachment to the child
   b. The ability to perceive the child accurately and to recognize and meet the individual needs and characteristics of the child; appropriate expectations of the child
   c. Disciplinary style
   d. Impulse control (affective and behavioral self-regulation)

3. Family functioning[a]
   a. *Structure and organization of the family:* Repetitive patterns of interaction (alliance, coalitions, subsystems; power hierarchy; separation of generation; boundaries between individuals; degree of individuality; cohesiveness; interdependency; enmeshment); clarity of roles and functions; rigidity and flexibility of system, openness to information
   b. *Communication:* Clarity–ambiguity; directness–indirectness; consequences of verbal and nonverbal communication; metacommunication (rules about what can be said, by whom, to whom, how), themes, preoccupations, avoidances, quantity
   c. *Affect:* Emotional tone, expression, intensity, variation, rules about expression; comfort level with feelings, responsiveness
   d. *Control and decision making:* Leadership style, flexibility, consistency, forms of reinforcement, cooperation, resistance, attitude to feedback
   e. *Conflict resolution:* Method and style; management of differences and disagreement; areas of difficulty
   f. *Developmental parameters:* Age-appropriateness of expectations, roles, intergenerational issues; management of autonomy and individuation; fit between developmental tasks of adults and children

---

[a]From Broder and Hood (1983, p. 142).

or psychological problems that impair their functioning. A psychiatric diagnosis per se does not necessarily mean a particular individual encounters significant difficulty in functioning on a daily basis as a parent. Consistent with the transactional model, many other variables mediate the relationship between the presence of a psychological or psychiatric disorder and an individual's functioning (e.g., the provision of appropriate treatment or the presence of social supports). Similarly, the significance of health problems, substance abuse, or problems with the law for a parent's functioning must be examined with reference to other variables. It behooves the clinician to gather specific information that explicates the relationship, if any, between these diagnoses or problems and a parent's ability to support the child's recovery.

The quality of a parent's current relationships is another important variable. As we maintained in the preceding section, children may suffer from exposure to any serious disharmony, discord, or violence of such relationships. The parent's time, attention, and psychological resources may be diverted from the child to the parent's own troubled relationships. Conflict between marital partners may be generalized to their inconsistency in parenting, which would compound the child's difficulties. Conflict between marital partners may be revealed in disagreements about how to handle other aspects of the maltreatment, such as whether to report the situation to the police.

Clinicians must inquire about the degree and quality of other social supports currently available to the parent. This information should include not only the actual number of supports but also whether the parent *perceives* them as supportive. What function do these supports play in the parent's life and what kind of help or assistance do they provide? For instance, does the parent have ready and easy access to alternate caregivers who will provide relief in caring for a maltreated child who behaves aggressively and sometimes outrageously? Does the parent have relationships with individuals with whom he or she can talk and receive a sense of validation of, and support for, his or her feelings, or does the parent feel socially isolated? Are these natural social supports, or does parent rely solely on crisis nurseries, child welfare personnel, shelters, or therapists for support?

Social and cultural factors influence the parent's response to the child's maltreatment. A substantial proportion of children engage in sexualized behavior after being sexually assaulted. Social and religious values that strongly condemn any kind of sexual behavior in children may be associated with the parent's overly punitive and harsh responses, which may exacerbate the child's feelings of stigmatization, shame, and guilt (Gil & Johnson, 1993).

A parent's current employment and financial status can affect that parent's responses to the child. Parents who are unemployed and living in poverty may feel inadequate about themselves and their ability to provide for their families. These feelings may be associated with increased depression or anger. Parents may regard their child's maltreatment as yet another example of their own parental inadequacy. Furthermore, a precarious financial situation may preclude a parent from hiring other caregivers to provide a much-needed break from the sometimes intense demands of managing a maltreated child's behavior, thereby compounding a parent's feelings of tension, anxiety, and frustration. Living in a crowded, unsafe, or even dangerous environment increases stress for the child and other family members. In some countries, limited financial resources restrict the range of services and treatment options available to parents and their children. Other parents may be living in regions where treatment services are undeveloped. Besides identifying these areas of stress, a clinician must ask how parents have handled these difficulties, paying particular attention to their success in ameliorating them. Such successes may highlight particular strengths in the parents and family and may serve as a basis for effective interventions in any subsequent treatment plan.

Finally, evaluation of the family system can provide important information about how the family has adapted to the child's maltreatment. Familial problems that existed prior to the maltreatment may continue exacerbating the child's adaptation. Wolfe and Wolfe (1988) report that sexually abused children who live in families where the expression of negative feelings is prohibited or not sanctioned may be at risk for developing internalizing problems such as depression or anxiety disorders. A family in which parents exhibit little leadership or executive functioning may be at risk for failing to provide the child with the high degree of consistency and structure needed after the disclosure of abuse. Information about these characteristics of family functioning may not only identify the presence of important moderator variables but also suggest potentially significant intervention targets.

We recommend a variety of methods of gathering information in these domains, including individual and joint interviews with parents alone and with the entire family. Observations of the interaction between parents or caregivers may afford the clinician important data about the status of the relationship and its strengths and weaknesses. A number of useful psychometric tests are also available. The parent's current level of symptomatology can be assessed through the administration of inventories like the Minnesota Multiphasic Personality Inventory–2 (MMPI-2) (Hathaway & McKinley, 1989) and the Symptom Checklist 90–Revised (SCL 90–R) (Derogatis, 1983). The Impact of Event Scale (Veronen & Kilpatrick, 1986) can be used to assess the extent to which parents are bothered by intrusive thoughts about the abuse. The Dyadic Adjustment Scale (DAS) (Spanier, 1976) and the Conflict Tactics Scales (CTS) (Straus, 1979) augment information about the marital relationship obtained from more informal interviews. The reader is referred to Wolfe (1988) and Wolfe and Wolfe (1988) for a more detailed discussion of these and other psychometric instruments.

Other parenting dimensions can be assessed through a combination of parental interviews, direct observation of parent–child interaction, and the administration of standardized tests such as the Parenting Stress Index (PSI) (Abidin, 1995) or the Child Abuse Potential Inventory (CAPI) (Milner,

1986). A number of works describe the assessment of parenting capacity and the evaluation of the risk parents may pose to their children in terms of abuse and neglect (e.g., Schutz, Dixon, Lindenberger, & Ruther, 1989). The reader is advised to consult the above references for more detailed and extensive discussions of these issues.

Given the heterogeneity of parents and families in which maltreatment has occurred and given the broad array of contributing factors, including those related to parental and family functioning, the clinician should approach family assessment with reasonable expectations. That is, to assume that one can identify all the factors that influence the functioning of parents and family is unrealistic. However, the attempt to enrich our understanding of the potential influence of parental and family factors places the child's assessment in a much broader and more meaningful context.

FOUR

Assessment of the Child

In CHAPTER 3 we described our five underlying assumptions about clinical assessment. We would like to add one other assumption: *Clinical assessments of maltreated children must have a developmental focus.* This assumption is critically important for two reasons. First, knowledge of normal growth and development helps determine the significance of a particular behavior; that is, is the behavior or symptom a "problem" deserving attention, or is it expected of a child of that particular age? To use a simple example, nighttime enuresis is common for 2-year-old children but much rarer for 12-year-olds. Unfortunately, such distinctions may not be so easily drawn for other behavior. Reports of normative data regarding children's sexual behavior are quite recent (e.g., Friedrich et al., 1991, 1992). Before the publication of these data, clinicians were hampered in determining the clinical significance of a child's sexualized behavior toward other children. However, we must emphasize that considering developmental parameters alone is insufficient in any clinical assessment. Returning to our example of sexualized behavior, we may determine that a child's sexualized behaviors are not displayed by the vast majority of his or her peers. However, there are many other variables (e.g., use of physical or psychological coercion to gain the other child's compliance, lack of empathy for the other child's feelings) that must be considered when deciding the clinical significance of a particular behavior or symptom. Although a solid knowledge and understanding of children's development does not provide the complete perspective, it serves as a necessary starting point from which clinicians can begin to evaluate the child's response to maltreatment.

Second, knowledge about a particular child's developmental level furnishes critical information that guides the choice and application of assessment strategies. Developmentally sensitive assessments are essential to obtaining useful information that can guide clinical decision making and planning. The clinician who is interviewing a child must have a basic knowledge of the development of children's cognitive abilities, memory, and language. For example, preschoolers have particular difficulty with the concept of time and may not be able to answer questions about calendar dates accurately (Friedman, 1981). Also, young children often need external cues or props to help describe their experiences.

PLANNING THE ASSESSMENT OF THE CHILD

After interviewing the parents or significant caregivers, the clinician should have considerable information regarding their perceptions of the child's response to the maltreatment. The clinician might contact other significant people in the child's life for their observations, which may suggest areas the clinician might address in the direct assessment work with the child. Collateral reports also provide an even broader description of the child's functioning in different settings. For example, a child may indeed be having significant difficulties at home. The classroom or day-care center may, on the other hand, provide the consistency, attention, and safety for the child that in turn is associated with much more adaptive functioning.

The clinician should attempt to confirm the parent or caregiver's observations of the child's functioning in these other settings. Some parents or caregivers, including parents of maltreated children, are somewhat biased in their perceptions of the child. Everson et al. (1989) report that among mothers who provided little or ambivalent support to their children, there was no significant correlation between their description of their sexually abused children's psychological functioning on the CBCL and the children's ratings derived from a psychiatric interview. Of course, one cannot discount the possibility that teachers or day-care staff may have their own biased perceptions. This possibility may need to be confirmed by observing the child in the classroom or day care. Similarly, although parents or caregivers may not have identified a specific area of the child's functioning as a problem, the clinician should consult these other individuals who have had close contact with the child to learn if they do see a problem in that area.

After explaining the purpose of his or her call to the teacher or day-care worker, the clinician may ask fairly open-ended questions about the child's functioning. More specific inquiries should follow to ensure that all areas of functioning (e.g., intellectual and academic functioning, relationships with peers and adults, affective and behavioral self-regulation, self-esteem) have been reviewed. Clinicians may also ask teachers to complete broad-scale assessment instruments such as the TRF of the CBCL. Frequently, the clinician will want to talk to the teacher or day-care worker again after the assessment has begun in order to share observations, ask about areas of concern that became apparent during the assessment, and clarify any of the collateral's responses to the assessment instruments. These people often play an important role in the child's recovery, and their involvement in the assessment process is often a good way to establish a collaborative alliance.

Before meeting the child, clinicians must provide the parents or caregivers with some guidance about preparing the child for the assessment. If parents do not raise this issue, the clinician should broach it. It is best not to give direct guidance or suggestions immediately. The clinician can sometimes learn more about the parents' or caregivers' typical ways of dealing with the child by asking how they think the child should be prepared for the assessment and what they would like to say to the child about the first appointment. Some caregivers and parents have no idea of what they should say and had not considered this to be a significant issue. Other parents are quite distraught about bringing their child to a mental health professional; especially for an evaluation of the impact of maltreatment, since many parents are often overwhelmed by feelings of guilt, remorse, or shame. Often they would prefer not to say anything about the assessment to the child. Still others fear having to be assertive in the face of their child's resistance, which may be another indicator of parenting difficulties.

The clinician can encourage the parents or caregivers to give the child a brief but direct rationale for the assessment. They may tell the child that he or she is going to meet with the clinician and inform the child of the clinician's name. The parent should discuss the reasons for the assessment with the child. They might say that it is an opportunity to spend some time with a person who would like to talk with the child about the maltreatment (or whatever word may be appropriate). This person will want to find out how the youngster thinks and feels about what happened. Some children respond well when the clinician is described as a "feeling doctor" as opposed to a medical or "body doctor." If the clinician works in a medical facility, parents can assure the child that no medical procedures will occur at this time (unless some are planned). Parents may also reassure the child by saying they have already met the clinician and by empathizing with the child's feelings of anxiety, fear, or anger. Regarding the timing of this discussion, younger children should be told about meeting with the clinician only a day or two before the actual appointment. A longer wait often generates overwhelming anxiety in the child. Older children (8 years and up) should be told several days prior to the appointment. This period provides them with the opportunity to ask more questions about the rationale for the assessment, the process, and any other concerns. However, these age guidelines should not be rigidly applied and need to be adapted to the child's idiosyncratic needs.

INTERVIEWING THE MALTREATED CHILD

As clinicians, we sometimes assume that children cannot or will not talk about the maltreatment they have undergone. We immediately rush them into the playroom with the expectation that this is the only way of gathering relevant information. However, although interviewing children takes considerable training and experience, the therapist can use interviews to gather considerable information. Interviews also allow the clinician to do an informal evaluation of the child's verbal proficiency and the kinds of alternate assessment strategies that might have to be used. If clinicians make no attempt to talk with a child about the maltreatment and other issues, they may never learn how adept the child might be in this area.

A detailed description of child development and its implications for assessment are beyond the scope of this volume. We refer the reader to other works that include comprehensive accounts of developmental research implications for interviewing maltreated children (Garbarino, Stott, & Faculty of the Erikson Institute, 1989; Steward, Bussey, Goodman, & Saywitz, 1993). We will, however, incorporate some of this information in our discussion of practical assessment strategies.

Stage 1: Introduction

Meeting the Child and Orienting Him or Her to the Assessment

Usually the clinician will meet the child and parents or caregivers in some kind of waiting or reception area. When greeting the child and introducing oneself, it is often useful to bend or crouch down to be more at the child's level. The clinician should then inform the child that they will be going to the clinician's office and that the parents or caregivers will be in the waiting room when the appointment is finished. Even at this very early point in the assessment process, the clinician can begin to gather some information about the child. Does the child respond appropriately by acknowledging the clinician's presence, for example establishing eye contact, responding to the clinician's greeting, or shaking hands? Was the family sitting together and interacting in the waiting room, or was one member, perhaps the child, sitting at a distance from other family members? How does the child separate from the parents/caregivers? Does the child become anxious and insist the parent accompany him or her to the clinician's office? Or does he or she separate from the parents with no any evidence of anxiety and interact in an overly friendly or indiscriminate manner? Is the child mute while walking to the office, or does he or she initiate or respond to social chit chat? Highly anxious children should be allowed to have a parent or caregiver accompany them to the interview. Also, there is nothing to be gained by insisting that a frightened, highly distressed child accompany you to your office. Such tactics may compromise the chances of forming a therapeutic alliance with the child and may reinforce the notion that adults are insensitive and unresponsive to the child's particular needs. After one or two sessions with the parent or caregiver present, usually the child allows that person to leave the session.

Once in the clinician's office, the child must be oriented to the assessment process. It is useful to say your name again and then to ask for the child's understanding of why he or she has been brought to the session. Have the parents or caregivers prepared the child as planned? Some parents may have provided an explanation. However, the child may be too embarrassed or anxious to talk about the reasons, or the child may have many fantasies or misconceptions about the assessment. We have heard children explain that they have been brought to an outpatient program at a pediatric hospital because they were "sick" and needed "shots," or that they were "bad" children and the clinician would decide whether they should be taken away from their parents.

After determining the child's understanding of the assessment, the clinician must clarify its purpose. This is particularly important for those children who claim to have no idea of why they are there or for those who harbor misconceptions. Even with most children who have a clear understanding of the referral reasons, the clinician should confirm their account. We recommend strongly that the clinician talk directly about the assessment's purpose, that is, that the child is there because he or she has been maltreated in some way. The clinician may begin by saying, "I understand from your parents [or foster parents or social worker, if appropriate] that somebody touched your private parts [when speaking with sexually abused children]." An equally straightforward approach should be taken toward children who have been maltreated in other ways. Clinicians may acknowledge that the child has been hit or use whatever phrase may be appropriate to the details of the child's experience. Similarly, the clinician may acknowledge episodes of neglect ("I understand that you didn't get enough food") or psychological maltreatment ("I understand that people yelled a lot at you and called you names"). The clinician should then clarify his or her role by saying, "I see other kids who have had the same kinds of things happen to them. My job is to find out how kids think and feel about these things and see if there is anything that I or other people can do to help the kids feel better."

There are several reasons why we believe it important to raise the maltreatment issue at such an early phase. First, direct statements like these set the stage for establishing a therapeutic alliance with the child who now better understands the reasons for coming to see the clinician. At this initial meeting, the therapist begins to set some expectations—that is, that the maltreatment will be a principal focus for both the clinician and the child. Second, by saying such statements as, "Someone touched your private parts," or, "Someone hit you," in a neutral, nonanxious way, the clinician begins modeling the direct expression of these sensitive and painful issues. This approach may be especially important for a child whose parents or caregivers have never talked directly about the maltreatment. Other parents might have become terribly distraught when their child disclosed maltreatment details. Often such children become reluctant to talk about the maltreatment in order to protect their parents from these painful feelings. Exposure to another adult who begins modeling a different way of dealing with these issues exposes the child to an adaptive model of coping with the feelings and beliefs about the maltreatment. Also, the child is reassured that he or she can deal with these issues with an adult who can tolerate the child's distress and will not fall apart. Third, the clinician begins to desensitize the youngster. The use of phrases that refer directly to the maltreatment exposes the child to this material, so his or her anxiety can begin to abate. Fourth, by bringing up the subject of the maltreatment so directly and quickly, the clinician begins to convey an expectation that the child can eventually handle this topic. Finally, telling the child early on that the clinician has seen other children who have undergone similar experiences begins to counteract the child's sense of isolation and stigmatization. This can be done in a concrete way, especially for younger children. For instance, if they are displayed on a wall or bulletin board the clinician can point out pictures made by other children who have been similarly hurt.

Rather than asking about the maltreatment, the clinician should inquire first about the child's feelings about the assessment, especially now that the child better understands its purpose. The clinician should empathize with feelings such as anxiety or anger and then provide the child with some control over initiating a discussion of the maltreatment (Friedrich, 1990). Some children immediately launch into a detailed discussion about what happened. However, most children need further preparation and the opportunity to form a relationship with the clinician before they feel sufficiently comfortable to communicate their experiences, whether verbally or through other means. Adapting Friedrich's (1990, p. 151) suggesstions about engendering a therapeutic component in the interview, the clinician might say, "You're right, it is hard to talk about this, especially with someone you've just met. Most kids want to get to know me better before we talk about what happened. Would you like us to talk about other things and do some other stuff before we talk about how you were touched [or whatever phrase might be appropriate for the specific type of maltreatment]?" If the answer is yes, the child may be told that at a later time they might discuss whether he or she is comfortable enough to talk about these issues. Most children feel relieved that they are not expected to divulge this information so soon.

On occasion, we inadvertently replicate some elements of the original maltreatment in our clinical assessments. In response to the desperation of referral sources such as parents or child welfare staff, clinicians may feel compelled to develop a quick formulation explaining the child's symptoms and identifying possible courses of action. Consequently, clinicians may place considerable pressure on the child to provide a full account of the actual maltreatment during the first few assessment sessions. To the child exposed to previous coercive interactional patterns with adults, such as being physically or psychologically forced into sexual activity and/or to keep it secret, the clinician's misguided attempts may be yet another example of the untrustworthiness of adults. This coercive style confirms the child's internal working model of others as untrustworthy and insensitive and exacerbates his or her feelings of powerlessness. Sometimes clinicians make false promises to persuade the child to open up about the maltreatment. Statements like "If you tell, everything will be fine" or "Daddy won't go to jail" may have little basis in reality. For many maltreated children, their worlds fall apart after they disclose abuse or neglect and as a result some perpetrators are incarcerated. The child feels let down again by adults who have not kept their promises or commitments. These feelings reduce the likelihood of the child's active participation in the evaluation and subsequent therapy and increases the youngster's reluctance to openly discuss aspects of the maltreatment.

As clinicians, we must remember that like many adult clients, children coming to see a mental health professional are embarrassed, anxious, and sometimes overwhelmed by feelings of shame, guilt, and stigmatization. Assessments that respect the child's sense of privacy and his or her embarrassment and need to have some control over the assessment process are more likely to actively engage the child in the evaluation. The clinician's sensitivity to this issue contributes to the therapeutic atmosphere of the assessment. The child begins to learn that some adults can identify and empathize with his or her feelings and will treat him or her with respect and consideration. For many chronically maltreated children, this is a novel experience that begins to modify the child's internal working models of others as insensitive and uncaring and himself or herself as unworthy of respect.

Before actually interviewing the child, the clinician should clarify other aspects of the assessment. Many of these children have lived in unpredictable, chaotic, and sometimes threatening environments. They consequently anticipate the same kind of adverse events during the first session with the clinician. By orienting the child to the structure of the assessment, some of his or her anxiety about what will happen is alleviated and the child receives a reassuring sense of predictability. The clinician should tell the child how he or she would like to be addressed (e.g., Doctor, Mr., first name) and where they will be spending the session. Using a clock for younger children, the clinician can indicate how much time they will spend together and that they will rejoin parents or caregivers in the waiting room (or other previously designated locale) at the session's end. The clinician should also point out that washroom facilities are available and that all that is necessary is for the child to say that he or she needs to use them. By the end of the first session, the child should have some idea about how sessions work.

Inquiring about Other Topics

Now that the child is oriented to the assessment's purpose and structure, the clinician can begin to inquire about topics other than the maltreatment. This inquiry serves several purposes. First, it allows the clinician to establish some rapport with the child. The clinician can focus upon the child's strengths by asking, "What are some things you do best?" These discussions are less threatening and enable children to talk more openly and easily. They begin to counteract feelings of low self-esteem. Second, a child's responses and presentation in this interview phase may suggest he or she has traits (e.g., self-esteem, verbal skills, intellectual status) that have moderated the maltreatment's impact. The child's responses also may help to identify potential targets of intervention or alternate assessment strategies. For example, does the child display good attention and concentration, or is the behavior more consistent with a diagnosis of an attention deficit disorder? Can the child articulate ideas or feelings about a particular topic, or does evidence of poor verbal skills suggest the need to consider less verbally oriented assessment strategies? Later we will present a framework to organize this information.

Recreation and Interests. Previous interviews with the parents or caregivers may have led to the identification of some of the child's strengths and interests. The clinician might begin the child's interview by inquiring about these areas so as to start building rapport. The child's strengths may include hobbies, sports, pets, or even more mundane interests such as favorite television shows. The major goal is to get the child talking about personal strengths and interests and for the clinician to display enthusiasm and a genuine curiosity. Rushing the child through this phase of the interview detracts from the rapport that can be established and may convey a lack of genuine interest by the clinician. This line of inquiry also allows the clinician to see the child at his or her best and provides useful information about the child's abilities and interests or lack thereof, particularly compared with that of his or her peer group.

School. Our review of the impact of maltreatment indicates that many maltreated children have significant problems at school in terms of their academic performance, social relationships, and behavior. Focusing upon the child's problems in adapting to school may again be too threatening to the child, resulting in sparse and unelaborated responses. These responses reflect the child's attempts to protect himself or herself from even greater threats to his or her self-esteem should these problems be fully and openly acknowledged. Consequently, the clinician may want to focus first upon more positive aspects of school by asking what the child likes and does best there. Similarly, the clinician might ask the child to identify which people in school he or she likes most. Is there anything about school that seems to provide a sense of satisfaction or pride? More troublesome aspects can then be addressed by asking what the child dislikes about school and why these situations or relationships are problems. Besides paying attention to the content of the responses, the clinician should listen closely to the underlying affective tone. For example, when describing a fairly dismal academic record, does the child sound genuinely sad or distressed? Does the child attempt to defend against such feelings by minimizing the difficulties and displaying little emotion?

Peer Relations. The child's descriptions of peer relationships yield important information regarding the child's ability to establish and maintain healthy relationships as well as the characteristics of the child's internal working models of relationships. The clinician may want to begin this inquiry by asking about the depth and nature of the child's peer relationships. Does he or she have no friends, one friend, or many friends; or does the child claim friendships with nearly everyone? If the child has a best friend, what specific activities do they do together, how often do they have contact, and what do they like about one another? When disagreements arise, how do they settle conflicts? Does the child have conflicts with other children, and, if so, why do these problems arise? Some children may externalize and blame others for their peer difficulties, assuming little, if any, responsibility for these problems. Has the child ever been disappointed by peers, and how frequently has this happened? The child's responses may reveal an expectation that others, including children of the same age, are unreliable, untrustworthy, and quite threatening figures. Alternatively, does the child describe himself or herself in fairly negative ways? Does the child convey an expectation that no one will ever want to be his or her friend because of these negative characteristics? Sometimes, by asking children to describe the "perfect friend," similar themes may be revealed.

Family Relationships. First, children should be asked to describe the composition of their family, including pets. Then they can be encouraged to describe pleasant family relationships. They can be asked to describe the fun they have together as a family unit, with their mother and father separately, and with their siblings. Ask children to identify what they like most about living with their family. Does the child provide an account that includes specific details of these positive aspects, or is the account vague and devoid of detail? Although other factors such as verbal skills can certainly play a role here, the clinician might start speculating about the veracity of a child's glowing descriptions if few details are supplied. The clinician must also assess whether the child's affect is congruent with the descriptions of these positive relationships. Also note whether the positive relationships are with parents as would be expected in younger children in particular, or whether they are with extended family, friends, or even pets.

After inquiring about these more positive aspects, the clinician might begin asking about some of the more troublesome characteristics of family life. Are there any changes the child would like to see the parents or family undergo? Sometimes asking the child to pretend that he or she has a "magic wand" and could change parents or family in any way helps younger children respond with sufficient detail. The clinician should ask the child what kinds of changes he or she would like in each parent or significant caregiver, siblings, and the family as a unit. At this point, maltreated children sometimes begin talking about their abuse or neglect or about other aspects of parenting, such as not receiving sufficient emotional attention. If the clinician believes the child can now cope with a more detailed inquiry about the maltreatment (to be discussed in a later section of this chapter), he or she ask whether the child is ready to talk about it at this point. If the child responds affirmatively, the clinician may go on with this kind of questioning.

Other more general inquiries that should be asked of every child include the expression of feelings by family members. For instance, who gets angry in the family, what do they get angry about, and how do they express their anger? Who in the family becomes sad and, how can the child tell if someone is sad? Such questions may elicit material regarding the maltreatment.

Plans for the Future. The therapist should preface questions in this area by saying that he or she appreciates that most people change their minds about what they would like to do in the future as they grow up. (The clinician does not expect the child to provide a definitive preference or choice.) Again, it might be best to start with more neutral inquiries: What kinds of activities or job would the child like to do as an adult, and what is the specific appeal of each? The child may then be asked about any thoughts regarding other aspects of adult life, especially relationships. Does the child think he or she will marry or have children? What would be the advantages and disadvantages of being married or having children? Again, the child's responses may provide some interesting information about expectations of relationships. Some children will maintain adamantly that they will never have children because they are too much "trouble" and not worth the effort. Such attitudes may be a reflection of their parents' or caregivers' feelings.

General Health. The clinician should not forget to ask the child about his or her general physical well-being and specific problems such as enuresis, encopresis, disturbed sleeping and eating habits, and somatic complaints such as abdominal pain. A child's general statement about not sleeping well may serve as a springboard for more specific inquiries. Questions can be asked about any particular fears the child experiences when going to bed, intrusive or recurrent thoughts or preoccupations while attempting to fall asleep, and the presence of any frightening dreams. Such symptomatology may indicate significant anxiety or even posttraumatic stress disorder.

If the child has good verbal skills and becomes actively involved in this phase of the assessment process, the clinician will generally spend a session discussing these topics. At the end of the first session, the clinician should very briefly summarize for the child, what has been learned taking care to emphasize the child's strengths as well as areas that are causing distress or difficulty. The clinician should also help the child understand the next step in the assessment process, perhaps saying that the child will be coming back to talk further and do some other activities with the clinician. Finally, the clinician might thank the child for attending and participating.

Stage 2: Interviewing the Child about the Maltreatment

Preparing the Child and Beginning the Inquiry

It is not a good idea to start the inquiry about the maltreatment near the end of an interview. The clinician and child need sufficient time to explore these issues gradually. Furthermore, strong feelings may be elicited in the child. Ending the interview without providing sufficient opportunity for the child to calm down, at least to a certain extent, does that child real disservice. This is especially so if the child must return to an environment such as the classroom, where the demands for sustained attention, concentration, and well-regulated behavior are quite stringent.

Such a discussion can open with the clinician saying something like, "I'd like to talk with you now about what happened when you were hit [or whatever phrase might be appropriate to the specific maltreatment]. I know some things about it, but it would sure help me if you could tell me more about it." The clinician should then reiterate this discussion's purpose: "As I told you when we first met, I'm really interested in your feelings and ideas about what happened to you. This may help us think of some things we can do to help you and your family feel better about what happened." Children need this explicit rationale, especially those who believe that interactions with a therapist may well result in abusive or exploitative episodes. For example, a boy who has been sexually abused by an adult male may become anxious when a male therapist takes him into a private office and begins to talk about sexual matters. Discussions about sexuality may in fact have preceded the incidents of sexual abuse by the perpetrator. Without a clear explanation of the rationale for these conversations, the child may misinterpret the clinician's actions in accordance with his internal working model; that is, adult males, especially those who talk to him in private about sex, cannot be trusted. After explaining the rationale, the clinician can ask if the child feels comfortable enough to begin talking about the maltreatment. If the child is ready, the clinician provides some further ground rules: the child should do it gradually, use whatever words or terminology are comfortable, and understand it would be perfectly acceptable for the child, in response to the clinician's questions, to state that he or she does not want to answer that particular question, rather than saying, "I don't know." The clinician should also inquire about any fears the child might have about the maltreatment or about describing it. It is important not to provide the child with any false reassurances that "everything is going to be okay."

To start this phase, ask the child to give an open-ended account of what happened. Rather than firing all sorts of specific questions, give the child the opportunity to tell his or her story without interruption, apart from gentle encouragement like "Go on" or "What happened next?" Nonverbal signals of clinician discomfort or anxiety while listening may result in the child prematurely terminating the description of the incidents to save the clinician from further discomfort. Managing one's personal reactions to these often horrific stories is critical; this issue is discussed in Chapter 12.

As in any clinical interview, the clinician must attend to the child's account on several different levels. The clinician must listen for the content. When compared with what the child had told other people, are there any significant discrepancies? Are significant details omitted, or is the child now disclosing new information? Does the child provide a fairly elaborated and detailed account, or is it sparse and devoid of detail?

Besides listening to the content of the account, the clinician must attend closely to the process, or how the child describes what happened. The child's general emotional demeanor and any changes in the types of feelings and the manner in which they are expressed merit close attention. What kinds of feelings and emotions accompany the description? Can the child express feelings associated with the maltreatment, or does he or she attempt to constrict the affect and thereby provide a matter-of-fact account? Do particular segments provoke different emotional reactions? For instance, a child may become especially restless and fidgety, leaving the chair and moving about the room when feeling anxious. Another child might "close down": he or she stops expressing any more feelings and terminates eye contact with the clinician. Others may become oppositional and defiant to deflect attention from a particular aspect of the account. We have seen children who seem to become sexually excited when talking about aspects of the sexual abuse. Children's thinking processes should also be carefully evaluated in this phase. Does their speech become less coherent, do they evidence a deterioration in attention and concentration, or do they begin to provide tangential responses or comments as a function of different aspects of their account of the maltreatment? Again, such information may provide clues about those aspects of the incidents that are particularly troublesome or distressing.

After the child provides an open-ended account of the maltreatment, the clinician may inquire about specific aspects of the incidents, including the emotional, cognitive, and behavioral sequelae. We have already reviewed Finkelhor and Browne's (1985) model of the traumagenic dynamics of child sexual abuse. Although this model was developed to help understand the impact of child sexual abuse, we believe that three of the factors–powerlessness, betrayal, and stigmatization–can be incorporated in interviews with children who have experienced other forms of maltreatment. The first factor, traumatic sexualization, is relevant to sexually abused children. Table 4.1 shows an outline of these factors and some possible areas of inquiry. It is only a rough guide, and the clinician must adapt the vocabulary and structure of the questions to suit the particular child's developmental level. Interviewing the child who can talk about such issues in this systematic manner may provide the clinician with a rich source of data and deepen an understanding of the child's experience.

Semistructured and Structured Interviews

Pynoos and Eth (1986) developed the Traumatic Event Interview Schedule, which can be used with maltreated children. After an expectation has been established that the maltreatment needs to be described, the child is encouraged to draw a picture of what happened and to tell a story about it. The interview then moves on to a more explicit discussion by the therapist asking the child to review any sensory experiences (e.g., feelings or odors) connected with the maltreatment experience. The clinician promotes and encourages a full description of what happened and asks the child to identify the "worst moment" of the event.

Vicky Wolfe and colleagues have developed a useful structured interview technique, the Children's Impact of Traumatic Events Scale–Revised (CITES) (Wolfe et al., 1989). This instrument is designed to help gather information about a child's perceptions, attributions, and feelings about his or her sexual victimization. The CITES has nine subscales, six related to impact (betrayal, guilt, helplessness, intrusive thoughts, sexualization, and stigmatization) and three related to attributions about the abuse (internal versus external, global versus specific, and stable versus unstable). The child is asked to respond "very true," "somewhat true," or "not true" to 54 items. Wolfe and Wolfe (1988) note that the scale may be especially useful in obtaining information from sexually abused children who are reluctant to divulge information about these issues in a more open-ended format.

TABLE 4.1. Areas of Inquiry Using Finkelhor and Browne's Traumagenic Dynamics

1. *Traumatic sexualization* (to be used for sexually abused children)
   a. Increased salience of sexual issues
      - Nature of the sexual abuse?
         - Pleasurable/reinforcing aspects of the abuse?
      - What kinds of sexual behavior does the child display now?
         - Frequency?
         - Onset?
         - Degree of pleasure/reinforcement?
      - Nature of sexual fantasies and feelings?
         - Frequency?
         - Onset?

   b. Confusion regarding sexual identity
      - Fears *re* future sexual desirability?
      - Fears of being gay?

   c. Confusion regarding sexual norms and standards
      - Is sex equated with affection?
      - Is sex used to obtain rewards and attention?

   d. Sexuality and anxiety
      - How did the child feel when being abused?
      - Worst fear?
      - How does the child feel now when thinking about the abuse or sexuality?
      - Does the child want to have sex in the future? Under what conditions?

   e. Fears regarding body integrity
      - Is the child fearful he/she was hurt or damaged, especially genitalia? (e.g., sexually transmitted diseases, HIV)
      - Fearful of implications for future sexual functioning?

2. *Powerlessness*
   a. Coercive aspects of the maltreatment
      - Degree of coercion (psychological/physical) used by the perpetrator?
      - Does the child perceive the above aspects as coercive?

   b. Helplessness
      - Could the child have done anything to stop the maltreatment?
      - Anticipated consequences of taking action?
      - Feelings *re* not being able to do anything to stop the maltreatment?
         - Anxiety?
         - Despair?
         - Depression?
         - Anger, identification with the aggressor?

   c. Perceived effectiveness/consequences of having taken action (e.g., disclosure)
      - Accidental versus purposeful disclosure?
      - If the disclosure was purposeful, what were the child's motives in disclosing?
      - Outcomes of the disclosure? (Did the maltreatment stop? Perpetrator incarcerated? Dissolution of the family?)

(continued)

TABLE 4.1. *cont.*

3. *Betrayal*
   a. Premaltreatment relationship with the perpetrator
      - Describe the relationship before the onset of the maltreatment. Positive and negative aspects?
      - Feelings toward the perpetrator?

   b. Feelings about the perpetrator after the onset of the maltreatment
      - Extent of: loss? sadness? anger? hurt?
      - How does the child express these feelings?
      - Have these feelings been generalized to other people? (e.g., can't trust any men?)
      - Child's feelings *re* the future of the relationship? Does he/she want it to be reestablished (under what conditions)? Does he/she want the post-maltreatment relationship changed in any way?

   c. Extent to which the child feels tricked or taken in by the perpetrator
      - Was the child suspicious of the perpetrator? For how long? Why?
      - How did the perpetrator involve the child in the maltreatment?

   d. Environmental response to the child's disclosure
      - What did others do or say when they heard the disclosure or were informed about it?
         - Parents/caregivers
         - Siblings
         - Members of extended family
         - Peers
         - Other community members (e.g., teachers, church people)
      - Response of the wider community?
         - Legal/justice system
         - Child welfare system
         - Medical/mental health system
      - Child's reactions to the above responses?

4. *Stigmatization*
   a. Stigmatizing aspects of the maltreatment
      - Child's perception of attitudes/feelings *re* the maltreatment conveyed by the perpetrator? (e.g., shame, secrecy, disgust)
      - Child's perception of the reaction of others in acknowledging the child was maltreated?
      - Child's own attitudes/feelings *re* the self?

Alleviating Anxiety

Raising the maltreatment issue generates considerable anxiety in many children, even if they had provided an initial disclosure to representatives of a child welfare agency or the police. Children become anxious for many reasons. As reviewed in Chapter 2, discussing maltreatment details or even being exposed to these stimuli via the clinician's questions can evoke this kind of anxiety. Some maltreated children may have been threatened by the perpetrator or family members about disclosing the abuse. Threats may range from further maltreatment, extreme or even life-threatening punishment, or the loss of love and emotional abandonment by the family. Other children may have been told that the perpetrator might have to leave the home or be incarcerated, or that no one would believe their accounts. Some maltreated children have been imbued with the notion that it is wrong to reveal personal family matters to others, especially if they have been threatened with the breakup of the family postdisclosure.

Children may become anxious when being interviewed about the maltreatment because of expectations about what others, including the clinician, might think of them. As we have seen, some maltreated children make internal attributions about the maltreatment, for example, that it is their fault. The resulting negative self-image may have been compounded by perpetrators who reinforce this notion. Youngsters may have been told they are "bad" children who deserved the neglect, psychological maltreatment, or physical abuse or that they are "perverted" because they participated in sexual activity or "wanted it." When asked to reveal some maltreatment details and the associated feelings and thoughts, many abused children believe their failings and weaknesses would be plainly revealed if they do so, and that others will think of them in the same negative way they perceive themselves. Furthermore, acknowledging these negative self-perceptions is a great threat to a child's already shaky sense of self-esteem and elicits even more anxiety. Friedrich (1990) notes that some sexually abused individuals fear that simply talking about the abuse will result in revictimization.

What can the clinician do to alleviate some of the anxiety that is apparent in these interviews? First, the clinician should attempt to gauge the child's feelings about discussing the maltreatment before actually initiating such a conversation. The child may be asked what he or she thinks the discussion will be like and to identify some of the easy and more difficult aspects. Asking, "What's the worst thing that could happen if you talk about this?" or, "What's the worst thing I or someone else could think about you?" helps the child identify those fears. If the child identifies a negative reaction from other people or the clinician, the clinician can assure the child that he or she has heard the accounts of many other children and will not think negatively of the child. The clinician can use alternate media to ascertain the child's fears and anxieties, such as asking the child to draw a picture of what would happen if the maltreatment was discussed and of how the child would feel or of how others would react.

Second, the clinician should remain very alert to any overt or covert manifestations of anxiety throughout these interviews. Labeling feelings by simple comments such as "You look pretty upset right now," validating the normalcy of these feelings, and commenting on how other children have shown similar reactions in this context may attenuate some of the child's distress. The clinician should attempt to understand the basis for the child's anxiety and inquire even further about particular fears or negative expectations that might underlie this response. By providing a deep sense of empathy and conveying the notion that the child is not necessarily crazy or disturbed for harboring these feelings, the clinician demonstrates that some adults can treat the child's worries with sensitivity and concern. This approach begins the process of modifying the child's negative internal working models of others and of the self as unworthy of this kind of response.

Third, the clinician must be patient and adopt a gradual approach when interviewing. Even though the clinician may have told the child that he or she will not think negatively of the child, some children, especially those with little trust in adults, may need to see concrete examples of this promise. Therefore, they may disclose information and their thoughts and feelings about the maltreatment gradually while paying keen attention to the clinician's verbal and nonverbal responses. Children may even engage in provocative or oppositional behavior to determine the clinician's trustworthiness (i.e., whether the clinician will respond to such provocations abusively or adopt a firm yet respectful way to handle this behavior). The clinician can bring this dynamic into the open by commenting upon the functions this behavior serves (i.e., it enables the child to determine, before he or she divulges sensitive information, if the clinician can be trusted). Then the clinician might suggest some concrete ways by which to prove his or her trustworthiness, rather than allowing this behavior. The following case illustrates this approach.

> A 9-year-old boy who was severely sexually abused by his mother's boyfriend over many years was referred for clinical assessment. Historical information revealed that this child had been exposed to other forms of maltreatment, including some physical neglect and abuse, in his very early years. Jeff's presentation in the initial assessment sessions suggested a youngster who had little, if any, trust in adults: he was reluctant to talk about his past and became defiant in an effort to determine if the clinician would accept him when he behaved in this manner. The clinician empathized with Jeff's fear of disclosing too much too quickly but at the same time placed firm but nonabusive limits on some of Jeff's acting out. Jeff agreed that he did not want to talk about the maltreatment, since he expected the clinician, like so many other adults in his life, to discount his feelings and treat his account with contempt. He could articulate that he expected the clinician to reject or even hurt him if he became unruly in the assessment sessions.
>
> The clinician suggested to Jeff that they develop a "trust meter." This was a chart on which Jeff indicated whether the clinician had been trustworthy each session. The clinician and Jeff developed some specific criteria

that Jeff could use in evaluating the clinician's reactions (e.g., not laughing at Jeff's accounts of other problems or issues, paying attention to Jeff as evidenced by not yawning, looking directly at Jeff while he was talking, and not hitting him if he became defiant and oppositional). They also agreed that the clinician would have to prove his trustworthiness according to these and other criteria in five sessions before Jeff would even start talking about the maltreatment. Fortunately, the clinician met these criteria, and Jeff gradually began to talk about the abuse and neglect he had experienced.

As we can see, rushing the process with a youngster like Jeff or insisting he talk about his experiences would have just confirmed his internal working model of others as insensitive, uncaring, and disrespectful of his needs. Clinicians must maintain realistic expectations about the amount of information that can be gathered in any assessment. The goal is to gather sufficient information to develop a working understanding of the child and a set of recommendations regarding interventions that, hopefully, will be useful. Because the child may have a high level of anxiety or use of defenses such as repression or dissociation, the clinician may have to enter into a therapeutic relationship with the child before more information is revealed. Further, it is important to note that if a child was very young and preverbal at the time of the maltreatment, the child may never verbally recall memories.

Fourth, the clinician should guard against giving false reassurances about the benefits of such a discussion. In the short term, many children will probably feel worse after talking about these issues; they may remember more maltreatment details, and their defenses may not protect them fully from the onslaught of pain and distress associated with these memories. The clinician should acknowledge that this is indeed a painful process and that many children do not immediately feel better after discussing material more openly in the assessment phase. The clinician should emphasize that the assessment is just one part of a potentially longer process and over time will hopefully afford the child some relief from pain.

Putting Closure to the Discussion about the Maltreatment

At the end of the discussion about the maltreatment, the clinician must put some closure to it for the child. Briefly summarizing what has been learned and emphasizing the normalcy and understandable nature of the child's anxiety or other affects may alleviate some of the child's distress. The child may be complimented for displaying courage in talking about these painful issues and may also be asked about any worries associated with the discussion. Again, sending a highly distressed and disorganized child out of an interview into environments where behavioral and affective self-regulation is necessary does not benefit the child. The child may become more fearful talking about the maltreatment in the future. Finally, the child should be informed about plans for subsequent assessment sessions.

Interviewing about Presenting Problems

Just as the clinician wants to gain an understanding of the child's perceptions of the maltreatment, so is it important to adopt the same kind of phenomenological approach to the assessment of the child's presenting problems. The child should be given the opportunity to talk in a more open-ended way about these problems. For example, the clinician may say, "You told me that you had been having some nightmares about what happened to you. Please tell me more about them." Subsequently, the clinician asks more specific questions about the problems. Perhaps the clinician requests a more detailed description of what the child actually does or feels and whether the child can identify any precipitants of these feelings or actions. The clinician also asks about the child's understanding of other people's concerns about his or her problems, the child's own desire to change them, what has helped in the past, and what might be useful now. The child's responses to these inquiries are affected not only by anxiety and a reluctance to speak openly about them but by developmental variables. For example, very young children do not yet have the cognitive capacity to engage in introspection. Therefore, they will probably not be able to give an account of the precipitants associated with their problems. This fact again underscores the importance of gathering data via different modalities and from other sources.

The clinician should ask about other aspects of the problem behavior. If the child is physically aggressive toward others or engages them in inappropriate sexualized behavior, the clinician should ask about the other children's identities, how many children are involved, and whether the child can appreciate or understand their reactions. The last point may be especially important in understanding whether the child has empathic appreciation of the effects of his or her behavior upon others. The child should be asked about the presence of aggressive or sexual fantasies associated with this behavior, even though the role of such fantasies in children's sexualized behavior is still a point of controversy (Hall, 1993). The reader is referred to Gil and Johnson (1993) for a much more detailed description of the assessment of children's sexualized behavior, including the use of interviews.

The clinician should attempt to ascertain the meaning of the particular problems for the child. Turning to our example of sexualized behavior, it is usually insufficient just to obtain a report from parents about the type or frequency of such behavior. We need to find out what the sexual behavior means to the child and why it might be so important (Berliner, 1989): Does the child ever think about sex? How does the youngster feel when he or she has sexual feelings? Do they bother the child? How does the child feel when thinking about another person having sex? Why do people have sex? When shouldn't people have sex? The same principle applies to interviewing the child about other behavior problems, such as physical aggression: How does it feel when the child wants to hit people? How does the child feel after hitting someone? When shouldn't people hurt one another?

Children may show the same kind of anxiety and reluctance to talk openly about these problems as they did when they were asked about the maltreatment. Behavioral and interpersonal difficulties pose a real threat to their already low self-esteem, and a public acknowledgment of them makes them feel even worse about themselves. They expect others may regard them negatively if they talk openly about their problems, especially those that are particularly embarrassing (e.g., sexualized behavior, encopresis). Children may be fearful about their family's reaction if their parents or caregivers find out how truly "bad" or "crazy" the children believe themselves to be. They may expect their parents to abandon them, send them away, or punish them severely. The clinician can use the same kinds of strategies to allay children's anxiety about discussing the presenting problems that were used in the interviews that were used to focus upon the maltreatment.

The clinician who has conducted comprehensive interviews with children who are able and willing to talk about these issues has probably amassed a considerable amount of data. However, the clinician should attempt to confirm or refute some of his or her tentative hypotheses by using other modalities that do not rely so heavily upon verbal skills. This course is particularly applicable to children who do not have good verbal skills or those whose accounts may be significantly affected by other factors. It is to these assessment methods that we now turn.

PLAY ASSESSMENTS

The verbal skills of many children, especially young children, are limited. Moreover, our preceding review of the developmental outcomes of maltreatment suggests that the language of maltreated children is further compromised. Although we have maintained that the clinician should first try to interview the child to determine whether an interview will be a profitable assessment modality, many maltreated children cannot participate fully in interviews. As well, many harbor real fears about discussing their experiences. Faced with these obstacles, the clinician must turn to other strategies to gather information.

A basic assumption of assessment and therapy is that both require a medium of exchange or communication between the client and clinician. Words and verbal interchanges serve this function for most adult clients. Play may partially serve this function for child clients. Children's play provides an opportunity for them to communicate with others about important topics, such as internal, psychological events or events or experiences that are manifested through observable play behavior. For the child, play may serve as a safer medium through which these issues can be addressed. By talking about the maltreatment to which a small doll was exposed, rather than about his or her personal experiences, the child can communicate this information in a metaphorical and therefore safer manner. Similarly, by portraying a character in a play scene as extremely angry toward an abusive parent the child feels less threatened than if he or she talked directly about the anger elicited by a parent's abusive actions. Engaging in play scenarios in which characters express sadness about never having the kind of parents they always wanted may be somewhat more tolerable than openly acknowledging such pain. In general, play allows children to deal with threatening or anxiety-provoking material as if it were someone else's problem, thereby placing much-needed psychological distance between the child and the material.

When we discussed interviews with children, we focused upon two broad domains: the content, or what the child said; and the process, or how the child said it. The same organizational scheme can be applied to evaluating the play of maltreated children. The play may include examples of the child's own experiences of maltreatment, such as parental dolls who physically or sexually abuse, neglect, or psychologically maltreat child dolls. Thematic development in the play may provide clues to some relevant issues associated with the maltreatment. Play characters may express feelings about the maltreatment and evidence responses that have some relevance to the child's reactions, such as retaliating through physical aggression or adopting a very passive, victimlike approach.

Of particular interest for clinicians who see abused and neglected children is posttraumatic play (Terr, 1990). In this type of play, the child ritualistically constructs the same scenario, acting out a series of events that have the same outcome every time the play is enacted. Terr (1990) reports that by controlling the reenactment of this frightening and traumatic event, the child tries to gain a sense of mastery and empowerment over it. However, the rigid reenactment of the same ending (e.g., the child is physically abused and sent to the hospital) may not provide the child with any alternate resolution of this situation, which then reinforces the child's sense of helplessness and lack of control over an adverse situation. Furthermore, posttraumatic play is characterized by a lack of enjoyment or freedom of expression.

The process of the play, or the manner in which the child plays, is another valuable source of information. First, the child's involvement of the clinician in the play may yield some information about the child's relationships. Does the child engage in solitary play where the clinician is relegated to being on the periphery of the action? Does this style persist even when the clinician attempts to become more actively involved? Or is the child extremely dependent upon the clinician—for example; asking for help in mundane tasks such as getting a toy from the cupboard or requesting that the clinician make most, if not all, of the decisions about what to do in the playroom? Does the child behave in a provocative and oppositional manner, such as refusing to clean up or even leave? These relationship patterns may reflect previous or current maladaptive ways in which the child interacts with other individuals. Second, children's play may reflect their typical ways of handling difficult or painful material. For example, some children engage in compulsive play, in which they spend a great deal of time arranging the furniture in a doll house or insist upon using rulers when drawing. Such compulsive strategies may suggest underlying anxiety and a desperate attempt to control the overt expression of these feelings. As significant issues emerge in play and generate intense anxiety and conflict, the child may disrupt the play, for example stopping the play and shifting to a new activity. At the other extreme are children who cannot manage their impulses and become behaviorally out of control. They may be overstimulated by some of the material or themes and cannot regulate their affects. The impulsive, scattered play of some children may reflect other problems such as an attention deficit disorder.

The choice of play materials may be clinically significant. Are the child's choices appropriate to the child's age? Although immature choices may be manifestations of developmental delays, children may make the same choices because of significant emotional needs. For instance, a 10-year-old physically neglected child may spend a great deal of time nurturing herself or himself by nursing on a baby bottle because these needs have never previously been met (Mills & Allan, 1992). But the actual use the child makes of these materials may be of greater significance than the particular things chosen. Finally, the clinician should assess the degree of verbalization the child exhibits during the play. Does the child spontaneously verbalize while playing and can he or she move from play to a verbal mode of interaction? The child who moves comfortably from using play to more direct verbal discussion of the issues exemplified in the play may evidence an ability and willingness to use both for communication.

There are several ways of using play to gather more information about a child. Free-play situations expose children to a minimum of directives from the clinician. In this type of play, some maltreated children may quickly begin to reenact episodes from their own experiences of abuse and neglect. If the child does not communicate the feelings of the characters in the play about these experiences, the clinician should ask the characters how they feel and what they think about the maltreatment. The clinician might say, "I want to ask the little girl a question. How does she feel when her father hits her on the head like that?" Other inquiries may be addressed via the metaphor of the play and in the third person to gather even more information along the lines of the traumagenic dynamics outlined in Table 4.1. The clinician should guard against asking too many questions too quickly, since doing so may have a somewhat disruptive effect upon the play's spontaneity.

Some children avoid enacting significant themes in play to avoid feeling anxiety and pain, just as they avoid the clinician's interview inquiries. Consequently, they gravitate toward certain activities to avoid painful issues. They may want to play endless board games that, after a relatively short time, provide little information. Rather than allowing this behavior to continue, the clinician might take a more active role and provide situations or scenarios to which the child is asked to respond. There is a historical tradition for this approach. David Levy (1939) was a psychoanalyst who promoted "release therapy." He believed that the expression of feelings (catharsis) in certain situations could be therapeutic. He would set up conditions or situations, such as play with small dolls, to resemble the situation in which the trauma occurred. Although we will discuss the use of structured play therapy in subsequent chapters, this approach may have some real relevance for assessment. The clinician might ask the child to "make up a story about a family," using small dolls. Sometimes this approach is all that is needed for the child to reenact maltreatment scenarios and to express associated thoughts and feelings. However, other children may reenact bland stories devoid of clinical content. Again, this type of response reflects a child's attempts to avoid such painful material. What can the clinician do in this situation? The clinician can take the lead and present play scenarios to which the child is invited to respond. Using small dolls, the clinician might introduce this approach by stating, "I'm going to act out a story for you using these dolls. All I want you to do right now is just sit back and watch and listen." Following this explanation, the clinician would enact scenarios in the doll play that are similar to the child's own maltreatment experiences. Once a scenario is provided, the clinician may ask the child to respond by stating, "Show me what happens next." The child may be asked to show or express how the child character in the play feels about being maltreated. Questions that evaluate the child's beliefs about the maltreatment (e.g., "Why does [the name of the doll] think she was hurt like this?") may be asked via the play. Clearly, though, the use of this kind of approach, in which the clinician takes the initiative and presents these scenarios, is inappropriate for a forensic/legal interview. The use of this suggestive questioning should be used only after child protective and judicial authorities have investigated the child's allegations.

Buchsbaum et al. (1992) describe a "narrative story stem technique" that includes components similar to the directed-play assessment format we have just described. Using doll play, the interviewer begins a story (the "story stem"), which the child is asked to complete. According to Buchsbaum et al. (1992), in their study the content of the maltreated children's stories included themes of interpersonal aggression, neglect, and some sexualized behavior, as well as their representational models. The doll play also revealed the use of defenses such as avoidance, idealization, and identification with the aggressor. The appendix accompanying this article describes story-stem narratives that may be of interest to the clinician who wishes to add this useful technique to an assessment repertoire.

Toys and equipment for play assessment do not have to be expensive or elaborate. Essential items include small; bendable doll figurines; a doll house; puppets; domesticated and wild toy animals; assorted cars and trucks; a few table games to permit relief from emotionally laden activities; and art materials such as paper, crayons, felt pens, pencils, and paint.

PSYCHOLOGICAL TESTING

Psychological tests have been used for different purposes in the assessment of maltreated children. They have been used to evaluate allegations of child sexual abuse by examining how groups of sexually abused children perform on tests compared with nonabused children. Given the very mixed findings of the ability of tests to discriminate between sexually abused and nonabused youngsters (e.g., Friedrich, 1990; Waterman & Lusk, 1993), mental health professionals must be extremely cautious and judicious in the use of psychological testing to validate a child's allegations of sexual abuse. Although we are not aware of any data on this issue pertaining to other forms of maltreatment, we suspect strongly that the same conclusions may well be applicable.

The second purpose of psychological testing maltreated children is to gather more information about their response to the victimization and to identify those variables in the child that may influence the impact of such experiences. Psychological testing may be more useful here. Given the limitations of this volume, we cannot provide the reader with an exhaustive list of all the psychological tests that are clinically useful in assessing maltreated children. What we would like to do is to alert the reader to the potential uses of these tests.

Cognitive and Academic Testing

Knowledge about a child's cognitive and academic functioning is important for a number of reasons. First, these are areas that might have been significantly impacted by the maltreatment. Second, intellectual functioning and academic achievement may serve as important moderators of the association between the maltreatment and developmental outcome. Third, difficulties in the academic and cognitive areas may merit clinician intervention. A maltreated child with significant academic delays will probably experience considerable frustration and even lower self-esteem, increasing the probability of even more symptoms. Fourth, knowledge of a child's strengths and weaknesses in this area may suggest the use of particular therapeutic strategies. For example, a child with low verbal abilities and skills may not be an appropriate subject for an approach that places heavy emphasis upon verbal interchange.

A number of scales and tests may be used to evaluate a child's functioning. The Wechsler Intelligence Scale for Children–III (WISC–III) (Wechsler, 1991), Stanford–Binet Intelligence Scale–fourth edition (Thorndike, Hagen, & Sattler, 1986), Kaufman Test of Basic Abilities (Kaufman & Kaufman, 1983), and the McCarthy Scales (McCarthy, 1972) are widely used measures of intellectual functioning. The Vineland Adaptive Behavior Scales (Sparrow, Balla, & Cicchetti, 1984) yield information about the child's developmental status and adaptive functioning. Academic achievement can be assessed through the administration of tests such as the Wide Range Achievement Test–revised version (Wilkinson, 1993) or the Wechsler Individual Achievement Test (Psychological Corporation, 1992). The clinician must also remember to evaluate or refer the child for consultation regarding other developmental problems such as attention deficit disorders or speech–language delays. Similarly, problems such as sensory deficits, other neurological conditions, or fine and gross motor difficulties deserve a thorough investigation by qualified professionals.

Child Self-Report Measures

In previous chapters we reviewed parental-report measures of children's behavior. A number of child self-report measures are used to evaluate a wide range of symptoms and problems, including anxiety and fears, depression, and self-esteem. The Fear Survey Schedule for Children–Revised (FSSC-R) (Ollendick, 1983; Scherer & Nakamura, 1968) is used to identify a child's specific fears and patterns across five areas but does not provide information about fears specifically related to maltreatment experiences such as sexual abuse. To remedy this situation, Wolfe and her colleagues (Wolfe et al., 1989) developed the Sexual Abuse Fear Evaluation (SAFE) subscale, a 27-item scale embedded in the FSSC-R. The SAFE subscale comprises two factors, the Sex-Associated Fear scale (e.g., watching people kiss on TV, talking or thinking about sex, being tickled) and the Interpersonal Discomfort scale (e.g., mean-looking people, people not believing me, being lied to by someone I trust).

We have already discussed the CITES-R, an abuse-specific measure designed to assess specific sequelae of sexual victimization (Wolfe et al., 1989). Incorporating some of the other more recent abuse-specific measures may well improve clinical practice. Mannarino et al. (1994) developed the Children's Attributions and Perceptions Scale (CAPS) to assess the unique attributions and perceptions related to the victimization experiences of sexually abused youngsters. The scale consists of 18 items and 4 subscales: Feeling Different from Peers, Personal Attributions for Negative Events, Perceived Credibility, and Interpersonal Trust. Mannarino et al. (1994) note that as the items do not make any reference to sexual abuse, the measure is not as abuse-specific as it could be. The scale is administered in an interview format, and subjects are instructed to respond based on a 5-point Likert scale. As discussed in Chapter 2, Mannarino et al. (1994) found that 7- to 12-year-old sexually abused girls scored significantly higher than nonabused controls on the total CAPS and three subscales. This pattern reflected a greater sense of feeling different from peers, heightened self-blame for negative events, and reduced interpersonal trust. In Chapter 1 we mentioned that Briere (1996) has also developed the TSCC, a brief child self-report measure that can be used to assess several dimensions related to the experience of trauma.

Other self-report measures have been developed to evaluate different dimensions of the child's functioning. The Children's Manifest Anxiety Scale–Revised (CMAS-R) (Reynolds & Richmond, 1978) and the State–Trait Anxiety Inventory for Children (STAIC) (Spielberger, 1973) yield information about the child's level of anxiety, although again neither was specifically developed for use with maltreated children. Instruments such as the Piers–Harris Children's Self-Concept Scale (Piers & Harris, 1969) and the Perceived Competence Scale for Children (Harter, 1982) have been designed to assess children's self-esteem. The Children's Depression Inventory (Kovacs, 1983) is a commonly used measure of a child's level of depression.

Although these self-report measures may provide some useful clinical information, there is danger in relying exclusively upon them. As we have already noted, no single assessment modality or measure is infallible. A problem we have encountered with these measures is that some maltreated children respond in socially desirable ways, thereby rendering an underestimation of their problems. This problem occurs even though others involved with the children report numerous behavioral and interpersonal difficulties. The same phenomenon has been reported in the literature; in Chapter 1 we described how younger maltreated children may deny problems that pose a real threat to their self-esteem. If a clinician begins to see an exaggeration of positive qualities in the self-report measures of a child who is, by the report of others, encountering significant problems, the possibility that the child is engaging in this defensive maneuver should be considered. This conclusion may be supported by other data, such as the child responding, during the interview, that he or she has no problems whatsoever.

Projective Techniques

Projective assessment has a long history of use with disturbed children, particularly from a psychodynamic and psychoanalytic perspective. Unlike structured measures (e.g., self-report inventories and measures of intellectual and academic achievement), projective techniques present ambiguous perceptual stimuli. The child is asked to draw a picture, complete sentences, tell a story, or define a visual image in amorphous stimuli such as ink blots so that the typical defenses he or she has erected against the painful affects and cognitions associated with past experiences can be subverted. Although not every mental health professional has undergone the specialized training necessary to administer and interpret these measures, they offer the clinician another perspective on the maltreated child.

Friedrich (1990) provided a valuable discussion of the use of projective assessment with sexually abused children. We would like to follow his lead and extend his discussion to children who have experienced other forms of maltreatment.

Projective Drawing

Drawings may be difficult for very young children to produce, since they do not yet have the necessary visual–motor control. Similarly, somewhat older children with delayed visual-motor development may be unable to produce drawings. They may find the process so aversive that they refuse to draw or do so in a cursory manner. Moreover, one should remain aware that many of the following techniques do not have normative data and that their validity and reliability as clinical instruments have not yet been established empirically.

Draw-a-Person with Inquiry. Drawing human figures has long been a standard part of child assessment. However, the clinician should be extremely cautious about overinterpreting the figure's graphic representation, especially about relying exclusively upon the symbolism of the drawings (Friedrich, 1990; Gittleman, 1980). Supplementing the drawing with an inquiry may serve as a catalyst to elicit more direct material. We have found the following procedure helpful in assessing maltreated children. The child is instructed to draw a picture of a whole person and, after completing the picture, he or she is asked to draw a picture of himself or herself. The clinician may have concerns about how the child views individuals of the opposite sex, and if the two drawings are of the same sex, the clinician can ask for a third drawing of a person of the opposite sex. After the child completes the drawings, the clinician asks the child a series of questions. Table 4.2 summarizes the inquiry which was developed by Dr. Bob Robinson of Alberta Children's Hospital a number of years ago. Some maltreated children begin to talk quite directly about their own experiences of abuse and neglect during the inquiry, especially in response to questions like, "What makes the person [in the drawing] scared?" This is the case in the following example:

> Six-year-old Amanda had been physically abused and neglected by her father, her sole caretaker. Although she had disclosed some of this information to child welfare authorities, Amanda was reluctant to discuss this material, especially her feelings, in the clinical interviews. Her responses to the inquiry regarding the drawing of herself in the Draw-a-Person exercise suggest that the physical assaults have elicited some painful feelings:
>
> (Sad?)"If someone punched her."

TABLE 4.2. Draw-a-Person Inquiry

1. What is the person's name?
2. How old is _____? (referring to the name the child has given the figure, including the child's own name in the drawing of the self)
3. What is _____ doing?
4. What is _____ thinking?
5. What would make _____ feel:
   Happy?
      How would _____ show it?
   Sad?
      How would _____ show it?
   Angry?
      How would _____ show it?
   Scared?
      How would _____ show it?
   Worried?
      How would _____ show it?
6. If _____ could have three wishes, what would they be?
7. If _____ could be any animal he/she wished to be, which would _____ most want to be? How come?
8. If _____ could be any animal he/she wished to be, which would _____ least want to be? How come?
9. If _____ were the only person on an island and could only have one person with him/her, who would _____ want to be there?

Note. Developed by Dr. Bob Robinson, Section of Psychology, Alberta Children's Hospital, Calgary, Alberta, Canada.

(Angry?) "Somebody beating her up. Punch and kick her, push her down."

Amanda gave a more specific and personalized account of her own experiences when asked to identify three wishes. Her comment on her third wish was similar to the actual abuse she had undergone and had disclosed to the child welfare authorities, although she continued to describe the the the incidents in the third person (i.e., "she"):

"To be a grown-up, then she wouldn't have to be bossed around. Her father gives her a spanking on her bum with her pants up when she's bad."

Following Amanda's lead, the clinician took the opportunity to ask for more details about these incidents but used the third person ("What else happened to her?"). Amanda responded with the following statements:

"Her father hit the side of her head with his bare hand. He yells at me, hits me."

Notice that Amanda has switched from the third to the first person in the last statement. She has progressed from talking about her experiences in a somewhat indirect manner to referring directly to them. The clinician finished this part of the inquiry by asking Amanda how she felt when she was hit:

"Sad, scared. I see monsters, nightmares."

One of this young girl's presenting problems were anxiety-based symptoms, including nightmares.

The drawing and the inquiry may reveal other aspects of the child's self-image, worries, anxieties, and aspects of fantasy life, as was the case with the following child:

A 10 year-old girl, Linda, had been taken as a toddler from her family, in which she had been seriously physically neglected. She was adopted by another family 5 years later. Her biological younger sister, whom she had not seen since she was adopted, remained with Linda's natural parents. Although Linda had said little about her sister when she was interviewed, her anxiety and concern emerged in the responses to the inquiry concerning her drawing of herself:

(Happy?) "If I got my sister back."
(Show it?) "I don't know."
(Sad?) "If she was dead."
(Show it?) "Like anyone would, crying."
(Angry?) "If someone beat her and made her go to the hospital."
(Show it?) "Punch his lights out."
Three wishes: 1. "Have my sister back."
2. "Going to Disneyland with my sister."
3. "To give her a Barbie doll or any kind of doll she wants."

Linda's feelings of loss conveyed in these responses emerged more fully in subsequent therapeutic sessions.

Besides its content, clinicians must scrutinize the process of the drawing. Was the drawing done in a haphazard, quick manner that may reflect a child with poor self-esteem who has little confidence in his or her abilities? Alternatively, did the child adopt a meticulous, obsessive approach that reflected a lack of tolerance for any imperfection? When asked to do the task, did the child immediately protest, claiming that he or she couldn't do it? The child's verbal language may be characterized by a lack of coherence and thus difficult to follow. Children with weak verbal skills may may show poor syntax and vocabulary and little elaboration of ideas or details.

Kinetic Family Drawing. In this technique, the child is asked to draw a picture of his or her family doing something together. Again, the content may reveal information pertinent to the child's perspective of the family. For instance, are family members actively engaged with one another, or are they disconnected from each other? Does the child depict himself or herself as on the periphery of the family? Do siblings receive more attention? Sometimes the child's choice of which family to draw can be revealing. We have seen a number of maltreated children in foster homes who refuse to draw their natural families, preferring to depict their foster families. When foster children do not draw their own natural families, we usually ask why this is so. Some children have told us that drawing their family and thinking about them is too painful or that they now regard the foster family as their "real family." As with the Human Figure Drawing, the clinician can then ask questions like, "Which person in the family gets the maddest?" "Which person gets the saddest?" "Which two people get along the best?". Sometimes, when a child is asked to draw an ideal family, important clues emerge about the changes the youngster would like to see effected or the fantasies that she or he harbors about family life.

Draw the Maltreatment. Some children who cannot furnish a detailed verbal account of their maltreatment are much more able to draw episodes of their victimization. They may furnish considerable detail, and the clinician can inquire about what is happening in the picture. Addressing the child's depiction of himself or herself in the third person may be somewhat less threatening to the child, who then may be more able to answer questions about his or her thoughts or feelings. Again, it is important to observe closely how the child does this drawing. Some children absolutely and adamantly refuse to do it, reflecting their need to avoid the painful material. If they do participate, their attention and concentration may be quite impaired because of their anxiety. They may also attempt to avoid the task by asking to go to the washroom or asking the clinician extraneous questions. Children who have approached the task of making other drawings in a more organized and thoughtful fashion may show a significant change when asked to draw a picture of their own victimization. Their anxiety may increase, resulting in a haphazard or chaotic picture.

Draw Your Feelings about the Maltreatment. A child who did not show his or her personal reactions in the preceding drawing with any degree of specificity may now be asked to draw how he or she looked or felt while being victimized and to label this graphic representation verbally, another clue to the child's ability to express internal states verbally. Themes of helplessness, inadequacy, and powerlessness often emerge in these drawings. These themes contrast with the feelings of strength, power, or even identification with the aggressor that emerge when the child is asked to draw how he or she would have liked to look when the maltreatment began.

An 11-year-old boy, Doug, was referred for a clinical evaluation after his disclosure of sexual abuse by his natural father on several occasions 3 years earlier. Doug maintained that his father, who was divorced from Doug's mother, anally raped him during Doug's visits to the paternal home. At the time of assessment, Doug was physically aggressive with other children at school and had attempted to touch the genitals of several female classmates. The frequency of these behaviors had increased over the last several years.

In the clinical interviews, Doug divulged that he had not disclosed the abuse earlier because his father had strapped his bare buttocks with a belt while telling him that even "worse things" would happen if he ever told anyone of the abuse. Doug described himself as "pretty wimpy" during these assaults. He believed he should have either done "something" to stop his father or disclosed the incidents sooner.

The first figure (Figure 4.1) is Doug's depiction of what he looked like when he was being sexually assaulted. When asked to verbally label the feelings portrayed in this picture, he described himself as feeling "very, very bad." Although he did not possess good verbal skills, Doug reflected upon his drawing and then told the clinician that the picture depicted his feelings of sadness.

The clinician then asked Doug to draw a picture of how he wished he could have looked like when the abuse began (Figure 4.2). This massive, heavily muscled figure is in stark contrast to the much smaller, weak-looking self-portrayal. In response to the clinician's questions about the second drawing, Doug began to talk about his fantasies of being a powerful figure and of how he would eventually demonstrate his strength by hurting others, rather than being the passive, helpless victim of his father's assaults. Doug had compensated for profound feelings of powerlessness by seeing himself as being able to assault others.

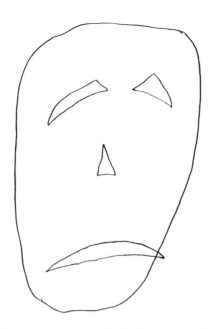

FIGURE 4.1. Doug's depiction of his feelings during his sexual assault.

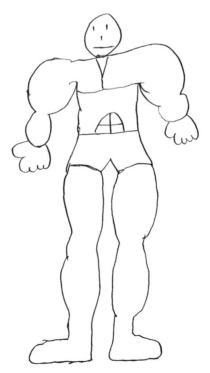

FIGURE 4.2. Doug's depiction of how he wished he had looked before the abuse began.

Draw Your Body. Some children who have been physically and sexually abused may have been physically injured or harbor fears that their bodies were damaged by the abuse. These realities and fears may be accompanied by somatic complaints. Children's depictions of their bodies may provide some information relevant to this dimension.

Draw the Perpetrator. This drawing task can help the clinician understand how the child perceives the perpetrator, perhaps as a threatening or menacing figure. Some children may depict the perpetrator more positively, reflecting their underlying ambivalence about the relationship. Some children absolutely refuse to draw the perpetrator at all, because to do so elicits overwhelming anxiety. Asking the child to draw what should happen to the perpetrator may provide the youngster with the opportunity to express his or her ideas about this issue. Some children may be so angry that they want the perpetrator incarcerated for life or even executed. Others want the perpetrator to "get help."

Drawing of Dreams and Other Symptoms. Rather than talking about a frightening dream, a maltreated child may find it more tolerable to represent it graphically. This kind of drawing may serve as a springboard for the clinician to ask about other aspects of the dream, such as what "the worst part" of the dream was, or what might have preceded or followed in the dream, if these aspects were not depicted. This inquiry not only serves to evoke more content; it also provides an opportunity for the child to begin to express some underlying affects and emotions associated with the maltreatment.

We have also asked children to depict graphically some aspects of their presenting problems. For example, asking children who are physically or sexually aggressive to draw a picture of other children's reactions is one more way of gathering information about the child's ability to appreciate the impact of his or her actions and the extent to which the child's feelings of empathy are developed.

Projective Storytelling

The clinician has a considerable choice of projective storytelling tasks. The TAT, conceived by Murray (1938, 1943) and developed by Bellak (1993), is widely used with adults and some children. Bellak (1993) also developed the Children's Apperception Test (CAT) for youngsters aged 3 to 10 years. A more recent measure, the Roberts Apperception Test for Children (RATC) (McArthur & Roberts, 1982) is sometimes preferred by clinicians because the pictures are more realistic, contemporary, and active (Friedrich, 1990). Caruso (1987) developed the Projective Story-Telling Test to evaluate maltreated children. Its pictures often elicit stories related to physical and sexual abuse. Friedrich (1990) noted that the child who is preoccupied with these issues is more likely to project them onto these cards than to respond to the more ambiguous stimuli of the CAT or TAT. Sometimes stories are transparent reflections of aspects or issues in a child's life.

> Jack was an 11-year-old boy referred for assessment after he had been apprehended from his father's care. His father, who had physically abused Jack since he was an infant, was the primary suspect in the death of Jack's twin sister when the children were 2 months old. Jack returned to live with his mother after being apprehended. He produced the following story to Card 3BM (a slumped-over figure) of the TAT:
>
> "Well, this is a boy and he got beat up by his father and he's on the staircase crying. He'll go to school, tell the teacher, tell Social Services, and have a happy life. He moved to his mother, and they have a happy relationship."
>
> The story's description of the abuse, disclosure, and subsequent course of events was identical to Jack's own experiences. It reflects his fantasy of a conflict-free relationship with his mother. This desire for love and commitment from parents, which he had never previously received, was reflected in his story to Card 6BM (an older woman and younger man):
>
> "It's a cold winter day and it's snowing and there's a lady and a man. They have one kid who is 11 [Jack was 11 years old at the time]. It's a blizzard and he's outside. And he gets lost. It's very late and he still hasn't come home and everybody's worried, so they phone the police and everybody goes out to find the kid. They find him and everything's okay."

In an interesting study, McCrone et al. (1994) administered a projective story-telling task to grade 6 children enrolled in the Minnesota Mother–Child Interaction Project. The maltreatment group comprised 43 children who had been physically abused, sexually abused, or neglected or had parents who were psychologically unavailable. These children were asked to tell stories to two cards from the Tasks of Emotional Development Test (Cohen & Weil, 1971) and two from the TAT. Compared with a group of 53 nonmaltreated children, the maltreated group evidenced significantly greater negative expectations of relationships as measured by their stories to these cards. They attended selectively to the cards and described negative aspects of relationships to the near exclusion of the positive aspects depicted in the cards. Defenses such as projection, introjection, displacement, splitting, and preoccupation were quite prevalent in the maltreated children's stories. Furthermore, maltreated children frequently told overelaborated stories characterized by unintegrated use of detail that added complexity, but not necessarily coherence, to the story. A smaller group of maltreated children, particularly the boys in the group, told impoverished stories that included little, if any, detail. McCrone et al. (1994) suggest that both the overelaborated and the impoverished styles were evidence of defensive exclusion, which diverts attention away from a source of upset and involves the deactivation of internal processing. Although defensive exclusion minimizes distress, in new situations it limits a child's attention to what is happening in relationships and prevents individuals from experiencing their feelings. The adolescent in the following example produced impoverished stories:

> Joseph, 14 years of age, was administered the TAT as part of a comprehensive assessment. He had been apprehended from maternal care following neglect and physical and sexual abuse. The last included forced intercourse with his mother and a younger sister. Joseph was normally an immature but talkative person of average intelligence. His responses to cards averaged three to four terse sentences each, including inquiry. In the 12 stories he produced, running away "solved" the situation in 7 and deaths occurred in 5. His response to Card 13B (a child sitting in a doorway) typified his stories:
> "Poor kid has nothing to do so he sits in the sun twiddling his thumbs. (How does he feel?) Bored. (What will happen?) He'll get sunstroke and die."

Another example of defensive exclusion is manifested in the idealization characteristic of some stories; interpersonal conflicts are magically resolved without any elaboration or reference to realistic processes. This strategy again allows the child to avoid confronting or acknowledging painful interpersonal difficulties and conflicts. The following example illustrates this defensive maneuver.

> Jeff (first referred to earlier in this chapter) told the following story to Card 4 (a woman holding onto a man) of the TAT:
> "A guy wants to go to war and she doesn't want to let him. He breaks away from her arms and goes to war. He never comes back, but his wife lives happily ever after."
> This story reveals Jeff's significant difficulty with loss. Instead of fully acknowledging the situation, he imposes an idealized ending: the wife, who initially did not want the man to leave, is not bothered by feelings of sadness or grief. Instead, she "lives happily ever after." This ending reflected Jeff's reluctance to talk about the feelings of sadness and loss related to his history of never having had relationships that met his profound needs for affection and nurturance.

Rorschach Test

The Rorschach is one of the oldest projective tests and is still widely used today. There are various scoring and interpretive systems, but the most widely used today is Exner's (1993). The Rorschach test can provide a comprehensive description of a client's personality organization and functioning, including reality testing, perception of the self and relationships, and typical ways of handling feelings and stress. As such, it may be a useful instrument to use in the broad assessment of maltreated children.

Friedrich (1990) maintains that Rorschach responses may be useful in the diagnosis of dissociative phenomena. He argued that dissociation may be more a likely diagnosis when the clinician notices increasing regression across the series of cards or when a child provides a response, particularly of a mutilation or sexual nature, and then denies ever having made this response during the inquiry.

Although it is not common, sometimes children will provide personal responses to the cards that are clear references to their own experiences of victimization. This is the case in the following example.

> Ten-year-old Bob had been sexually abused by his natural mother and her male common-law partner. His mother forcibly had sexual intercourse with him when he was 8 years old. At the same time, his mother's partner raped him. The rape was associated with intense pain and bleeding from his anus.
>
> Throughout the assessment, Bob expressed his concerns that his body had been physically violated and irreparably harmed. His preoccupation with these issues emerged in the following response to Card II of the Rorschach:
>
> "When my bum was bleeding. Here are the two sides of my bum and the white part in the center is the hole [anus], and this red stuff looks like blood."
>
> Bob's preoccupation with the sexual aspects of his mother's assaults was reflected in this response to Card VI:
>
> "It looks like my mom's private part when she opened it. Here's the slit and the hair."

OBSERVATIONS OF THE CHILD

Sometimes the simple act of sitting quietly and watching a child behave or interact with others is a revealing exercise. Observing the child's behavior while he or she is interacting with family members contributes to a comprehensive assessment and can occur in the waiting room, interview or play room, or at home. Schutz et al. (1989) provide a comprehensive outline of observational targets. These targets include dimensions such as positive emotional warmth and attachment; differentiation of the child from the parent; accuracy of parental perceptions of the child's emotions, behavior, and verbalizations; reasonableness of expectations; and effectiveness of communication. The therapist must observe the child's response closely and also evaluate parental responses in these domains. For example, cleanup is a common but useful natural observation time. The child's willingness to tidy up in response to the clinician's request in the play room and parental requests in the waiting room can be compared. Also, it may be useful to observe the child in both unstructured (free play) and structured interaction with parents (Schutz et al., 1989). A parent and young child might participate in teaching tasks such as matching shapes or puzzles and cooperative tasks such as building a house of blocks. The therapist might instruct a parent to teach an older child to sew on a button or play checkers or to engage in a cooperative task such as recreating a construction model. Drawing a specific picture or choosing and reading a book together are other structured tasks that may be employed profitably to gather information about the parent–child relationship.

Although time consuming, observation in environments other than the clinician's office may be especially useful. For instance, classroom observations may yield information about relationships with peers, the youngster's ability to manage academic and behavioral demands in a structured setting, and the quality of the child's relationship with important adults like teachers. After completing his or her observations, the clinician might confer with teachers to learn whether the child's behavior and presentation were typical and to clarify any remaining questions. Similarly, observations at a daycare center or a baby sitter's home are a source of useful information. The therapist may have to speak with the caregiver to determine if the observed behavior is typical of the child in that setting.

Besides making observations of the child with parents and in other settings, the clinician should also note the youngster's mental status, as outlined in Table 4.3. The child's physical appearance, relationship with the examiner, behavior, cognition, perception, speech, affect, and insight and judgment should all be evaluated. Particular attention should be paid to those areas in which difficulties are apparent or the child seems to be showing an unusual response.

ASSESSMENT OF ATTACHMENT ORGANIZATION AND INTERNAL WORKING MODELS

In Chapter 2 we argued that children's attachment organization and, in particular, their internal working or representational models partly determine their response to others and their feelings and beliefs about themselves. It is important to assess attachment organization in any comprehensive evaluation, given its important role in the etiology and maintenance of problems in these and other areas. Therapy may have to address such difficulties. The strange situation has demonstrated its utility as an aid in classifying attachments in infancy, but it was never intended for use as a clinical instrument. Attachment classifications derived from the strange situation originated from

TABLE 4.3. Mental Status of the Child

1. Physical appearance

2. Relationship to the examiner
   a. Nature of the relationship; common presentations include:
      (1) Fearful and anxious
      (2) Closed and guarded, wary
      (3) Indiscriminate
      (4) Aggressive/sexualized
   b. Working alliance (extent of cooperation with the assessment)
   c. Social skills

3. Behavior
   a. Activity level
   b. Degree of organization (e.g., impulsive, compulsive, messy)
   c. Reactions to:
      (1) Limits
      (2) Failure
      (3) Challenges

4. Cognition
   a. Intelligence
   b. Attention and concentration
   c. Thought processes (e.g., organization, coherence)
   d. Problem-solving ability
   e. Thought content (major themes, general knowledge, delusions, etc.)

5. Perception
   a. Orientation in time, space, and person
   b. Short- and long-term memory
   c. Dissociation

6. Speech
   a. Vocabulary
   b. Syntax
   c. Articulation, fluency, and expressiveness
   d. Comprehension
   e. Specific disorders

7. Affect
   a. Emotional tone
   b. Range and intensity of affect
   c. Appropriateness to content
   d. Awareness and control of affect

8. Insight and judgment
   a. Regarding own problems, motives
   b. Regarding consequences of own behavior and actions

research studies of the behavior of nonclinical samples in a single laboratory session. The therapist needs to determine whether the intensity and persistence of the attachment pattern are beyond age-appropriate norms and whether it interferes with other areas of functioning in order to determine its clinical significance (Lieberman & Zeanah, 1995). The clinical value of the strange situation is also limited by the intensive degree of specialized training required for specific coding practices.

The usefulness of the strange situation paradigm with older children, unlike with infants, is problematic. There is a rapid development in the child's perceptual, cognitive–representational, social, and communicative abilities that expands the types of behavior serving the attachment system, and there is less reliance upon proximity seeking and other behavioral responses as the child grows older (Cicchetti, Cummings, Greenberg, & Marvin, 1990). Attachment organization in older children is expressed through other modalities, such as verbal interaction, nonverbal cues and signals, and internalized representations of attachment figures. Internal working models become more accessible to symbolic representation with advances in children's language and cognitive capabilities (Solomon, George, & De Jong, 1995). Although evaluation that incorporates more overt behavioral expressions is still important, measurement of representational models using alternate means such as language, thought, and play becomes an important component of the comprehensive assessment of school-aged children. Rutter (1995) also notes that the strange situation depends on brief separations and reunions having the same meaning for all children. Therefore it may be difficult to apply the procedure in different cultures, as in Japan, where infants rarely leave their mothers in ordinary circumstances.

No one particular strategy or test has been identified as the assessment procedure of choice to be used in the clinical evaluation of school-aged children's attachment organization. There is not even a strong consensus about what constitutes a secure versus insecure or disordered attachment organization in older children, as there is for infants. Despite the lack of clarity, clinicians face the daily task of assessing the attachment organization and representational models of maltreated school-aged children. How do we go about doing this?

Some general principles might be useful to guide our evaluations. First, attachment disorders are relational disturbances (Lieberman & Zeanah, 1995). Consequently, the evaluation should include an assessment of the relationship between the child and the parent or current caregiver. Although a child may be in foster care and the disordered or insecure attachment originated in the context of the relationship between the child and his or her parent, vestiges of the attachment relationship may be observable in the relationship with the current caregiver. Observations of the child's interaction patterns are of immeasurable help in gathering this kind of information. Second, a major component of attachment organization that must be assessed is the older youngster's representational models. We have argued that the modalities through which the internal working models are expressed expand. Thus, representational models are more accessible for assessment and must be incorporated in any evaluation. Third, the clinician must rely on multiple measures in different environments, since there is no one test or procedure that yields all the answers. The following is a tentative guide for the assessment of attachment organization.

Early Relationships and Attachment History

The child's early relationships and attachment history as outlined in Table 3.3 are a useful beginning point for this assessment. Specific questioning may provide valuable information about the nature of children's early relationships. However, the information is often unavailable, especially for children who no longer live with their natural parents. Sometimes a review of child welfare files or the records of agencies that provided intervention to the family may yield some relevant data.

Relational Aspects of Current Attachment Organization

Although information about early relationships and attachment history may be useful, we cannot assume a complete continuity between earlier and later attachment organizations. Children's attachment patterns and internal working models can undergo some modification from these earlier developmental periods. Therefore, an assessment of a child's current attachment organization, including the child's actual interpersonal behavior, is necessary. Carson and Goodfield (1988) outlined three major areas that can be assessed in examining attachment potential: reciprocity in which the child can both give emotionally and respond to others' affection, separation response to either possible or actual loss, and the ability to explore the environment and take the risks necessary to learn and master new tasks. They outlined a series of questions for caregivers that they have found useful in assessing these three dimensions of attachment (Table 4.4) (Carson & Goodfield, 1988, pp. 118–119).

The therapist also may want to consider using observations of child–parent interactions during reunions to gather information about the child's current attachment organization. As part of an assessment session, young school-aged children and parents may be separated for approximately 1 hour for individual interviews and then reunited in the clinician's presence. Videotaping reunions and carefully reviewing them may prove to be especially useful for clinicians who want to sharpen their ability to discriminate among some of the more subtle differences in reunion behavior.

TABLE 4.4. Questions in Assessing Current Attachment of Child

---

1. Can the child give emotionally, let others matter to him or her, and respond to affection?
2. Can the child tolerate emotional intimacy or does he or she seek objects as an expression of caretaking? Are objects more important than emotional responses from others?
3. Does the child mold with the primary caretakers (excluding those who have trouble doing this because of temperamental characteristics)?
4. Does the child show affection spontaneously or initiate a hug, kiss, or touch?
5. Does the child seek affection indiscriminately or show selective preference for adults?
6. Does the child look to others in seeking help, show pleasure in receiving attention from others, or receive satisfaction from adult intervention?
7. Does the child cling, allow adults to have body space, or get enough gratification from adults to separate even briefly?
8. Can the child engage in unsupervised, age-appropriate play and get along with peers, or does the child require adult involvement and intervention?
9. Can the child explore the environment and be curious so that he or she can learn in school and take pleasure in new challenges and tasks?
10. Can the child assimilate and use new information, learn from experience, and retain information?
11. Does the child show empathy and respond to the emotions of others?
12. Can the child enjoy successful and pleasurable experiences without engaging in negative behavior afterwards, allowing him or herself a good time?
13. Does the child imitate other children's behavior, which is seen to be reinforced by adult approval? Can the child spontaneously initiate behaviors based upon his or her sense of self and utilize his or her behavior as a way of getting positive recognition?

Note. Adapted from Carson and Goodfield (1988, pp. 118–119).

What should clinicians look for in these reunions? Main and Cassidy (1988) identified four main patterns of attachment derived from the first 5 minutes of reunion of 6-year-old children with their mothers. Children judged *secure* responded to their mother's return in a confident, relaxed, and open manner. *Anxious–avoidant* children maintained a neutral coolness, including an avoidance of interaction with the mother. Children classified as *anxious–ambivalent* exhibited elements of avoidance, sadness, fear, and hostility and were clearly ambivalent about seeking proximity to the parent. Children classified as *disorganized–disoriented* in infancy took control in one of two ways when they were 6 years old. First, these children took confrontational control and overtly rejected the mother in a punitive way ("controlling–punitive"; Lyons-Ruth, Alpern, & Rapacholi, 1993, p. 583). In the second pattern, children attempted to care for or comfort the mother by providing helpful directions ("controlling–caregiving"; Lyons-Ruth et al., 1993, p. 583). The child may at first appear as overly bright and enthusiastic at reunions and seems to feel responsible for making the parent feel happy (Goldberg, 1991).

Despite the apparent usefulness ability of reunion behavior in discriminating among different types of attachment organization, one might question the validity of the reunion context for older school-aged children who have become accustomed to separations from their parents after many years at school and participation in other out-of-home activities. Their responses to reunions after brief separations may not be valid displays of their particular attachment organization.

Representational Aspects of Current Attachment Organization

A number of different strategies have been developed to assess the attachment organizations of older children from the representational perspective. Although these measures were developed as research tools in studies that did not include clinical samples, they may have some clinical applicability. We hope these measures serve as catalysts for the initiation of clinical–empirical research in which their validity and reliability would be examined rigorously.

Narrative Story Stem Technique

Earlier in this chapter we described the use of this strategy, in which children are asked to complete stories using dolls. The results of some work by attachment researchers may be helpful in developing story stems for clinical assessment. Cassidy (1988) presents six story beginnings in which self-esteem, family conflict, and outside threat are enacted in the mother–child relationship. Bretherton, Ridgeway, and Cassidy (1990) developed five attachment-related story beginnings and then asked 3-year-old children to use the dolls to show and tell what would happen next. Bretherton et al. (1990, pp. 300–305) describe the administration details of the attachment story protocol, the required materials, and the content of the five story beginnings. This information may be particularly useful as a starting point from which clinicians can adapt the material for use with older children. For example, in the Departure story, the examiner depicts a mother doll and father doll facing a grandmother doll and two child dolls. In the story, the parents are going on a trip and say good-bye to the children, who remain at home with the grandmother. The examiner then asks the child to use the dolls to show what happens next. Solomon et al. (1995) modified Bretherton et al.'s (1990) doll-play story-completion task by encouraging 6-year-old children to select a doll to represent the "self" and to construct a pretend family. They provided subjects with a flat surface upon which furniture was arranged into rooms. Bretherton et al.'s (1990) Departure and Reunion scenarios were used as the story-completion tasks.

The results of these three studies are quite consistent. Children with a secure attachment organization acknowledged the importance of the relationship with the mother in the doll play and described a warm, positive, direct, and supportive relationship with her. The doll protagonist was depicted as accepted and valued despite flaws. Solomon et al. (1995) found that secure children were more likely to give "confident" stories from which two major themes emerged. In the first, the "danger and rescue" story, the child telling the story introduced dangerous or frightening events originating outside the family, usually during the Separation, but the situation was resolved safely by the Reunion's end. The second theme was characterized by the child displaying confident, comfortable autonomy (e.g., the child makes an elaborate lunch). The characters expressed pleasure in the reunion, with an explicit acknowledgment that a separation had occurred.

Avoidant children dismissed the importance of the relationship, portrayed the doll protagonist as isolated or rejected, or sometimes gave no response to the story stem or did so only after several "I don't know's or prompts. These children characteristically denied experiencing separation anxiety by negating, canceling, or "undoing" the separation itself (e.g., the child tried to accompany the parents on their trip). They also avoided the reunion or showed casual disinterest in the parents' return. The stories' narrative structure was characterized by a stereotypic depiction of household and baby-sitting activities; there was an empty, affectless quality to some of their stories.

Children with an ambivalent–resistant attachment organization were significantly more likely to give "busy" stories (Solomon et al., 1995, p. 454). They did not express fears directly about separation; rather, these fears and other negative feelings were reserved or displaced onto other story characters. The stories featured fun and pleasurable activities, and the overall quality was of a happy mood and busy activity. Reunion stories were characterized by delay and distraction. Reunions began but were never thoroughly completed because of obsessive and irrelevant actions by the child or other characters. These time-consuming and distracting activities constantly interrupted the story line (if one was detectable) and resulted in a digressive narrative structure.

Controlling children (i.e., those who had been disorganized–disoriented in infancy) were significantly more likely to give "frightened" stories consisting of two types: "chaotic" and "inhibited" (Solomon et al., 1995, p. 454). In the first, children enacted chaotic and dangerous events but, unlike the content of the stories of secure children, events were unresolved and led to the disintegration of the self and/or family. The behavior of parental figures or other adults was often frightening or abusive. The children in these stories were helpless to control their behavior or the frightening events. Solomon et al. (1995. p. 454) describe the narrative structure of these stories as "chaotic" and "flooded." Catastrophes arose without warning and dangerous people or events were vanquished, only to surface repeatedly. The children depicted punishments as abusive and unrelenting. "Inhibited" stories were markedly constricted, and the children appeared frightened in the testing situation. They seemed extremely uncomfortable with the task and did not want to enact the story. Children who were controlling gave odd responses that did not seem to make much sense or were disorganized, such as throwing the doll on the floor.

Klagsbrun–Bowlby Adaptation of Hansburg's Separation Anxiety Test

Hansburg (1972) originally developed the Separation Anxiety Test (SAT) to measure adolescent separation anxiety. Klagsbrun and Bowlby (1976) adapted it for use with children aged 4 to 7 years. The test features six photographs of children undergoing separation from their parents. The separation experiences range from a parent saying good-night to a child to a picture of parents leaving for 2 weeks. The subject child is asked how the child in the picture feels about the separation and then what the child would do. Wright, Binney, and Smith (1995) modified the SAT for 8- to 12-year-old children by producing a new set of photographs to provide older children with more age-appropriate separation situations and settings. They also used older (10 years old) models in the pictures.

Main, Kaplan, and Cassidy (1985) scored the SAT responses obtained from 6-year-old children for "emotional openness." High-scoring children could imagine the pictured child expressing appropriate negative feelings and offered appropriate reasons for these affects. High scores also indicated these children could maintain a balance between expressing and containing feelings. Typically, children who attained high scores on emotional openness had been classified, at the age of 12 months, as secure with their mothers. Shouldice and Stevenson-Hinde (1992) also found that the responses of 4½-year-old children who were rated as secure were more capable than other children the same age of expressing feelings in a balanced and moderate manner on the SAT. The former handled distress aroused by separation with low levels of defensiveness. Children who had been classified in infancy as avoidant with their mothers tended to give responses ranging from silence and the inability to express feelings spontaneously to an outright denial of feelings. This closed emotional expression was replicated in the study conducted by Shouldice and Stevenson-Hinde (1992). According to Shouldice and Stevenson-Hinde (1992), ambivalent children were significantly more likely to express anger in their SAT responses than were other children. This finding is consistent with the hypothesis that these children had learned to overexpress their needs to provoke a parental response (Kobak & Sceery, 1988). Other children classified as disorganized–disoriented in infancy, showed a marked disorganization of responses, such as making irrational responses to the separation (e.g., the child would feel "good" during the separation from parents; Main et al., 1985, p. 88) and using incoherent speech patterns (Shouldice & Stevenson-Hinde, 1992). Some who also gave disorganized responses became depressed, and one even began to hit a stuffed animal; these responses were also typical of children who had received disorganized/disoriented classifications as infants.

Main et al. (1985, p. 88) asked children how they would respond to the most severe separation experience in the Klagsbrun-Bowlby (1976) adaptation of the SAT: "This little girl's/boy's parents are going away on vacation for 2 weeks; what's this little girl/boy gonna do?" Main et al. (1985) hypothesized that for children with a secure attachment organization, the representational models of the attachment figure would be accessible. Therefore, these children could imagine more active ways of dealing with the separation than could insecure children, who would see these figures as inaccessible. The highest score was given if the child actively persuaded the parents not to leave or accomplished the same end through another means. A high score was also given if the child expressed feelings such as anger or distress directly. A slightly lower score was given if the child found an alternate attachment figure with whom to stay, and a middle score was given to youngsters who played with objects but in an imaginative way that made them feel better. Lower scores were reserved for unelaborated play. Low scores were given for complete silence or "I don't know." Any response that decreased the attachment figure's accessibility (e.g., killing the self or the parents) was given the lowest score. There was a strong positive relationship between the scores on this question and earlier attachment security to the mother but not to the father. Secure children had many unique ideas regarding possible actions in response to the 2-week separation. Avoidant children typically "did not know" what the child might do, and disorganized–disoriented children became silent, depressed, irrational, or occasionally self-destructive (Main et al., 1985, p. 96).

Family Photograph

Main et al. (1985) devised another simple but ingenious task for 6-year-old children that can be used in clinical settings. The examiner merely showed the child a photograph of himself or herself with the parents, which had been taken earlier in the day when the follow-up assessment session began; no other inquiries or questions were directed to the youngster. Children judged to be secure in response to the photograph readily accepted the photograph, smiled, or showed interest. They casually let go of the photograph following an inspection of a few seconds. These were most often children who had received a secure classification with their mothers at 12 months of age. Youngsters who most often avoided the photograph, refused to accept it, or actively turned away from it had received an avoidant classification in infancy. Others became depressed or disorganized while viewing it. Main et al. (1985, p. 90) describe one child who had been playing cheerfully with the examiner but then immediately took on a depressed presentation and bent silently over the family photograph for 12 seconds. Children such as this had most often been previously categorized as disorganized–disoriented as infants. The foster parents of children who no longer have contact with their parents can be asked to bring a photograph of the child and natural parents, if one is available.

Fluency of Discourse

The fluency of the conversation between parents and child in the reunion episode has also been used to assess attachment organization (Main et al., 1985). Children most likely to have been classified as secure in infancy displayed fluid discourse as older children. Individual speech was characterized as fluid if the child and parent spoke directly and had little difficulty in accessing or expressing information. Parent and child answered each other directly with little pause. Dyads on which the child had been classified as avoidant in infancy demonstrated restricted discourse when the child was 6 years of age: there were frequent pauses between adult and child conversational turns, topics were restricted to impersonal or inanimate objects with little elaboration, and the parent frequently asked rhetorical questions. Disorganized–disoriented dyads engaged in dysfluent and disorganized discourse. Their discourse was marked by false starts and stumbling by the parent, false starts by the child, a focus on relationship-related topics, and the parent's passive response to the child attempts to steer the conversation.

Family Drawings

Kaplan and Main (1985; cited in Bretherton et al., 1990) compared the family drawings of children with the latter's attachment classifications. Secure youngsters' drawings showed family figures close to each other but not overly so. Arms tended to be held out in an embracing position. The figures were well individuated, and not all were smiling. Avoidant children's drawings had an aura of falseness: all family members were smiling, but there was a greater distance between figures. Children classified as controlling–disorganized showed a mixture of characteristics of the drawings of secure and avoidant children as well as many bizarre elements. The controlling/disorganized children added strange marks and unfinished objects or figures or scratched out parts of the drawing. These children sometimes added over-bright and cheery elements like rainbows or hearts without integrating them into the overall design.

This fairly detailed description of previous attempts to measure and describe the attachment organizations of older children is meant to stimulate clinicians to start thinking of the assessment of this important aspect of maltreated children's functioning in creative and critical ways, to refine previous attempts, and to develop new ones. We hope that clinically oriented research reports will appear soon that either confirm or refute the applicability and utility of these suggestions and lead to more valid and reliable ways of assessing attachment organization.

ASSESSMENT OF DISSOCIATIVE IDENTITY DISORDER/MULTIPLE PERSONALITY DISORDER

Putnam (1993) reports that children normally display a range of dissociative behavior that peaks at 9 to 10 years of age and then declines through adolescence to low levels in adulthood. Careful observation is required to determine the presence of dissociation and to distinguish normal, age-appropriate dissociation from that used for coping with maltreatment. As well, children generally have a generally poorer sense of continuity about their behavior than do adults (Putnam, 1993). Therefore, children are not particularly reliable reporters of their own experience. Consequently, assessment of dissociative behavior in children is likely best approached by careful and extended observation of the child. Parents, foster parents, child-care workers, and teachers can be trained to monitor the child carefully and observe any range of behavior that suggests the presence of dissociation. Table 4.5 is an outline of observational behavioral targets for identifying the presence of dissociative identity disorder/multiple personality disorder (DID/MPD), as described by Lewis (1996, pp. 313–315) and Lewis and Yeager (1994, pp. 732–734). We strongly recommend these excellent reviews of the symptoms and behaviors characteristic of childhood dissociation disorders.

As indicated in Table 4.5, a range of types and levels of intensity of behavior may be manifested by children who are dissociating. Lewis (1996) and Lewis and Yeager (1994) suggest that a clinician be alert to the possibility of dissociation if there is a family history of dissociative disorder and if the magnitude of different types of medical, behavioral, and psychological symptoms is high. A combination of perplexing forgetfulness, episodic trance states, mood fluctuation, and violent or self-injurious behavior might

TABLE 4.5. Dissociative Symptoms in Childhood

1. Extreme changes in moods, behavior, preferences, and demeanor
2. Trancelike states—in fantasy world and oblivious to surroundings; sometimes labeled as "daydreaming"
3. Amnesia for actions and events occurring during the absent time while in the trancelike state; may deny responsibility for actions during these times; sometimes labeled pathological liars
4. Vivid imaginary companionship extending beyond 6 or 7 years of age; companions are relatively continuously present and, while defending the child, may be demeaning
5. Wide variety of physical complaints; medical records of numerous physician and hospital visits for symptoms that seem to defy medical explanation
6. Hysterical paralysis
7. Sleep disturbances and nightmares; sudden losses of consciousness; tend to have undergone neurological evaluations for these symptoms; symptoms may have been diagnosed as a seizure disorder
8. Auditory hallucinations; in severely dissociated children the voices may give orders; symptoms sometimes diagnosed as schizophrenia
9. Inner hierarchies of entities who serve specific functions sometimes present
10. Sometimes withdrawn and depressed but may present with severe behavioral problems; commonly receives diagnosis of attention-deficit/hyperactivity disorder or sometimes of bipolar mood disorder; symptoms often diagnosed as conduct disorder

Note. Adapted from Lewis and Yeager (1994, pp. 732–734) and Lewis (1996, pp. 304–310).

also be present. Symptoms may include observed changes in abilities, knowledge, preferences, and demeanor. Trancelike states may be present that are often labeled by others as daydreaming. These states involve spontaneous blank staring; the child seems unaware of his or her surroundings. The child may experience amnesia for the duration of the episode; when it is over, the child will resume activity as if nothing had happened. The youngster also may deny performing actions that others had observed. This was the situation in the following case:

> Megan was a 9-year-old child placed in a residential treatment facility because of out-of-control and outrageous behavior in her home. According to Megan's mother, a stepfather had left the home when Megan was approximately 3 years old. He reportedly had been harsh and degrading with the child before that time. Megan reported few negative memories of this man. Her behavior in the residence and at school was highly unpredictable, with no apparent precipitants to the marked shifts in her presentation. She often strongly denied her behavior and absolved herself of responsibility for her actions. Megan's presentation in the assessment was also confusing. During a period of play observation, Megan chose to play

checkers but seemed confused and angry during the game. After making a move, she would vehemently deny making it on her next turn and argue with the clinician to be allowed to change it. Initially this behavior seemed manipulative, but over time it was clear that Megan did not remember making the moves. Combined with many observations by other individuals, this behavior served as confirmation that Megan often dissociated. In later months, she demonstrated two distinct personality states that allowed her to cope with previous maltreatment and her expectations that others would degrade and humiliate her. Megan varied from appearing as a young and gentle girl to a tough adolescent who wore thick makeup and verbally and physically attacked others.

According to Putnam (1993), the confusing and variable presentation evident in this case example is not atypical. These children often receive diagnoses of behavioral or other difficulties before their dissociative behavior is identified. When medication has been used to treat these other conditions (e.g., epilepsy, attention deficit, schizophrenia) the results are often equivocal or poor (Lewis, 1996; Lewis & Yeager, 1994; Putnam, 1993).

Another behavior that may suggest the presence of dissociation is vivid imaginary companionship (e.g., the child plays alone but assumes decidedly different roles and voices). The imaginary companions of normal children appear only at times of stress, are comforting and benevolent, and tend to disappear by the time the children are 6 years old. In contrast, the imaginary companions of children who dissociate tend to continue until the children pass the age of 7 years and sometimes into adolescence (Lewis, 1996; Lewis & Yeager, 1994). These imaginary companions are consistently present and may act as strong defenders, absorbing the child's pain but also belittling the youngster. The child may have auditory hallucinations in which voices sometimes give the child orders. Sleep disturbances and nightmares, a variety of physical complaints; and, possibly, hysterical paralysis may occur. Some dissociative children have elaborate hierarchies of entities who fill specific functions in their lives.

A diagnosis of multiple personality disorder should be considered if the child displays one or more distinct personality states that periodically take full control of the child's behavior (Putnam, 1993). According to Vincent and Pickering (1988), multiple personality disorder in childhood has only recently been recognized. They suggest that in contrast to the adult presentation, these alternate personality states in children tend to be less clearly delineated, have more fluid boundaries, and are less likely to fully dominate the body for extended periods. Finally, although some dissociative children may just be withdrawn and seem depressed, many display severe behavioral problems. As the above listing shows, a number of dissociative symptoms are present in many other types of behavioral and psychological childhood disorders. To identify dissociation or diagnose multiple personality disorder, behavior must be reliably and repeatedly observed over time. Moreover, the accurate diagnosis of dissociation depends upon gathering diverse types of data from multiple sources. As noted by Lewis (1996, p. 309), "At present, there are no psychological, medical, or neurologic tests to identify or confirm the diagnosis of DID/MPD."

Lewis and Yaeger (1994) and Lewis (1996) describe some innovative assessment strategies. These include developmentally sensitive questions designed to reveal the presence of symptoms and behaviors of dissociation (see Table 4.6). Lewis and Yaeger (1994) and Lewis (1996) report that several of these questions were suggested by adult patients suffering from DID/MPD. These patients believed the questions would have helped them to reveal their symptoms when they were youngsters. Lewis and Yaeger (1994) and Lewis (1996) recommend that clinicians look for evidence of dissociation in children's journals, schoolwork, and drawings. Different drawing styles and types of spelling and handwriting reflect alternate personalities.

A number of checklists and screening instruments for dissociative disorders in children and adolescents have been developed. The need to ensure that observations of a child's behavior are made by persons thoroughly familiar with the child is an underlying principle of the Child Dissociative Checklist (CDC), a 20-item instrument (Putnam, Helmers, & Trickett, 1993). The adult who completes the measure circles the response on a 3-point scale (2 = very true, 1 = somewhat or sometimes true, 0 = not

TABLE 4.6. Questions Regarding Dissociative Symptoms and Behaviors

1. You know the way people can switch channels on a TV set? Well, some kids, if they are in trouble and need to be especially big or strong, or if they want to play around like a baby, can switch and become big and strong, or they can be little like a baby. Can you ever do that? (If the answer is "yes," ask: "When?" "What is it like?")
2. Many kids who have been through a lot or have been hurt are able to space out and go to a special place in their heads and not feel it. Can (could) you do that?
3. Many children who have been through a lot or who feel lonely can talk with someone in their heads. Can you do this? (If "yes," ask: "What does the voice sound like? Is it a man's voice? A woman? A child? An animal? Are there ever two voices talking to each other? Do they ever tell you what to do or not to do?")
4. Many children, when they are lonely and upset, have a make-believe friend or toy they talk with. Can you do that?
5. Have you ever been told that you said or did something and you could swear you had not done it? (e.g., saying something? talking something? hurting someone?)

Note. Adapted from Lewis (1996, pp. 313–316) and Lewis and Yeager (1994, p. 736).

true) that best describes the child's behavior on a given item over the past 12 months. The items tap several domains of dissociative behavior: dissociative amnesias; rapid shifts in demeanor, access to information, knowledge, abilities, and age-appropriateness of behavior; spontaneous trance states; hallucinations; identity alterations; and aggressive and sexual behavior. Malinosky-Rummell and Hoeir (1991) and Putnam et al. (1993) demonstrate that the CDC readily discriminates between normal and traumatized children. The vast majority (95%) of children with formally diagnosed dissociative disorders score 12 or higher, whereas only 1% of controls achieve this level. However, the CDC is not a diagnostic instrument and does not systematically inquire about the DSM-III-R/DSM-IV criteria for dissociative disorders. Like any assessment strategy, it should be incorporated into a set of measures in order to attain as rich and accurate an understanding of the child as possible. Steinberg (1996) has been prepared a comprehensive review of testing methods for assessment and diagnosis of dissociative symptoms in children and adolescents, including the CADC (Reagor, 1992), a 17-item checklist for clinicians and the Child Dissociation Problem Checklist (Peterson, 1991), a 45-item checklist. Lewis (1996) describes the development of the Bellevue Dissociative Disorders Interview for Children, an interview protocol that covers the major signs and symptoms of dissociative disorders. She notes that interviewers have the freedom to move flexibly from one topic to another rather than having to adhere to a structured interview, a format many anxious children are unable to handle. We recommend that clinicians interested in augmenting their assessment skills review these valuable references.

FORMULATION OF THE TREATMENT PLAN

After assessment interviews with parents or caregivers, contacts with collaterals, and the individual assessment of the child as outlined above, the clinician should have amassed a vast amount of information. At times, integration of the data and formulation of a treatment plan can be daunting. It is crucial to maintain a focus on the child and his or her needs and to develop a conceptualization or formulation of the problem. Accomplishing both not only permits an understanding of the child but may suggest viable interventions likely to benefit the child and the family. Besides being a means of communicating with others, producing a report or a written outline after developing this conceptualization challenges the clinician to organize his or her thinking about the case clearly.

Developing a treatment plan involves three major steps, which are outlined in Table 4.7. Before any interventions can be considered, the clinician must determine the clinical significance of the presenting problems.

TABLE 4.7. Three-Step Treatment Plan Formulation

Step 1: Determine clinical significance of presenting problems
1. Review findings from the child
   Mental status
   Attachment organization and internal working models
   Emotional and behavioral self-regulation
      Externalizing problems
      Internalizing problems including dissociation and PTSD
   Language development
   Cognitive development and adaptation to school
   Development of self
   Peer relationships
   Coping and defense mechanisms
   Determine if localized or developmental effects are present that require attention and intervention

2. Review findings from the family for problems that may require intervention
   Family functioning premaltreatment and postmaltreatment
      Marital relationship and family functioning
      Individual functioning of parents
      Nature of attachment to the child
      Poverty and stability of supports
      Single parent
      Parenting and discipline
      Accurate perception of the child's needs; appropriate expectations
      Impulse control
   Support of child postmaltreatment
      Acknowledgment of maltreatment
      Belief in child, feelings toward child
      Adequacy of parenting
      Protection from more maltreatment

3. Review of environmental problems that may require attention and intervention
   Cultural–societal toleration of maltreatment
   Community reaction to the child and family
   Supportive milieu for the child and family
   Provisions of appropriate services

Step 2: Formulate the problem
1. Develop a conceptualization about the mechanisms contributing to the emergence of clinically significant problems (e.g., internal working models, classical conditioning, learned helplessness)

2. Consider the moderating variables that are compensatory or potentiating for maltreatment impact across the child, family, environment, and maltreatment factors.

Step 3: Develop an intervention plan
Consider and set priorities regarding treatment interventions to remediate the impact of maltreatment and prevent further maltreatment. Examples of some possible interventions follow:

(continued)

TABLE 4.7. *cont.*

1. Child
    Need for protection, apprehension
    Foster home or residential placement
    Community youth worker involvement
    Short-term symptom-focused therapy
    Long-term therapy for developmental impacts
    Group therapy (e.g., abuse, anger management)
    Speech therapy, occupational therapy
    Special school class, tutoring, etc.
    Day treatment to address school and emotional needs
    Pediatric consult (e.g, regarding ADHD)

2. Family
    In-home support (e.g., homemaking, behavioral management training)
    Parenting training
    Day-care placement and subsidy
    Low-income housing
    Public assistance
    Family therapy
    Marital therapy
    Individual therapy
    Anger management training
    Drug and alcohol treatment programs

3. Environment
    Community education
    Family or individual meetings; communication with extended family
    Support in further police interviewing
    Court support to child and family
    Public health nurse involvement

First, the clinician should review the findings derived from the assessment of the child. The clinician must determine if effects arising from the maltreatment, are localized or developmental and if they require attention or intervention. The clinician must remain alert to the presence of other problems that are not necessarily associated with the maltreatment, since they too may require intervention.

Then the clinician must examine the findings regarding the family, including both premaltreatment and postmaltreatment behavior across several domains of functioning. These domains include marital and family functioning, individual functioning of the parents, and parenting abilities and skills. Parental support of the child postmaltreatment requires particular attention. Finally, the clinician should consider broader environmental factors that may present difficulties and require attention. These factors include extended family, peer, and community reactions to the child's maltreatment and broader ones such as poverty. The appropriateness of current services and those provided in the past to the child and family need to be evaluated.

Once clinically significant problems have been identified and understood, the clinician may proceed to the second step in developing a treatment plan tailored to the specific child and family. This step has two parts. First, the therapist must develop a conceptualization about the mechanisms that are contributing to the emergence and maintenance of clinically significant problems. Of course there may be more than one mechanism operating. Once the mechanisms of impact are identified, the clinician must consider moderator variables. In this way, strengths and weaknesses across the child, family, environment, and maltreatment domains can be evaluated.

Step three, development of an intervention plan, begins once the clinician has developed a formulation of the problem. The formulation serves as the basis of the plan. If the child initially shows symptoms of a posttraumatic stress disorder and the therapist adheres to the model that was hypothesized to underlie these symptoms in Chapter 2, then exposing the child to the aversive stimuli related to the abuse so that the anxiety can be extinguished will be a major component of the individual treatment. Some children may require individual therapy so that their attributions and cognitions about the maltreatment may be reexamined and reformulated. On the other hand, children with strong feelings of stigmatization may benefit more from group therapy, where they can learn that their experiences and feelings are shared by others. Some children's distress may be a function of their parents's anxiety or the deterioration in parenting skills associated with the discovery of the abuse. In these situations the child may not require individual therapy; rather, interventions must be directed at parents. Even with children who have been seriously affected by abuse or neglect, individual treatment may not be the treatment of choice. In our experience, young children (below 5 years of age) do not have the requisite verbal or cognitive skills to benefit from this approach. Second, their psychological well-being is so dependent upon their parents and the family environment that intervention should be focused on helping the parents become the primary agents of change. We have also occasionally encountered children who absolutely refuse to participate in any therapy. Working with parents may be an alternative and helps them cope better with their children's behavior.

Current opinions about the most effective approach may depend, in part, more upon personal beliefs than upon any empirical data. We lack an extensive pool of rigorous treatment outcome studies that compare the efficacy of different approaches (Finkelhor & Berliner, 1995). Moreover, the question "What kind of therapy is the most effective for maltreated children?" may be too broad. It is most unlikely that one treatment modality will meet the needs of all maltreated children. There is considerably heterogeneity in their functioning and in the variables that moderate the impact of diverse forms of maltreatment. Consequently, treatment effectiveness will vary as a function of this diversity.

Although the focus of this book is individual child therapy, we emphasize throughout that children should never be treated in isolation. Even if they are no longer residing in an abusive or neglectful home and are in an excellent alternate living arrangement, therapists must still engage these latter caregivers in a collaborative alliance and enlist them as allies in the treatment process. Therapists must work with other significant individuals who exert a powerful influence over the children's lives. Similarly, a child participating in individual or family therapy may benefit from group therapy in the course of his or her treatment. Adhering rigidly and solely to one therapeutic modality limits the comprehensiveness of the services that can be offered.

Recommendations about interventions should be built upon the child's and family's strengths. For example, children with good verbal skills who, during the assessment, demonstrated a facility in talking about their experiences may benefit from verbally oriented therapy rather than a nonverbal, play therapy approach. Matching the interventions to the needs of the child and the family is crucial; mismatching may lead to the conclusions that the treatment modality was ineffective, that the modality was incorrectly used, or that the child or family undermined treatment, when none of these statements are really the case (Looney, 1984). The therapist should pay particular attention to those areas where intervention can be accepted by the family and is thus likely to produce helpful change.

Individual psychotherapy may be the principal intervention or one of several components of a treatment plan. Localized effects may require relatively short-term, structured individual child therapy with parental support. Pronounced developmental effects may require the consideration of long-term individual child therapy; apprehension from home; specialized foster home or residential placement; family therapy; and various medical, educational, occupational, and speech therapy interventions. In many cases, the therapist cannot implement such a myriad of interventions simultaneously; they need to be prioritized. Assuring the child's immediate physical safety may be the priority, followed by the introduction of psychotherapeutic interventions as the child and family can tolerate and respond to them. The transactional model can help in prioritizing interventions and may reveal indications that some interventions cannot be undertaken until certain factors change. This was the situation in the family described below and earlier, in Chapter 3.

Three children were in the care of George, who was stepfather to two and father to one of them. Concerns about multiple types of maltreatment in the family arose shortly after the mother deserted the children 4 years previously. Various assessments and interventions had been provided to George and the children. George was always agreeable to input but seldom actively benefited from in-home support and parent training. He remained passive and noncommittal and was isolated with no support in the community. When interviewed, the children minimized their concerns and were hesitant to engage with the clinicians or provide information. Given George's borderline cooperation, child welfare personnel chose not to remove the children from his care. Early assessments indicated that the children were doing poorly in all areas of functioning and were suffering from a number of developmental effects. Child welfare personnel exerted increasing pressure on the clinicians to see the children in individual therapy to address these problems. The clinicians took the strong stance, however, that individual therapy would be inappropriate while the children remained in George's care. They reasoned that therapy would be only a small part of their experiences and would do little to change their expectations about others, particularly since George could barely provide basic care for the children. He could not support them in school and peer relationships, let alone give the support they needed to profit from therapy. The clinicians believed that continued maltreatment would likely occur without active intervention from child welfare services and that the children would continue to deny and minimize their experiences. Consequently, the children would have had grave difficulties addressing these issues in therapy.

Despite the children's obvious and increasing needs, the clinicians used the transactional model and also considered the parental and environmental factors in recommending that therapy be initiated only after the children had been removed from George. Eventually George placed the children in care. Once out of the situation, all three children reported significant emotional, physical, and sexual abuse as well as neglect. One of the children reported George's maltreatment only after being permanently removed from George's care. The boy frankly stated that he had not acknowledged the abuse sooner because he feared coercion and more maltreatment if he reported the maltreatment and then was returned to George. After being removed, the children engaged in individual long-term therapy and group therapy.

Interventions may be carried out at the level of the child, the family, and the wider community. It is important that any potential treatment plan be formulated in a way that is practical and workable for the child and family. Often, a clinician may formulate a multifaceted and comprehensive treatment plan only to discover that various components are not available; too expensive; or possibly too overwhelming for and are rejected by, the family.

FEEDBACK SESSION
WITH PARENTS OR CAREGIVERS

In providing feedback to parents or caregivers, the clinician presents a formulation about the nature of the child's problems and how they might be alleviated to permit healthier development. It is crucial to provide information in a relatively simple and straightforward fashion. The clinician cannot assume that every parent will understand most psychological and developmental terms. Even those parents who have been in therapy or are well educated and verbal may not be familiar with terms used by the clinician. It is often helpful in this presentation to give examples of the child's behavior that illustrate the findings. The therapist should identify strengths in the child's and family's functioning so that therapy can build upon these assets while bringing areas of difficulty to the attention of the child and the rest of the family.

Following a review of the child's and family's response to the maltreatment, the clinician might describe what methods of intervention might be useful. The treatment plan should follow logically and simply from the findings so that parents or caregivers can understand why a particular intervention has been recommended. Parents and caregivers must be engaged in an alliance with the clinician so that they can support the child's therapy at both logistical and emotional levels (strategies for engaging parents are described in Chapter 6); they need to feel they are a necessary part of the child's therapy. This goal may be achieved by having parents or other caregivers become active participants in setting goals. These goals should be as specific as possible. The therapist should tell parents what the specific expectations are for their involvement in the child's therapy and what they must do to complement the therapist's work. The therapist should negotiate a schedule for sessions so that the child can attend therapy reliably.

The clinician may have to provide the parents or caregivers with some specific guidance and suggestions during the feedback session that will help them limit or contain particularly troublesome behavior by the child, such as physical or sexual aggression. Restrictions regarding the child's unsupervised contact with other children, substitute activities that may be used to redirect the child's negative behavior, rewards for the child for appropriate behavior, and a clearly defined person to whom caregivers can report problem behavior by the child may be essential (Gil & Johnson, 1993). Similarly, caregivers may require immediate specific instructions on how to deal with stealing and hoarding food by a severely neglected child. These plans may need to be written so that parents or caregivers can refer to them daily. Such a specific plan also decreases the caregiver's, child's, and clinician's anxiety.

The clinician should tell the parents or caregivers some of his or her expectations regarding the child's progress in therapy and what feelings and reactions of their own may emerge over the course of therapy. The parents or caregivers will have greater trust in the clinician if she or he discusses what difficulties and regressions may be expected before they occur, during what parents had expected to be a smooth and easy process. The involvement and roles of other professionals need to be clarified, with perhaps a larger case conference being called to discuss these issues.

Finally, a discussion about the length of therapy and its cost is necessary so that parents or caregivers can give informed consent for the child's participation. The cost will include time commitment and/or monetary investment. The clinician should briefly explain how the end of therapy is determined by referring to its specific goals, so that parents do not feel they are committing to a seemingly endless involvement. The therapist should invite questions and comments from the parents or caregivers throughout the feedback session. It is often useful to ask whether the formulation is congruent with their perceptions and expectations. Also, encouraging feedback about how the treatment plan can be altered or fine tuned to make the recommendations even more viable helps to engage parents in the treatment process. Despite feedback sessions during which parents seem to understand clearly all that is said, they are often overwhelmed by the content and volume of information they receive. The clinician should not assume they will retain all this information. Consequently, the clinician may need to review the issues and explanations over the course of therapy. The therapist's willingness to provide even more information as the parent's or caregiver's understanding of the child increases is helpful.

After providing feedback for parents or caregivers, the clinician may also wish to provide the child with formal individual feedback. The amount of detail and depth of this feedback will vary depending on the child's developmental status and needs. Again, the clinician should encourage and welcome feedback from the child.

FIVE

Principles and Goals of Treatment

IN THIS CHAPTER the reader will be provided with a conceptual basis for some common treatment goals and strategies applied to maltreated children. They are derived from our understanding of the sequelae of maltreatment and the mechanisms of impact described in Chapters 1 and 2, as well as from the principles and techniques of assessment described in Chapters 3 and 4. Without an understanding of the theoretical bases for treatment modalities, the same clinical technique may be applied indiscriminately to every maltreated child, regardless of the idiosyncratic needs of the child or the family. Although it is important to have a large repertoire of specific strategies and interventions, it is equally important to have a theoretical understanding that guides our choice and application of techniques.

Before we discuss the specific goals of treatment and their rationale, we briefly review the basic principles of treatment that have guided our work in this area. The reader will realize quickly that they are consistent with the principles underlying our discussion of clinical assessment.

BASIC PRINCIPLES OF TREATMENT

Treatment Must Be Comprehensive and Ecologically Based

As we have already discussed, the clinician must be prepared to address the wide domain of problem behavior and areas of dysfunction associated with the maltreatment as well as the problems that predated the maltreatment. The clinician may have to intervene in many different settings and environments to provide truly comprehensive and individualized services to a child.

The child must never be treated in isolation from his or her family or caregivers and immediate environment. There are many factors, including those concerning the family and larger society, that contribute to or moderate a child's response to maltreatment. Although many maltreated children require direct treatment, intervention must also occur at the family level to maximize the child's recovery and growth. The needs of the families deserve attention and include "survival needs" (e.g., food, clothing, and shelter); crisis intervention; training in parenting skills; and more traditional individual, marital, or family therapy (Cicchetti & Toth, 1995).

This principle also applies to children who do not live with their families and will have no contact with them. Even in these cases, some adult is assuming responsibility for the child's care, whether it be a foster parent or the staff of a residential treatment facility. Although clinical work with these individuals might be quite different from the interventions directed at biological parents, the clinician must have some kind of regular and ongoing contact with them, since such contact facilitates delivery of the most effective and optimal treatment to the child. For example, communication with the staff of a residential facility provides the clinician with ongoing information about the child's response to treatment and alerts the clinician to any significant developments in the child's life at the facility that may have implications for the intervention. It also ensures a coordinated, consistent approach among all the individuals involved in that child's life. The same argument can be made for contact with other collaterals, such as teachers or child welfare workers.

Clinician contact with other individuals involved with the child may yield other benefits. Ongoing communication and consultation with a child welfare worker can help ensure that these broader systems meet the child's needs appropriately and sensitively. For example, changes in a child's placement must be thoroughly discussed with all the important and influential adults in the child's life. Some clinicians resent the time and energy that must be expended on these broad issues of case management and fear that contact with other professionals will in some way contaminate their relationship with their child client. However, we believe that failure to play this more active and broader role significantly limits the effectiveness of clinical work with child clients.

Treatment Must Have a Developmental Focus

Treatment Must Address Developmental Effects

Abuse or neglect can disrupt a child's ability to negotiate stage-salient developmental tasks and may have a significant effect upon the child's ability to handle future developmental tasks successfully. Therefore, clinicians must evaluate and treat, when necessary and appropriate, the developmental effects associated with maltreatment. As well, they must intervene to remedy those localized effects that do not have the same major developmental ramifications.

Treatment Must Be Developmentally Sequenced

As we have seen, one factor that contributes to the emergence of sequelae associated with maltreatment is the child's developmental level. A child's perception or interpretation of the meaning of the maltreatment may change as a function of his or her progress through different developmental stages (James, 1989). Therefore, therapy must be available to maltreated children at various points in their lives. For example, a child who has undergone serious maltreatment may do some very profitable work in therapy when he or she is 8 or 9 years old and then again as an adolescent. However, this child may have to return to therapy as an adult. This is most likely when the person confronts maltreatment-related issues reelicited by typical adult developmental tasks such as establishing romantic or sexual relationships with others or parenting one's own offspring.

Another way of thinking about this notion of developmentally sequenced treatment is to conceptualize it as a "family practice" orientation. The therapist functions as a primary care provider, much like the traditional family physician. Treatment is provided to clients for different reasons over time, and the therapist has an ongoing relationship with each client or patient. Although the client may not see the family physician for extended periods, the practitioner is regarded as a resource who can be consulted whenever difficulties arise. Cummings (1986) suggests there is no reason why clients cannot interrupt therapy when they are no longer under stress and then return to therapy when they need to. This model of practice speaks to an even larger issue. We need to divest ourselves of the notion that we "cure" people and have only one chance to help a client become problem free for the rest of his or her life, so that if our clients encounter difficulties several years after the termination of therapy, we have in some way failed in our jobs. According to Cummings (1986), this is "absolute sheer nonsense" (p. 429). Returning to psychotherapy is not necessarily a failure either for maltreated children or for the clinicians who treat them. The fact that some ask to return to therapy with the same clinician may speak well of the trusting and secure relationship established with the therapist. Of course, sometimes clinicians cannot help when clients request future services, since these clinicians may not have the relevant skills or expertise. Rather than providing direct services, the clinician might serve as a referral source to ensure that the individual gets appropriate help. We would also like to note that this model is not appropriate for all maltreated children, especially those showing more localized effects. Many of these children can be treated quite successfully and need not return for a subsequent course of therapy.

Treatment Must Be Developmentally Sensitive

Treatment and intervention strategies must be congruent with the developmental abilities and capacities of the child. For example, a therapeutic approach that places heavy emphasis upon verbal exchanges will not be effective with a child who displays compromised or deficient receptive and expressive language skills. Implementation of such an approach would engender more frustration and a greater sense of failure in the child, who is already suffering from a shaky sense of self-esteem. In Chapter 4 we described play therapy as a clear example of a developmentally sensitive treatment approach.

Use Directed or Nondirective Therapy with Maltreated Children as Required

There seems to be a common myth that child psychotherapy, especially play therapy, refers solely to a nondirective approach. The best-known proponents of this approach include Allen (1942), who considered certain transactions in the therapist–client relationship to be the crucial elements in successful "relationship therapy." This approach was elaborated and amplified by Axline (1964, 1969). As one of her eight basic principles of nondirective play therapy, Axline (1969, p. 73) postulates that "the therapist maintains a deep respect for the child's ability to solve his problems if given an opportunity to do so," and "the therapist does not attempt to direct the child's actions or conversations in any manner. The child leads the way; the therapist follows." However, this ability to eventually bring up emotionally sensitive material may not be true of all maltreated children. Contrary to Axline's assertions, some children in therapy may not take the initiative in raising issues related to their victimization.

An exclusive reliance upon nondirective play therapy may not be in the best interest of our young clients, although it certainly has a role in the treatment of maltreated children. It can be used to engage them in a relationship and establish some rapport. Some children will initiate metaphorical play spontaneously as a way of depicting their experiences and feelings regarding their victimization; the therapist needs to do little to help the child begin this process. However, other children are so frightened and anxious they cannot even use the psychological distance inherent in play to express their concerns, and they engage in activities that help them avoid confronting this material. Nondirective therapy may inadvertently strengthen these defenses. The child must be exposed, either directly or indirectly, to this painful material for the anxiety to be extinguished and to begin reformulating the meaning of the abuse or neglect.

Rasmussen and Cunningham (1995) cite other reasons for "focused play therapy" with sexually abused and abuse-reactive children. Many parents cannot afford the financial expense of long-term therapy. Other children may be at further risk for victimization if they do not learn specific self-protection skills. We incorporate the concept of directed play therapy in our subsequent descriptions of therapeutic techniques. Likewise, children may need directed help to develop more adaptive ways of coping with the aftermath of maltreatment (Rasmussen & Cunningham, 1995; Cunningham & MacFarlane, 1991; Gil & Johnson, 1993). They may engage in highly inappropriate behavior such as physical or sexual aggression. The hope that children will spontaneously or willingly raise these issues is naive, in our opinion. The therapist must be more directive to enable children to confront these often embarrassing patterns that in the past have brought them much condemnation. The therapist must have not only skills in both nondirective and directed therapy but also the flexibility to use different approaches when indicated. Rigidity in both thinking and practice does little to help these children.

Treatment Must Be Culturally Sensitive

Therapists must be sensitive to the child's cultural tradition and context when they are considering the appropriateness of different techniques and interventions. An excellent example of one program that is sensitive to clients' heritage is "Project Making Medicine," a training program at the University of Oklahoma (Edwards, 1995; Subia Bigfoot, personal communication, September 18, 1995). The program comprises 2 week-long training sessions for professionals who work with abused American Indian children. The program incorporates spiritual traditions as integral components that serve to reverse children's feelings of victimization. American Indian spirituality relies upon symbolism, and burning sage or cedar provides a cleansed atmosphere for the therapeutic work. Cleansing with smoke or herbs also assists these victimized children to visualize their innocence. According to the program director, Dr. Dolores Subia Bigfoot, an overall goal is to have therapists validate and honor their clients' participation in these and other ceremonies, even if the therapists themselves do not use such ceremonies in therapy sessions (Subia Bigfoot, personal communication, September 18, 1995).

COMMON GOALS OF THERAPY

The basic principles discussed above provide us with a general orientation to psychotherapy with maltreated children. We now discuss some common goals of therapy, with particular attention to their rationale and implications for clinical intervention. We wish to make it clear, however, that this discussion can serve only to provide the clinician with general guidance in choosing possible treatment goals and interventions. Although the goals described below are clearly not applicable to every maltreated child, they are derived from our previous discussion of maltreatment impact and some possible mechanisms that might be responsible for outcome. Each child requires an individualized treatment plan that identifies specific goals and interventions.

Helping Children Acknowledge the Maltreatment and Express the Associated Feelings and Cognitions

The ultimate goals of psychotherapy with maltreated children are to help them develop healthier and more adaptive ways of coping with the feelings associated with the victimization and to reformulate the meaning of these experiences. However, for a child to attain these goals, the youngster must first acknowledge (either directly or indirectly) that the abuse or neglect did indeed happen and then begin identifying and expressing the feelings and cognitions (e.g., attributions regarding responsibility) connected to the maltreatment; uncovering the abuse or neglect is a means to this end. Apart from being a prerequisite to these two goals, acknowledging and expressing feelings serve other purposes. First, doing so diminishes the likelihood that the child will develop more intractable and serious symptoms and difficulties in the future. Second, these actions relieve some of the child's distress and anxiety. We now discuss these two purposes in more detail.

In Chapter 2, we described the development and use of defense mechanisms by maltreated children, especially from the perspective of internal working models and attachment theory. Chronically maltreated children may develop multiple working models of relationships and of the self and are unable to integrate discrepant and incompatible information from different models. "Representational" defenses prevent them from being overwhelmed by negative and intolerably painful feelings. They may overidealize their maltreating parents to avoid confronting the fact that their parents may not care about or even love them. Thus, incompatible information from different models is kept apart by the reliance upon overidealization or other defenses such as projection, displacement, dissociation, introjection, and splitting. But, as we have seen, the models and feelings excluded from consciousness still exert a potent and sometimes malevolent influence upon the child's adaptation to the world.

Thus, these defenses are adaptive in the short-term because they protect the child from intolerable feelings of pain and distress. The defenses may have deleterious long-term effects, however, since they exclude from awareness those models and feelings that in turn affect the child's perception of reality, interpretation of events, and subsequent behavior. To gain some control over these unconscious influences, the child must first become aware of their existence and the operation of his or her defensive strategies. Sometimes parents will resist therapy for their child out of the belief that all the child needs to do is to "forget about it." The danger with this approach is that the feelings and cognitions engendered by the maltreatment remain. Maladaptive coping strategies then emerge that compound or magnify the youngster's distress and lead to even more future difficulties. Crittenden (1992b) asserts that a central treatment goal is to help these children discard these defensive strategies so that they can be more open to new information about relationships and themselves. To do this, the child must become cognizant of his or her discomforting and painful feelings and able to tolerate them without resorting to maladaptive defense mechanisms.

What does this mean for our work with chronically maltreated youngsters? What we are proposing is that children need to be able to acknowledge and express these often conflicting feelings about those who have hurt them and about themselves. Consequently, children may need intensive assistance from therapists to acknowledge the feelings connected to their maltreatment and to aspects of their relationships with others that are a problem. In a subsequent chapters we will describe specific techniques that can be used to facilitate the emergence of these split-off and previously denied representations and feelings. Sometimes the relationship the child establishes with the therapist provides an excellent opportunity to bring these models and feelings into awareness. For example, a child may become angry because the therapist cannot meet all of his or her massive dependency needs. The therapist can help the child relate this reaction to previous experiences with others; in this way the therapeutic relationship serves as a bridge to these earlier, negative internal working models. The child becomes aware that distorted reactions to a therapist are based upon these internal working models rather than upon an accurate perception of the therapist's true qualities, the child is thus challenged to reevaluate and modify these preexisting beliefs and expectations. By uncovering these experiences and the attendant feelings and cognitions, revising distorted beliefs, and developing mechanisms to better cope with the internal working models and affective states, the child no longer has to rely upon maladaptive coping strategies and defense mechanisms that engender even more difficulties. "Resolving" histories of abuse or neglect does not mean forgetting them. Rather than being disavowed, denied, or dissociated, abusive or neglectful episodes remain in the child's memory but lose their power to significantly disrupt his or her current functioning or developmental course. The episodes of abuse or neglect are integrated into the child's life in their proper perspective. As Crittenden (1992b) notes, the most important feature is not the content of what is remembered but the actual process of accessing and integrating information. In other words, children must learn to process information without distorting or excluding it. In turn, such children are rendered more open in the future to new information and more willing to experiment with alternate responses and interpretations of their experiences.

Besides reducing the likelihood that these children will develop even more serious symptomatology, exposing them to stimuli (e.g., memories, feelings, cognitions) related to the maltreatment is an important component of interventions designed to provide some relief from their current distress. As we saw in our discussion of conditioning theories in Chapter 2, many maltreated children develop anxiety-related symptoms, including posttraumatic stress disorder due to the pairing of previously neutral stimuli with stimuli associated with the maltreatment. These neutral stimuli then acquire aversive properties such that their presence elicits anxiety. The child learns to avoid stimuli associated with the maltreatment, including thoughts or feelings. Thus, if a child avoids thinking about the maltreatment, his or her discomfort is minimized. However, this defensive maneuver is not adaptive in the long term. If avoiding thoughts or discussion about the maltreatment is reinforced in the child, he or she never learns at what point, if any, the fears are no longer justified or adaptive. By not examining or talking about the maltreatment, the child eliminates the possibility of exposure to cues and affects. Therefore, the anxiety is not extinguished and the symptoms continue. We can derive a principal method of intervention from this conceptualization of anxiety: the child must be exposed to the feelings, cognitions, and memories associated with the maltreatment so that his or her anxiety can be extinguished. Forms of exposure range from more direct modes, by which the child talks directly about the maltreatment, to more indirect methods such as exposure to these themes via metaphorical play. Specific cognitive–behavioral techniques such as relaxation training or thought-stopping, may be useful in reducing a child's anxiety. These techniques may also help the child develop behavioral and emotional self-regulatory skills.

Helping Children Develop More Adaptive Ways of Expressing Feelings Regarding the Maltreatment

Besides acknowledging and identifying the feelings associated with their victimization history, children must learn to express these affects in adaptive and healthy ways. In Chapters 1 and 2 we reviewed how the ability to regulate feelings and behavior is often disrupted in maltreated children. For example, they display compromised internal state language. Rather than immediately expressing feelings through overt behavioral displays, words, for such children, serve to represent these affective states symbolically. The child's growing ability to use language to label and communicate emotions contributes significantly to his or her self-control and self-regulation.

A good example of this approach is helping children learn more appropriate ways of expressing their anger. The maltreated child may experience strong feelings of rage but may not have the ability to put these feelings into words. The child may express this anger through overt, behavioral displays such as physical aggression. These displays not only hurt others but invite retribution and rejection, which in turn exacerbate the child's negative self-esteem and feelings of isolation. Helping the child express this anger in more appropriate ways, such as through words, may lead to better emotional and behavioral self-regulation. Similarly, helping the child express feelings of sadness or despair regarding their betrayal by the perpetrator may prevent the formation of symptoms such as depression.

Helping Children Reformulate the Meaning of the Maltreatment

Uncovering the maltreatment provides an opportunity for a child to explore and possibly reformulate the meaning and implications of his or her maltreatment. Chapter 2 included an extensive discussion of the meaning (different types of attributions) the child may impute to the maltreatment and the role these attributions play in the child's subsequent adaptation to the trauma. Besides being exposed to the aversive stimuli, the youngster must have the opportunity to examine and revise the meaning of the traumatic event. In his discussion of psychotherapy with sexually abused children, Friedrich (1990) argues that uncovering the abuse provides the child with an opportunity to understand the experience. Maltreated children may well have to address important issues such as the following: "What actually happened to me?" "Why did the perpetrator hurt me?" "Was it my fault?" "How did I react to the maltreatment and why did I react that way?" "Does the fact that I was hurt mean that I can't trust anyone, or was this just an isolated experience?" "Will I be powerless in the future to prevent other assaults, or is there something I can do to protect myself?" It is essential that all maltreated children have the opportunity to explore these questions. Examining the meanings and implications of maltreatment may become a central task of therapy, especially for those children who have undergone chronic and repeated episodes of abuse and neglect. The therapist may have to help the child correct cognitive distortions such as the belief that he or she was ultimately responsible for the abuse. Children who were exposed to more isolated episodes of abuse and who now display localized effects also require the opportunity to explore these issues. However, they may not need as intensive assistance in this area as those who show more pervasive developmental effects. Bringing the maltreatment into the open is a prerequisite for the discussions and explorations that integrate these experiences into the child's life.

Modification of Internal Working Models

The notion that earlier relationships influence later ones is a basic tenet of attachment theory. Many children who have experienced chronic maltreatment from an early age expect the same or similar maltreatment in new relationships, and they may adopt some of the same coping strategies they learned at an earlier age. These new figures upon whom maltreated children impose their internal working models include a variety of people: teachers, foster parents, peers (e.g., friendships, subsequent romantic/marital relationships), and therapists. This notion of the child's tendency to impose an earlier model of relationships upon a therapist is, of course, quite consistent with Freud's conceptualization of the psychoanalytic phenomenon of transference (Bowlby, 1988b). Working from a traditional psychoanalytic perspective, Littner (1960) argues that maltreated foster children bring expectations and beliefs to new relationships. They often interpret the actions of new figures as hostile and negative and then behave in ways to provoke these individuals into rejecting or abusing them. Shirk and Saiz (1992) label this difficulty in experiencing others as positive and benevolent and in forming a positive working relationship with a therapist as an "attachment casualty": "In brief, children who are difficult to engage in therapy, whose affective orientation to the therapeutic relationship is negative, are hypothesized to have experienced unreliable, ambivalent, or hurtful early caregiving relationships" (Shirk & Saiz, 1992, p. 721).

A child may react to the therapist in ways characteristic of the earlier attachment patterns described in preceding chapters. The child with an avoidant attachment history may withdraw from the therapist, ignore overtures for interpersonal contact, and display little or no affect. By doing so, the child attempts to avoid the rejection, abuse, and hostility expected from the therapist, as well as the distress engendered when the child's need for security and comfort goes unmet. Other children, for example, those exposed to early inconsistent and neglectful parenting, may react to a therapist in the angry, aggressive but dependent and clingy fashion characteristic of those who formed ambivalent–resistant attachments to their early caretakers. Although the therapist, from his or her perspective, relates in a nonabusive and caring manner, the child may not initially perceive it as such and interpret it according to his or her own representational model. As noted by Littner (1960); Flaherty and Richman (1986); and Parker, Barrett, and Hickie (1992), the degree to which social supports and caring interactions will be perceived positively may depend partially upon internal working models derived from earlier years. We cannot assume that a maltreated child's psychological functioning will automatically improve if he or she is removed from an abusive or neglectful environment and then provided with what we regard as supportive and positive caretaking. The fact that changing the environment will not invariably eliminate all of a child's difficulties was demonstrated in two follow-up studies of children raised in institutions until they were at least 2 years of age. They were then either adopted or restored to a biological parent (Hodges & Tizard, 1989a, 1989b). At midadolescence, children were more likely to have formed strong and lasting attachments to adoptive parents than did adolescents to biological parents. However, both groups had more difficulties with peers, fewer close relationships, and were more oriented toward adult attention than were matched comparison adolescents. These results suggest the presence of long-lasting early institutional experiences. Although removing children from substandard and maltreating environments is necessary for their enhanced functioning, these children may require much more active and intensive assistance in accurately perceiving others' intentions as supportive and helpful.

There is continuity in development when interpersonal and other environmental experiences maintain already established developmental pathways or trajectories. In particular, continuity occurs when experiences are consistent with the individual's internal working model of self and others. For example, negative beliefs and expectations about relationships generated by repeated incidents of physical abuse will probably continue if the child is exposed to even further abuse. Conversely, positive experiences with others may engender some change or accommodation in the child's negative internal working model in a more positive direction. For a child whose experiences have been consistently unfavorable, introducing an element of discontinuity into that child's life through favorable, positive experiences is critical. It ensures that the deviation in the developmental pathway will diminish; new perceptions and interpretations of others and self emerge and may be associated with more adaptive functioning. Thus, besides being mechanisms for continuity, internal working models have the potential to be mechanisms for change. Psychotherapy, especially the relationship between the child and therapist, can be one opportunity to modify these negative internal working models by introducing some discontinuity into the child's life. The psychotherapeutic relationship, often so different from earlier ones marked by maltreatment and rejection, can counter the child's pessimistic and negative beliefs and expectations of others and self. In this way, *the therapeutic relationship is a medium for change.*

This perspective on the therapeutic relationship has formed the basis of different approaches to psychotherapy with adults and children. In an early work, Alexander and French (1946) describe this warm, positive relationship with the therapist as a corrective emotional experience that instills hope of something better in the client. Also, the theme of the curative aspect of the relationship between the therapist and the child has figured prominently in some schools of child psychotherapy (for a cogent review, see Shirk & Saiz, 1992, pp. 714–716). For instance, Axline's nondirective play therapy focuses upon qualities of the relationship, particularly the therapist's unconditional regard for, and acceptance of, the child, as the basis for change, rather than upon the development or implementation of specific therapeutic tasks or interventions (Axline, 1969). Shirk and Saiz (1992) note that within this tradition, the therapeutic relationship is believed to be the necessary and sufficient condition for change.

In the second major perspective on the relationship in child psychotherapy the interactions between the child and therapist are regarded as serving a different function. Rather than being the principal curative agent, the relationship or treatment alliance refers to "positive feelings the child had for the therapist that enabled the child to accept the therapist as an aid in overcoming emotional or interpersonal problems. In essence, the alliance was a means to an end. It referred to the affective quality of the relationship between child and therapist that enabled the child to work purposefully on resolving problems" (Shirk & Saiz, 1992, p. 715). In this perspective, it is assumed that there are specific therapeutic tasks or interventions the child must experience for change to occur. The therapeutic relationship serves to facilitate and encourage the child's participation in this treatment regimen.

We maintain that therapists should not assume a rigid and doctrinaire position that excludes either of these two perspectives. Therapists must have sufficient flexibility to develop and implement treatment programs that incorporate strategies designed to establish a therapeutic alliance with children and, at least with some chronically maltreated youngsters, to use the therapeutic relationship as a major agent of change. It is our contention that the relationship offers the therapist numerous opportunities to intervene and counter negative internal working models. This is especially so for the child's distorted perceptions of the therapist that emerge in the relationship. The creation of a generally warm, positive, and accepting therapeutic environment is a necessary basis for any successful psychotherapy. However, the clinician must attend to other aspects of the relationship: by intervening with some specific techniques in this particular domain the chances of successfully changing the child's internal working models are maximized. We describe these techniques in Chapter 7.

There are other conditions that maximize the benefits of the therapeutic relationship as a medium for change. A greater probability of changing maladaptive internal working models exists when children have multiple experiences or relationships that consistently counter these negative beliefs and expectations. The direct psychological treatment of maltreated children is just one component in an overall strategy to help reestablish progress along an adaptive developmental trajectory. We agree with Graziano and Wells (1992) that, although we must approach maltreated children's problems directly, develop effective treatment strategies, and evaluate them rigorously, psychological treatment constitutes only a "partial solution" to the problem of child abuse and neglect, albeit an important and significant one. An exclusive reliance on psychotherapy with maltreated children, whether based upon attachment theory or other theoretical orientations, is insufficient to fully ameliorate significant difficulties. Psychotherapy is not a panacea; it is one part of a comprehensive treatment plan in which interventions are directed at the level of the child, family, and factors in the broader environment. The failure to change or modify those aspects of a child's life that maintain or reinforce these negative beliefs and expectations (e.g., a child who continues to be maltreated while receiving therapy) will serve to attenuate or even obviate any positive outcomes of direct therapeutic involvement. As we have stressed throughout this book, the therapist must intervene directly with these other individuals and variables to ensure the child has positive experiences with others.

Some maltreated children do not exhibit impaired attachment patterns or negative internal working models of others and self. For example, a child who has always received consistent and appropriate care and is then sexually assaulted once by an adolescent babysitter may not manifest these developmental effects. This child may require therapy to address symptoms of a posttraumatic stress disorder, but the focus will not be placed upon the therapeutic relationship as the principal means of resolving this particular problem. Other youngsters may present with both developmental and localized effects. They need a number of different interventions, in some of which the therapeutic relationship is used as an instrument of change and others of which, specific anxiety-reduction strategies, for example, are used. The therapeutic relationship, although a potent strategy, is usually not sufficient by itself to counteract the diverse emotional and psychological damage associated with abuse or neglect. The therapist must be well acquainted with other techniques for treating a wide range of psychological and behavioral difficulties in children and be able to implement them. Consistent with the transactional model, ameliorating these localized effects may generate more positive internal working models of others (via the perception that others are sensitive to one's distress and willing to help) and of the self (via the perception that one can change and overcome one's difficulties).

Self-Perception

A common theme in the treatment of maltreated children is helping them change their perceptions of themselves and develop greater feelings of mastery and self-efficacy. Internal attributions, such as, "It was my fault that I was abused," contribute to the psychological distress of victims of interpersonal violence.

Some children may need to achieve a sense of mastery over their maltreatment to reduce feelings of fear, powerlessness, helplessness, and low self-esteem. For example, a child may have to review what he or she could have done or could do in the future to protect himself or herself from further maltreatment. Chapter 10 contains descriptions of some specific techniques that provide the child with the opportunity to transform feelings of passivity and impotence into those of activity and power. Furthermore, clinicians may have to help the child address more general issues of low self-esteem or an unintegrated sense of self associated with the operation of defense mechanisms such as splitting and dissociation. These mechanisms are particularly evident in children who have experienced chronic maltreatment.

These are some of the broad themes that confront many clinicians who work with maltreated children. At this point, we need to reiterate one of our central guidelines: the clinician must conduct a comprehensive assessment of the child and family in order to identify specific treatment goals and plans. Although these broad themes provide some direction about possible intervention targets and the mechanisms of change, a treatment plan must be individually tailored to meet the unique needs of the child and family.

SIX

Working with Parents and Caregivers

W E HAVE STRESSED throughout this book that the child's adaptation to maltreatment is influenced by multiple variables. One of the most important components of the assessment is determining the degree of risk for further maltreatment. Clearly, if a child is currently being abused or neglected or is at significant risk for further maltreatment, these areas require immediate and intensive intervention to ensure the child's safety. Working with abusive or neglectful parents to change these maladaptive patterns is a critical topic but one so vast that it exceeds this book's limitations. Rather, the focus will be on interventions with parents and caregivers that support the child's recovery and maximize the benefits derived from individual psychotherapy. First, we discuss some reasons for contact between a therapist and parents or caregivers. Second, we present concrete strategies that can be used to help parents support their children immediately after the maltreatment has been disclosed or discovered. Third, we discuss more long-term interventions with parents, alternate caregivers, and other important adults in the child's life. Subsequent chapters, although focused upon individual therapy, will include other suggestions for intervening with parents that support and amplify the therapist's efforts.

REASONS FOR CONTACT BETWEEN THERAPIST AND PARENTS/CAREGIVERS

Establish a Collaborative Alliance

As discussed in Chapter 3, individual psychotherapy with children whose parents do not support their participation is likely to result in premature termination of therapy. A lack of support may be reflected in responses that range from a parent's active refusal to bring the child to therapy sessions to more covert sabotage, exemplified by parental remarks to the child such as "therapy isn't all that important." These ambivalent and hostile attitudes erode children's trust in the therapist and the psychotherapeutic process and detrimentally affect their engagement and participation in therapy. It is crucial to engage the parents, even if they are not the focus of treatment: if parents or caregivers are hostile, treatment will usually break down. The child is then exposed to another unrewarding experience with adults who have been unable to meet his or her needs for support and assistance. To establish and maintain a collaborative alliance, the therapist must have regular contact with parents or alternate caregivers. In this chapter we describe a number of ways to establish and maintain this collaborative alliance.

Ensure That the Child Is Exposed to Multiple Experiences That Counter Negative Sequelae of Maltreatment

We have stressed this point throughout the book: psychotherapy is not a panacea for maltreated children: it is one component of a comprehensive treatment package. The failure to intervene at a broad level attenuates the chances of helping children recover. Contact with parents or caregivers gives the therapist the opportunity to provide these important individuals with helpful suggestions about managing aspects of the child's behavior or presentation that present problems and ensures a consistent approach among these various individuals. Achieving these goals increases the chances the child will be exposed to multiple experiences and interventions designed to counteract his or her maladaptive behavior patterns.

Supply Important Information about the Child's Functioning and about the Outcome of Therapeutic Interventions

It is vital that therapists gather ongoing information about the child's functioning, particularly in relation to the therapist's interventions. For example, the therapist may be exposing the child to stimuli related to the maltreatment too quickly, which may overwhelm the child's defenses and result in significant behavioral deterioration. Feedback from others, including parents or teachers, is essential to evaluate the outcome of interventions and make appropriate adjustments. As well, contact with parents or caregivers provides information about any significant events in the child's life that may have implications for therapy. Such events might include the death of an extended family member or changes in criminal proceedings related to the maltreatment (e.g., an adjournment of the case in which the child was scheduled to testify). Such important information allows the therapist to plan appropriate interventions, such as raising these issues in therapy. We now turn to a discussion of concrete and practical strategies therapists may use in working with these significant individuals.

SUPPORTING PARENTS OR CAREGIVERS IN THE IMMEDIATE POSTDISCLOSURE PERIOD

In Chapter 3 "family support" was identified as an important moderator of the effects of child sexual abuse in the empirical studies in which the variable was examined. Family support includes the family's belief in the child, emotional support (e.g., the parent does not blame the child), instrumental support (e.g., ensures the child receives appropriate medical/psychosocial interventions as well as appropriate responses to the child's symptoms/ behavior), and appropriate actions toward the perpetrator (e.g., notifying the police, protective services; cooperating in subsequent investigations). The earlier interventions can be instituted, the greater the potential for change. Consistent with one of the basic tenets of crisis intervention theory, individuals are more amenable to accepting assistance during the immediate stage of a crisis. They are more vulnerable, less defensive, and more open to suggestions. This model is particularly appropriate for those families experiencing an acute situational crisis resulting from the maltreatment (usually physical or sexual assault) of their child. In this section of the chapter we review those interventions and strategies that can be initiated with parents or caregivers in the period immediately after the child's victimization is disclosed or is in some way discovered. Three principal areas that might be addressed are education about some common themes and issues pertaining to maltreatment, assistance with parents' or caregivers' own reactions and feelings, and helping them directly support their children.

Educational Efforts

Using a psychoeducational approach, the therapist may give parents and caregivers considerable information. This approach may attenuate their anxiety and lead to more adaptive responses to their children's distress. Parents are often shocked or dismayed at the symptoms or problem behaviors children display in reaction to maltreatment. Informing parents that other maltreated children show similar behavior decreases some of this anxiety. They benefit from an explanation of the possible mechanisms leading to these problems. Other inexplicable behavior, such as a maltreated child's tendency to recant the initial disclosure, may be made more understandable by discussing some of the short-term adaptive functions of such responses (e.g., avoiding the consequences threatened by the perpetrator). The explanation may also prevent the adult from personalizing the behavior, that is, from thinking the child is recanting because the parent is inadequate. Education about the widespread prevalence of maltreatment such as sexual abuse may counter parental feelings of isolation and inadequacy.

Education about other aspects of the maltreatment can be of real benefit to parents. Parents and caregivers need a clear statement about the critical role they play in the child's recovery and the importance of family support for a positive outcome. Some parents believe their children will be irreparably scarred for life. The therapist can instill some hope by citing the evidence that such damage is not inevitable and that the parents can do much to facilitate a positive outcome. However, psychotherapy with many maltreated children, especially those exposed to years of abuse and neglect, is often difficult and arduous. Most do not show immediate improvement, and the behavior of some deteriorates during therapy as memories and feelings about their experiences emerge. Parents or caregivers with unrealistic expectations about the immediate benefits and improvements associated therapy are quickly disappointed. They begin to wonder about the usefulness of therapy, particularly when faced with a child who now presents even more challenging behavior. They have to be educated about the process of therapy and the sometimes slow pace of change.

As professionals, we sometimes assume that everyone has our specialized knowledge. This attitude pertains not only to information about maltreatment and the sequelae and mechanisms associated with it but also to the response of legal, child welfare, and medical/psychosocial systems to these cases. Becoming involved with these larger systems is often a confusing and perplexing experience for many parents or caregivers, and it exacerbates their anxiety and distress. The therapist can help these families by explaining the roles of various professionals who are or will become involved with them or their children. Sometimes parents assume that the involvement of child welfare authorities automatically results in the removal of their children. Although professionals must guard against giving false assurances, they should present the range of possible responses of agencies to the situation. A better understanding of the typical procedures that will be followed in child welfare agency and police investigations, court proceedings, and medical examinations can significantly reduce parents' anxiety, thereby allowing them to more adequately support their child.

Helping Parents Cope with Their Own Reactions and Feelings

The task of the therapist here is twofold. While validating and normalizing their feelings or reactions, the therapist must also help parents or caregivers learn healthy ways of expressing these feelings in ways that support the child's recovery. Parents should be informed that children are strongly influenced by their parents' attitudes and reactions to the victimization. They should also be told that catastrophic displays of emotion will just heighten the child's distress. In other words, although parents may have many strong and understandable feelings about their child's experiences, they must learn how to contain and express these feelings appropriately. What follows is a discussion of some common reactions of parents or caregivers and some interventions that can be employed.

Guilt

Some parents or caregivers feel extremely guilty about their child's victimization, especially if they have their own maltreatment history. When their children were younger or even not yet born, these parents might have promised themselves they would never allow their child to be maltreated as they had been. When the unthinkable happens, they are consumed with guilt and feel inadequate as parents. As was reviewed in Chapter 3, guilt feelings may contribute to the difficulty some parents have in placing firm and consistent limits upon their children's behavior. Other parents, out of a desire to protect their child from any future victimization, become extremely overprotective and severely restrict the child's activities. Unfortunately, children treated this way begin to regard themselves as even more powerless and inadequate and less able to protect themselves from future dangers. Parents with strong feelings of guilt may take the child out of treatment because the child's participation serves as a powerful reminder of the child's problems and the parents' role in their development. Parents may even feel guilty about pressing charges against the perpetrator, especially if that individual is a family member. The child may interpret the ensuing reluctance as a reflection of parental skepticism about the disclosure or a wavering parental commitment to protect the child from further assaults.

What can therapists do to help these parents who feel so guilty? Some parents truly knew nothing about their child's victimization yet still feel guilty. They may have failed to identify behavioral cues as indicators of maltreatment. However, these behaviors were probably so subtle that they would have escaped the notice of the most sensitive and astute observer. Parents should be told that their guilt is unjustified. However, some will probably still continue to feel guilty. They should be told that there is much they can do to make amends and expedite recovery. Other parents have actively contributed to their child's maltreatment or have not adequately protected their youngster. Rather than automatically absolving their guilt, the therapist should affirm their feelings of remorse and contrition. Concurrently, the therapist should inform them that these feelings of guilt and acknowledgment of their inadequacies as a parent may reflect an authentic sense of commitment to the child and a solid base upon which to build. Rather than focusing exclusively upon guilt, the therapist should assist the parent in identifying and implementing more appropriate parenting strategies (e.g., alternate child-care arrangements, or a better choice of partners). These actions will decrease the probability of future occurrences of maltreatment and strengthen the parent–child relationship. Within limits, guilt can be a potent motivator that helps parents to make healthy changes in the relationship with their children. However, therapists must not allow parents who feel extremely guilty to become immobilized in their efforts to set firm and consistent limits. Children who act out as a result of their maltreatment do not need parents or caregivers who ignore or excuse inappropriate behavior. What they need at this time of crisis are parents who, although sensitive and empathic to their underlying affects and dynamics, help them contain this behavior and develop healthier ways of functioning.

Anger

Parents whose children have been maltreated are understandably angry and outraged. In fact, the absence of anger is a worrisome sign: one might begin to question the parents' commitment to the child or their ability to empathize with the child's experience. In Chapter 3 we described how parents' unmodulated and extreme displays of anger may invalidate children's feelings of ambivalence toward the perpetrator. Children also may become anxious that their parents will be unable to control this rage, to the point that the parents might take action that might well lead to the parents' incarceration. Children may become reluctant to talk about their maltreatment to avoid evoking such strong and frightening responses in their parents.

Parents benefit from the opportunity to ventilate their unmodulated anger when the child is not present. They may be encouraged to identify individuals in their natural environment with whom they can talk about their anger. Although empathic with the parents' feelings, the therapist must educate them about the detrimental effects on children who are exposed to unmodulated displays of rage. Parents may be helped to develop healthy ways to express their anger and fulfill their desire for retribution, for example by cooperating with criminal investigation personnel and pressing charges against the perpetrator. After the parent has learned to control and express this anger more adaptively, joint sessions with the child and family may be particularly useful. The child may benefit from learning directly that the parent too is angry with the perpetrator, thereby validating the child's affects and experiences. We have used these sessions to encourage the family to develop healthy ways to express this anger together. One creative mother proposed to her 8-year-old daughter that they jointly draw some pictures that would depict their anger. Of course, many parents, especially in intrafamilial cases of physical and sexual abuse, may harbor ambivalence similar to their children's. They and their offspring can be helped to find ways of expressing these feelings.

Parents may feel some anger toward the child. They perhaps expected the child to protect himself or herself from the perpetrator or to have disclosed the maltreatment sooner. Again, they probably can benefit from information about the typical reasons why children cannot stop the abuse or disclose it sooner. Emphasis should be placed upon the feelings of powerlessness and helplessness children typically experience in these situations, even without overt threats or force. The parent may be angry with the involvement of child welfare agencies with the family, especially if they have previously had conflictual or negative previous experiences with such agencies. Educational efforts directed toward clarifying the possible (and potentially positive) role of child welfare services and the opportunity to ventilate this anger may attenuate some of the parents' rage.

Anxiety

Besides feeling guilt and anger, parents or caregivers usually experience considerable anxiety. They worry about the child's physical health. A child who has been physically abused may have serious medical problems. Parents will require clear and direct information about the child's medical status, most likely prognosis, and what they can do to help. Given the prevalence of problems such as HIV/AIDS and sexually transmitted diseases, parents of sexually abused children may share similar concerns and require information and guidance about these diseases.

Parents also worry about their child's current and future emotional and psychological well-being. Parents of sexually abused children may feel their child is tainted because of exposure to sexual activity and is now "spoiled goods." They may begin to wonder whether their child consented to the sexual activity, enjoyed it, or in some way initiated the sexual interaction with the perpetrator. Regehr (1990) notes that parents may project their own issues about sexuality onto their child. They require assistance to express these feelings and issues. For example, a father might become very concerned about a young son who did not immediately disclose sexual abuse by an adult male who was a family acquaintance. The father might begin to fear his son is gay, rather than realizing that there were probably many factors, including, possibly coercion or threats, that inhibited the child from disclosing sooner. The opportunity to discuss such issues and receive feedback or information from the therapist may help counteract parents' fantasies or distortions. Family sessions during which children have the opportunity to explain the reasons for their delayed disclosure may help parents gain a more accurate understanding of the issues. Prior to these joint sessions, both children and parents may require some individual work. The child will need assistance in identifying the reasons for the delayed disclosure, and parents can be encouraged to begin thinking about how they will respond to the child's statements in a constructive and supportive fashion. For example, parents may be prompted to empathize with their children's fear.

Parents may become anxious at the thought of the involvement of larger systems in their lives. Their child may have to testify in court, or child welfare agencies may take a more active role in their family. Parents' may feel less anxiety if they have more information about these agencies and the possible consequences for the child and themselves.

Denial

Some parents want to deny the maltreatment ever happened. This denial may be the result of their need to ward off their own feelings (e.g., guilt, anxiety, anger). Other parents deny the child's victimization because the perpetrator is someone they love, trust, or depend upon to meet their psychological and physical needs. In cases where the perpetrator is a family member, other family members or extended relatives may place considerable pressure on the parent to refute the child's disclosure and take no further action.

One of the most important things the therapist can do when confronted with this situation is to openly and directly acknowledge the parent's distress over these divided loyalties. The therapist should explore the possible consequences that might accrue if the parent acknowledged that the maltreatment happened. The perpetrator might be incarcerated and the family might go on public assistance, or there might be an emotional loss for the nonoffending parent. Some parents feel extremely guilty about not protecting the child. Denying the maltreatment may be another way to protect themselves from feelings of remorse, guilt, and inadequacy. A clear statement of where the responsibility for the maltreatment lies, that is, with the perpetrator, may alleviate some parental guilt. Others deny their children's victimization as a way of denying their own histories of abuse and the attendant feelings. Again, the therapist should inquire about the existence of these factors and empathize with the distress. The therapist should clearly describe the dangers in denying the child's experiences while simultaneously reinforcing the parents' critical role in their child's recovery. By quickly acknowledging any strengths the parent may have, particularly as they pertain to allying with and supporting the child, the therapist may further decrease the parent's reliance upon denial.

This topic of counteracting parents' or families' denial of maltreatment probably deserves its own chapter; however a more detailed discussion is beyond the scope of this book. We refer the interested reader to Friedrich's (1990) volume on psychotherapy of sexually abused children and their families. It contains an excellent chapter on treating the family, including useful strategies and interventions for establishing a therapeutic relationship and countering the family's reluctance to acknowledge the abuse. Although this chapter focuses specifically on sexual abuse, many of Friedrich's ideas and suggestions can be applied to other types of maltreatment.

Parents' Issues and Reactions
Based upon Their Own History of Maltreatment

Chapter 3 contains a review of some strategies that parents who themselves have a history of maltreatment may use to cope with the overwhelming feelings elicited by their children's victimization. They deny and minimize the child's experience, deal with it intellectually, or become so preoccupied with their own issues that they are physically and psychologically unavailable for their children. The last situation leads to a deterioration in such parenting skills as monitoring the child's behavior, supervision, limit setting, and emotional support. Parents' maladaptive strategies such as substance abuse further compromise their ability to provide emotional and behavioral support.

What can the therapist do to help these parents at this time of crisis? The goal in this phase is to provide them with sufficient support and guidance to enable them to adequately support their child. Expecting these parents to now fully resolve personal and sometimes longstanding issues related to their own maltreatment is clearly unrealistic. However, the crisis may well be a window of opportunity for the initiation of this longer-term process.

First, the therapist should empathize with the intense affects elicited by their child's victimization and reassure parents they are not "crazy" for experiencing powerful and sudden reactions. Individuals who experience symptoms such as intrusive memories are often uncertain about the reasons for their distress. Their perceived lack of control over their symptoms compounds their anxiety. The therapist can help by providing an explanation of the processes and mechanisms that lead to these reactions (e.g., by referring to conditioning theories in the posttraumatic stress disorder formulation described in Chapter 2). This knowledge may lead parents to the realization that they are not "crazy" and that others have gone through similar experiences.

Although these parents or caregivers may be experiencing significant distress, they still must be available to support their children. Therapists can facilitate supportive and appropriate parental responses by again explaining that their reactions will be a significant determinant of their child's adaptation to the maltreatment. Parents should be told that they must contain some of their own anxiety, anger, and sadness while in the child's presence and that prolonged and intensive affective displays will just overwhelm the youngster. The therapist should help parents choose some people who will be a source of support and to whom they can turn when upset. Parents can be referred for their own therapy, in which they can more fully explore and process some of these feelings. Unfortunately, waiting lists seem to be almost ubiquitous, and they may have to wait for lengthy periods before beginning their own counseling. The therapist can encourage parents to find alternate supports, such as good friends, clergy, and family physicians. If none of these sources is available, the therapist may have to continue providing this support. The therapist should be cautious about exploring the parent's own history of maltreatment and associated issues too deeply, especially if the individual is going to be referred to another therapist for counseling. Rather, the principal goal is to give the adult opportunities to express some of these feelings while concurrently promoting the parent's adaptive response to the child.

Parents who are highly distressed probably will need guidance and suggestions about how they can best help their child. The therapist and parent should identify *specific* statements or phrases the adult might use with the child, statements that will convey the adult's belief in the disclosure, acceptance of the child, ongoing willingness to protect the child from further maltreatment, and support for the child's recovery. Similarly, specific child management strategies should be identified and rehearsed (to be discussed in more detail below). For example, if a sexually abused child begins involving other children in inappropriate sexual activity, the parent or caregiver will need some concrete strategies to deal with this situation.

We cannot emphasize enough the importance of parents having a repertoire of strategies and responses. Although they may not always be effective in quickly calming a highly distraught or acting-out child, they will alleviate some parental feelings of powerlessness and lack of control. The therapist should encourage the parent to anticipate difficult situations that might arise by asking, "What's the worst thing the child could say or ask you about the abuse?" or, "What would be the most upsetting thing your child could do?" Identifying and rehearsing specific responses to these situations alleviates some parental anxiety, gives them skills to help the child, and reduces their feelings of inadequacy or ineffectiveness.

As well as these reactions to their children's victimization, parents or caregivers with a history of maltreatment may harbor negative feelings about their children's participation in psychotherapy. Some parents become jealous of the attention their child receives from the therapist, especially if they themselves are emotionally needy, dependent adults who had never been adequately parented themselves. Such feelings of jealousy may become so strong that parents may terminate their child's participation in therapy: it is too potent a reminder of the attention and nurturance they never received. Others are dependent parents who rely upon their children to meet their emotional needs. The child's close involvement with a therapist may be seen as a real threat, so parents end therapy prematurely to preserve their exclusive relationship with the child. The child becomes aware of the parental reaction and subsequently feels torn between feelings of loyalty to the parents and a growing attachment to the therapist. Regularly scheduled contact between the parents and the child's therapist or the parents' involvement with their own therapist may attenuate this jealousy. Furthermore, the therapist can suggest ways of strengthening the relationship between parents and child (to be discussed in a later section of this chapter). By so doing, the therapist makes it clear that he or she has no intention of usurping the parent's role in the child's life.

Helping Parents Support Their Children Directly

Besides managing their feelings appropriately to help their child, parents and caregivers can provide the child with more direct support on two levels. First, the parent's direct interaction with the child, such as talking with the child about the maltreatment and managing problem child behavior, contributes to the child's healthy adaptation. Second, the parent's ability to support the child via other agencies and systems may need to be addressed.

Talking with Children about the Maltreatment

Parents must be able to respond verbally to their children's initial disclosures of maltreatment in a way that conveys belief of the disclosure. Long interrogations that convey parental skepticism about its validity, or outright statements of disbelief, may well result in the child recanting the disclosure and developing even more symptoms. These reactions increase the child's level of guilt and reinforce feelings of stigmatization and low self-esteem. Therapists must coach parents in empathizing with the difficulty most children encounter when they disclose episodes of abuse or neglect. Statements such as "We know how hard it must have been for you to tell us, especially when he told you he'd beat you up if you ever said anything about this" may be very reassuring. Children require clear statements to the effect that the ultimate responsibility for the maltreatment was the perpetrator's and that the parents will now do everything possible to protect and keep the child safe from further harm. Again, family sessions wherein these issues are discussed afford parents the opportunity to convey these messages.

Parents must be able to empathize with the ambivalence many children feel about the perpetrator. As we have seen, feeling such empathy is often difficult for parents, who are often consumed with rage. However, they must be attuned to the possibility that their child may experience a real sense of sadness about losing the relationship with the person who hurt them. Parents must give the child the opportunity to express these feelings and to normalize and validate them. Many parents themselves harbor similar feelings of ambivalence and sadness about the perpetrator. Sharing feelings again validates the child's feelings and creates, in our experience, a closer relationship between child and parent.

Therapists should also warn parents or caregivers about providing children with a blanket reassurance that "everything is going to be okay now that you've told." For many children, disclosures are followed by even more stress and disruption. In response to children's inquiries about what will happen next, parents should be able to tell them about the most probable outcome, such as having to talk with police or child welfare authorities. Although the child cannot be provided with definitive answers about the consequences of this involvement, the parent should reassure the child that he or she will do everything possible to support the child through this process. Some children may have to undergo medical examinations because of physical or sexual assaults; the child should receive appropriate preparation for these procedures. Clearly, the parent or caregiver will have to use vocabulary and language appropriate to the child's developmental age and convey sufficient information that the child can understand. Giving too much information, as in describing all the details of a gynecological examination, will just overwhelm the child with anxiety. Parents must consider the child's developmental age when making a decision about the timing of this preparation. Telling a young child weeks in advance about an intrusive medical examination exacerbates the child's anxiety and confusion. The parent or caregiver must provide the child with the opportunity to express his or her anxieties or concerns after a medical examination or legal/forensic interviews have been completed. The child should not undergo a severe interrogation but should be gently asked about any worries or concerns. Parents or caregivers also may be highly distressed when their child must undergo this type of investigation and should have the opportunity to vent their feelings to other adults.

There are other things parents or caregivers can do to help their children. Sometimes maltreated children worry that others, including peers, will find out about what happened and ask them for information. Classmates may ask why a child who leaves school early to attend therapy sessions misses the last 2 hours of school every Tuesday afternoon. The parent or caregiver can provide some direct suggestions about what to say. The child should be informed that he or she has the right to privacy and that a vague answer about ongoing appointments may be appropriate. Other children may be asked by classmates for details of what happened. The child might politely respond with "I'd rather not talk about it." Of course, if people who have regular contact with the child continue to press for more details, the parent or caregiver will have to intervene and tell that individual to stop that line of questioning. Parents should understand they do not owe these other individuals an explanation. Parents, like their children, might have to assert their right to privacy.

Some maltreated children, especially younger ones, talk indiscriminately about their experiences to anyone who will listen. Unfortunately, other people such as classmates may then use this information to tease or taunt the child. It also may be a way for the child to obtain attention from others. The parent can help the child discriminate among people who should have this information and the conditions in which this information should be divulged. The parent should avoid using terms like "It's our secret," which reinforces the perpetrator's original instructions; rather, the parent or caregiver should teach the child that it is important and healthy to discuss the maltreatment openly with certain people and in particular contexts.

Some parents assume that their child has resolved all the feelings and issues associated with the maltreatment if the child no longer discusses these events. This assumption may be a mistake. The child may have stopped talking about it to spare the parent or family further distress or because he or she has remembered more incidents that are particularly anxiety provoking. Rather than just ignoring the issue, the parent should provide opportunities to the child to talk about the maltreatment if the child so chooses. For example, when alone with the child at home, the parent can broach this issue with the following statement: "You and I haven't talked for a while about what your uncle did to you. I was wondering if you want to talk any more about it." The parent must inform the child on a quite regular basis that he or she is willing and able to talk about what happened. By talking with a supportive adult, the child typically feels accepted, understood, and validated. Conversely, insisting or incessantly badgering the child to talk can represent another coercive experience, leading to even greater resistance to discussing these matters.

Parental Management of a Child's Problem Behavior

One of the most important ways parents and caregivers can help maltreated children in the immediate postdisclosure period is through active management of their problem behavior. Although some maltreated children may be asymptomatic, others show a diverse range of behavioral symptoms, from those based upon anxiety (e.g., nightmares, somatic complaints) to more externalizing behavior (e.g., sexually inappropriate behavior, physical aggression). As well as explaining the emergence of these symptoms, the therapist must help the parent develop some management strategies to alleviate the child's distress and acting out.

Externalizing Behaviors: Sexually Intrusive Behavior and Physical Aggression. Externalizing (or acting-out) behavior often poses the greatest problem for parents, especially if it has been generalized to other environments such as school or the neighborhood and if other people begin complaining to the parents or demanding they do something to control the child. Sexualized behavior is one of the more common sequelae associated with childhood sexual abuse. This pattern frequently merits the child's direct involvement with a therapist: in Chapter 9 an intervention approach with children, based upon cognitive–behavioral principles, is described. However, parents and other significant adults must receive some immediate guidance and assistance regarding the management of the sexualized behavior. We will review in some detail our approach to working with parents and families on this is-sue; we draw upon some of the treatment components identified by Gil and Johnson (1993). Many, if not most, of these principles and techniques can be applied to cases of physical aggression.

First, parents must be able to talk with the child about sexuality in gener-al. If they cannot do so, their ability to communicate about inappropriate sexual behavior will be severely compromised. There are several things the therapist can do to facilitate this process. Inquiring about the basis of the parent's discomfort may reveal a personal history of sexual abuse and that discussions about sex arouse considerable anxiety in the parent. The parent may benefit from therapy geared to addressing these issues. Another possi-bility is that the parent may have been raised in a family in which no one talked about sex. We have found that family sessions in which parents read sex education books to their children are particularly useful for both sets of parents. As the sessions progress, the parent's anxiety decreases and the parent has a structured format in which to talk about sex. With some ex-tremely anxious parents, we begin to read to the child in the parent's presence to desensitize both child and adult; all either of them has to do at this stage is sit and listen. When the parent feels more comfortable, he or she is re-quested to begin reading. The therapist may prompt the parent to encourage the child to ask any questions about the material and to respond ap-propriately.

After parents have attained this level of comfort, they may be more ready to talk with their child about the child's sexual behavior, particularly about their expectations in this regard. Similarly, parents must convey their ex-pectations about the use of physical aggression in the home. In our ex-perience, many parents have never considered what sexual values and mores they want to impart to their children. Consequently, the therapist must encourage parents to reflect upon this issue and make some decisions about what would constitute healthy or appropriate sexuality for their children. Cultural values often play an enormous role in parental conceptualizations of sexuality, and the clinician must remain sensitive to them. If it is a two-parent family, the partners must reach a consensus about acceptable sexual behavior. We have asked couples to discuss this issue at home and report on their success in the next session. Were they even able to talk about the subject? And if they did talk, were they successful in reaching an agreement? If they did not, the therapist must facilitate a discussion and assist them in achieving a consensus. Parental agreement is critical before children are included in these discussions. They need to know their parents are united on this issue and that limits and expectations will be consistently enforced by both. In subsequent sessions, parents can inform children of their values and expectations about sexuality. The therapist and parent may first have to rehearse what the parent will say, especially what words will be used to refer to sexual behavior such as masturbation. Besides identifying unacceptable sexual behavior and providing an explanation geared to the child's developmental level, parents should identify what they consider appropriate behavior. For example, we have seen many parents who have told their children that masturbating in private is an acceptable practice. We regularly caution parents about inducing excessive guilt or shame regarding sexuality.

If other children live in the home, they, too, should be included in these family sessions, especially if they are at risk for being victimized by the youngster who is demonstrating coercive, compulsive behavior that has proved refractory to normal limit setting and prohibitions. Family sessions are an opportunity for parents to articulate clear expectations and limits. Other children in the family should be given explicit permission (and told the actual words they may use) to inform parents if the child who has been maltreated attempts to engage them in sexual behavior or resorts to physical aggression. The danger of avoiding these explicit discussions is that by doing so the family is in effect in collusion with the often furtive nature of the child's sexual behavior, thereby placing other family members at risk for being abused. The family will benefit from an open discussion about personal boundaries and privacy in the home, such as ensuring that bedroom doors are closed when family members are changing clothes. There may have to be some clear limitations on the type of sexually explicit material that can be brought into the home. A number of sexualized children we have treated found such material to be very arousing and reported that this arousal preceded their coercive sexualized advances to others. Therapists sometimes must have to engage in intensive dialogues with parents who allow or themselves bring this material into the home, alerting them to the role such material may play in their child's sexualized behavior and suggesting they keep this kind of material securely out of reach if they refuse to get rid of it. However, the therapist should not assume that parents have complied even if they maintain otherwise. One father seemed genuinely surprised when he found that his 11-year-old son continued to watch the father's pornographic movies. The father explained that he had "hidden" the videotapes on the top shelf of his bedroom closet. When this resourceful boy discovered the tapes were no longer in the living room bookcase, he systematically searched the house and quite quickly found them. Although the father refused to part with them, he agreed to keep them in a locked toolbox and carry the key with him at all times.

Family sessions may also be used by parents to teach and even model nonsexual expressions of affection. Some sexualized children invade others' body space, for example, by pressing themselves, including their genitalia, against others. With the therapist's help, parents can propose alternate ways of giving and receiving physical affection, such as sitting closely beside each other or hugging that does not involve the same kind of body contact. Parents can be taught to give positive reinforcement to these healthier responses, just as parents would reinforce the prosocial, nonaggressive interactional patterns of children who had been referred for problems of physical aggression. The therapist functions like a coach for parents in sessions. He or she may prompt parents to discuss relevant issues, encourage family members to raise questions or express feelings or concerns, and clarify misconceptions.

Children who engage in coercive sexual behavior that does not meet the clear expression of parental expectations usually require external control of their behavior. There are two major components to this control: supervision and limit setting. A continuation of the behavior places other children at risk and provides even more reinforcement to the child (via physiological arousal or gratification of more psychological needs such as dominating others), while exposing the child to even further rejection and censure from others. Some require maximum supervision, even to the extent of never being left unsupervised with other children. Although this seems a drastic measure, parents may be told that it is necessary to prevent the child from doing something that would get him or her into trouble. A specific supervision plan should be developed and shared with all family members. The parents might tell the problem child that they are instituting this measure because they care about the child and want to ensure that he or she does not display such behavior again. We have found that such firm statements, accompanied by consistent monitoring, often attenuate children's anxiety about repeating harmful behavior and convey the parents' authentic commitment to their welfare. The level of supervision may be tapered off as the child demonstrates increasing ability to control the sexualized behavior. The specific behaviors used to make this determination should be clearly set out by the parents and understood by the child. The therapist may initiate this process by asking the family, "How will you know when he [the child] is doing better?" It is often useful for the parents, child and therapist to review and renegotiate these goals weekly. Children and parents need concrete evidence of their progress at regular intervals to maintain the hard work of therapy. Positive reinforcement of the child's progress often expedites change. The extent of supervision may be reduced as the child attains these goals.

The therapists can help parents set appropriate limits when their child behaves in sexually inappropriate ways. This is often a major task of therapy with parents who have had numerous problems over the years in setting consistent limits on other undesirable behaviors. The therapist can help parents identify the consequences of the child's sexualized behavior and learn how to deliver limits in a clear, nononsense tone of voice. Parents should be cautioned against appearing repelled by the child's behavior, inducing shame or guilt in the child, or devoting excess attention to the issue, for example, haranguing the child for hours. This tactic inadvertently supplies even more reinforcement and attention. Parents can be taught to reinforce the child's interactions with others that do not include unhealthy expressions of sexuality. Parents themselves often require a lot of reinforcement and encouragement, as well as practical guidance and concrete suggestions regarding behavior management to become firmer and more consistent with their children. In-home teaching services, if available, are often valuable in helping parents improve these basic parenting skills in their immediate environment.

This is but one area in which the therapist can provide assistance to parents or caregivers so they can learn effective ways of managing children's externalizing behavior. Therapists can help parents devise a similar plan to manage other types of externalizing problems, such as physical aggression. Parents learn to convey their expectations concerning this behavior directly to family members and to develop a plan that will ensure the safety of other children in the home. Consistent monitoring and supervision, limit setting, and reinforcement of prosocial, nonaggressive behavior complete the process. Patterson, Redi, Jones, and Conger (1975); Patterson (1980); and Alexander and Parsons (1982) incorporate social learning theory in the treatment of aggressive and coercive children by their parents, and the reader may want to refer to these works. Gil and Johnson (1993) and Friedrich (1990) provide comprehensive descriptions of the parental management of their children's sexually inappropriate behavior. Friedrich (1990) also include a five-part plan that parents might use to decrease their youngsters' compulsive masturbation.

Internalizing Behaviors: Posttraumatic Stress Disorder and Anxiety-Related Symptoms. One of the simplest things parents can do to help manage their children's anxiety is to learn to talk with them about their fears and worries, and we present here a short review of some helpful things parents might say. Parents might empathize with their child's anxiety, reassure the child that he or she is not "crazy," and that the parents will do everything to ensure the child's safety. However, parents must be warned against giving glib reassurances such as telling the child that "everything is going to be fine" when in reality the future is uncertain. They must sensitively and realistically acknowledge these challenges rather than denying them or reacting catastrophically to them, either of which will exacerbate the child's anxiety. Parents should begin to monitor their child's emotional state more closely and attempt to identify changes in the child's presentation that reflect escalating anxiety. Parents might then offer the youngster the opportunity to talk about the child's worries or even engage in breathing and relaxation exercises together.

Children may also be taught to identify the signs and signals that indicate their level of anxiety is rising, such as somatic complaints like abdominal pain, and then to request their parents' assistance. These reactions and feelings might be graphically delineated on an outline of the child's body to make them more observable and concrete. The therapist encourages the child to identify which adults (e.g., parents) the youngster would approach for help and what the child would say (e.g., "I feel really worried right now, and I'd like to talk to you") to gain their assistance. These adults are informed that the child might approach them, and they are provided with suggestions about how to best respond to the child's expressions of anxiety. Sessions between the parent and child in which they reach an agreement about when and how the child will approach a particular adult for help are especially useful. A child who has difficulty sleeping may benefit from measures such as having a night light and a well-defined bedroom routine.

Parents can provide practical and logistical assistance using child-focused techniques (e.g., helping the child "freeze" the perpetrator or assisting the child in tacking a positive dream picture on a wall); these techniques are described in Chapter 9.

Helping Parents Cooperate with Other Agencies

Parents's effectiveness as advocates for their children may be compromised by a lack of the practical skills and knowledge that are often necessary to secure outside services. As mentioned earlier, the therapist may help by educating the parent about the role of various professionals and agencies in helping their child recover and by identifying the possible range of outcomes. Parents, especially those who might have contributed to their child's abuse and neglect, may feel especially threatened and frightened at the prospect of dealing with other agencies. The therapist should empathize strongly with the parents' underlying fear and anxiety while coaching them in how to be effective advocates for their children. The therapist and parent might "brainstorm" all the questions the parent may have for physicians or child welfare staff and then rehearse asking these questions in an assertive but nonaggressive manner.

Service Delivery

Clinical services for parents in the immediate postdisclosure period may be carried out in many ways. The therapist might work on an individual basis with parents or in a group format. Some advantages of a group format include the greater number of parents the therapist can see and the fact that participants may benefit significantly from talking with others who are undergoing similar experiences, which usually helps reduce their sense of isolation and stigmatization. Winton (1990) investigated the effectiveness of a support group for parents whose children had been sexually abused. Although the parents' stress levels had not changed significantly at posttreatment, there were significant decreases in some of the children's dysfunctional behavior. Parents reported they found the group helpful and believed they had learned coping skills and had become more confident as parents. The group met weekly for 2 hours a week for 13 weeks; its focus was educational/therapeutic. In a more recent study, the effectiveness of concurrent 11-week cognitive–behavioral groups for 19 nonoffending mothers and their young sexually abused children was evaluated (Stauffer & Deblinger, 1996). Analyses revealed significant decreases in parental distress, less avoidance by parents of abuse-related thoughts and feelings, and more appropriate responses to their children's behaviors following participation in the group program and at a 3-month follow-up. Their children's sexual behavior showed a decrease across evaluations. Some parents also benefit from reading books or other materials that describe common reactions of abused children and parents and the ways parents can help and support their offspring (e.g., Hagans & Case, 1988).

Possibly more important than the type of modality in which information and assistance are delivered is the timing of the intervention. Services that can be delivered as quickly as possible after the child's disclosure may have greater impact because parents are more open to change at this time of crisis. The Child Abuse Program at Alberta Children's Hospital, Calgary, Alberta, Canada, has an Urgent Response Program by which parents are seen within 72 hours after contacting personnel about their physically or sexually abused child. Parents are provided with many of the services described above: education about typical responses of maltreated children, information about the role of various professionals and agencies, the typical course of investigations, the opportunity to express their own feelings about–and reactions to–the child's victimization, and concrete suggestions and guidance about how to deal with the child's behavior. Longer term clinical services are subsequently provided to those children and families who require them. The following is a typical case handled in this program.

Janet, the 37 year-old single mother of 14-year-old Brad and 9-year-old Cheryl, called the Child Abuse Program after Cheryl disclosed to her the night before that Brad had been sexually abusing her for the past 2 years. Janet was highly distraught during her phone conversation with the intake worker and asked for help in managing this situation. The intake worker informed her that child welfare authorities would have to be notified immediately. Although reluctant, Janet agreed to do this herself, and the case was assigned to a child welfare worker for investigation. The police also planned to investigate this matter. Given her level of distress, Janet was accepted for the Urgent Response Program and was seen 2 days after she called.

Janet was seen for two sessions that had a crisis intervention orientation. The therapist explained that his involvement was short term, that he would focus upon helping her and her family cope with the immediate stressors and demands of the postdisclosure period, and that another therapist would be assigned as soon as one was available for ongoing therapy if appropriate. After agreeing to this plan, Janet was invited to identify the concerns she wanted to address. She said the child welfare agency's involvement with her family was especially troublesome (at the time of this first appointment this agency's investigation had not yet been initiated). Janet had had no previous contact with child welfare services but was worried that her children might be removed from her, since she had read some sensationalized reports in the press about the child welfare agency "snatching kids." The therapist explained the mandatory reporting laws, the need to ensure the safety of children, and that Brad's removal from the family would depend on the risk he posed to Cheryl. The therapist also explained that the child welfare authorities might be able to provide useful services to the family, such as referring Brad to a treatment program for adolescent sex offenders sponsored by the child welfare agency. This information alleviated some of Janet's anxiety, although she remained dissatisfied with the slow pace of the investigation. No one had yet interviewed Cheryl, which was escalating the anxiety of both the daughter and mother. Janet and the therapist discussed various ways of approaching child welfare staff with these concerns. She subsequently contacted the assigned worker and expressed her concerns in an assertive but measured way. Fortunately, the worker was responsive and agreed to see the family sooner.

In the first session, the therapist raised the issue of Cheryl's safety, since Brad still resided in the home. Janet was concerned about protecting her daughter, particularly since Cheryl had told her mother that the assaults had always happened after school and before Janet returned home from work. With the therapist's guidance, Janet arranged for alternate child care for Cheryl after school at the home of a neighbor who was Janet's close friend and knew about Cheryl's disclosure. Janet and the therapist discussed other ways of ensuring Cheryl's safety, such as closely supervising and monitoring the two children.

Janet was extremely angry with Brad. Although she had not yet confronted him with his sister's allegations, Janet believed she must do this quickly. While normalizing and empathizing with Janet's anger, the therapist pointed out some drawbacks to confronting Brad at this time, such as the possibility of contaminating the criminal investigation and giving Brad the opportunity to force his sister not to talk with the authorities. Janet agreed to let the authorities confront her son, but she was finding it harder to contain her anger against him. She and the therapist identified several individuals in her natural environment with whom she felt she could talk when she felt especially angry. These people included some very good friends whom she trusted. Janet discussed how she would approach her friends and how she would tell them about Cheryl's disclosure.

Cheryl had been having nightmares for the past several months; the nightmares increased in frequency after her disclosure to her mother. Cheryl revealed to Janet that Brad had threatened to beat her up if she ever disclosed the abuse. The therapist incorporated this information in his explanation of why Cheryl's nightmares worsened after disclosing the abuse to her mother. He and Janet developed ways to help Cheryl with this problem. Janet kept reassuring her daughter that she had done the right thing in disclosing, and her mother, Janet, would do everything possible to ensure her safety, especially in the light of Brad's threats. Janet was encouraged to institute a more regular bedtime routine for Cheryl, bought a night light for her daughter's room, and asked Cheryl regularly if she wanted to talk about her fears.

After these two crisis interventions sessions, another therapist became available who assumed responsibility for the case. Cheryl began her own therapy to deal with a number of issues engendered by her brother's assaults, including feelings of powerlessness, stigmatization, and guilt about her brother's subsequent removal from the home and placement in a residential treatment program for adolescent offenders. Janet was an active collaborator in her daughter's treatment and received some individual sessions to deal with her own feelings of guilt about not having been aware of what had been happening to Cheryl.

Sessions for Janet and Cheryl were subsequently instituted with a family therapist to discuss Cheryl's anger about her mother's lack of awareness of her victimization. She felt her mother "should have known" what was happening, while Janet felt very guilty. Family sessions brought these feelings into a forum wherein they were directly addressed. Brad was eventually incorporated into the sessions after his own individual therapy had enabled him to accept responsibility for his behavior. He also had gained a better understanding from individual therapy of the basis and precipitants of his sexual assaults on his sister.

Although in the two crisis-intervention sessions with Janet many of the significant or long-standing issues in this family were not addressed or resolved, the sessions provided her with the support and guidance she needed to make and implement decisions that supported her daughter at this crucial time. For example, she fought for a quicker response by child welfare authorities, allowed the child welfare authorities and the police to confront Brad, and instituted alternate child-care arrangements to ensure Cheryl's safety. Although still terribly upset by her daughter's victimization, Janet felt some relief from her anxiety as she began expressing these feelings and discovered they were normal and expected reactions. Her feelings of powerlessness were countered by the concrete actions she took with the therapist's support, encouragement, and guidance.

PROVIDING PARENTS OR CAREGIVERS WITH CONTINUED SUPPORT AND ASSISTANCE

Parents and caregivers of maltreated children may require interventions after the immediate postdisclosure period, particularly if the children have been exposed to severe and chronic abuse and neglect and now display some of the serious developmental effects described in Chapter 1. These children frequently present formidable challenges to even the most skilled parents. A regimen of 1 or 2 hours of psychotherapy per week, although useful, is often insufficient to remedy pervasive and profound developmental effects. Maltreated children require multiple and repeated experiences throughout their daily lives, that is, a therapeutic milieu, in order to have any significant chance of recovery. Involving parents or alternate caretakers (e.g., foster parents) and other adults who have significant contact with the child (e.g., teachers) and ensuring their collaboration and cooperation in a comprehensive treatment program are all essential. Just as the therapist functions like a family physician to the child, the same kind of orientation to the parents or caregivers may be necessary. There are some adults who require support and guidance from the therapist as well as consultations, at different periods while caring for a maltreated child. For example, the maltreated child's entry into adolescence may pose particular difficulties for parents or caregivers. These difficulties result from changes in the child's behavior, the feelings and issues elicited in the adult(s) by these changes, or an interaction of the two. The therapist's reinvolvement is expedited for everyone if the therapist, parent, and child had already established a relationship characterized by trust and respect. Although some parents may become overly dependent upon clinicians, the therapist should not automatically dismiss their request for reinvolvement. Their need to return to therapy is not necessarily pathological or indicative of a failure to have helped the individual when therapy first began. We must never forget that raising these children is often hard work with few rewards; adults who assume these responsibilities require and deserve generous and competent support and assistance.

This section of the chapter includes a review of some selected interventions that may be used with parents who care for these children. The focus is not upon those interventions designed to change abusive or neglectful parental behavior. Instead, we describe strategies that enable parents and caregivers to complement and support the therapist's work. The last section of the chapter contains a review of consultative services provided to school staff and representatives of the child welfare and legal systems.

Interventions to Enhance or Consolidate the Parent–Child Relationship

Since a principal focus of this book is the relevance of attachment theory for treating maltreated children, we review here some strategies to enhance the relationship between parents or caregivers and children. As abused and neglected children are at significantly higher risk for forming insecure attachments, a major goal of psychotherapy is the remediation of insecure attachment patterns. However, because parents or caregivers have much more extensive contact with the child and more opportunities to intervene with this problem than the therapist, they must be enlisted as integral and crucial allies in the treatment process. Some of the work done with parents and their infants who have been maltreated or who are at risk for abuse and neglect has some relevance for our work with parents of older children. Besides suggesting practical strategies, this work offers a conceptual basis for interventions. We briefly return to the literature to see what insights we can derive for clinical work.

The goal of infant–parent psychotherapy is to change or modify the parent's mental representations (i.e., internal working models of self and others). This change is considered a necessary precursor for a change in parental behavior and the infant's subsequent development of a secure attachment. As we saw in Chapter 2, this work is based upon the premise that parents' unresolved and unacknowledged early memories and feelings, especially those regarding relationships with their own parents, operate outside consciousness but continue to affect interactions with their own youngsters. The therapist sees mothers and their children in joint sessions. The therapist uses observations of the parent–child relationship to explore the mother's feelings and, perceptions about and reactions to the child and how unresolved historical issues may have influenced the mother's current parenting attitudes and practices (Crittenden, 1992b; Fraiberg, Adelson, & Shapiro, 1975; Lieberman, 1992).

These theoretical ideas have been translated into intervention programs. For example, providing psychotherapy for the mothers who participated in Project STEEP (Steps toward Effective, Enjoyable Parenting) was thought to influence them in two ways (Erickson et al., 1992). First, therapists attempted to help the mothers develop a cognitive and emotional understanding of how their conceptions and assumptions, based upon their experiences with their own parents, influenced their current parenting practices. Second, the psychotherapeutic relationship challenged the mother's negative internal working model of the self and others and it afforded them a "secure base" from which they could explore painful and sensitive issues. To change these internal working models via the therapeutic relationship, therapists were as consistent and predictable as possible when relating to their clients. They made a real commitment to the mother, even in the face of the parent's unwillingness to participate in the program. For example, the therapists always showed up when they said they would and would not end a mother's program participation because she had missed some appointments. The therapists identified and affirmed strengths in both the baby and the mother and empowered the mother by helping her develop skills that would allow her to solve her own problems. The therapists sought to demonstrate their commitment and sensitivity by listening carefully and empathically to the mother's concerns and accurately reflecting their feelings. Within the context of the therapeutic relationship, the clinicians modeled more adaptive ways for the mothers to handle interpersonal disagreements. The therapists would directly articulate their frustration or even anger with clients while maintaining their commitment by refusing to reject the parents. After a solid psychotherapeutic alliance had been established, the therapists began identifying the functional patterns and defense mechanisms evident in the parent's relationship with the therapist and the child.

Erickson et al.'s (1992) report on the preliminary evaluation revealed some mixed results. Compared with control subjects, the STEEP participants displayed a better understanding of their child's needs and better life management skills, reported fewer symptoms of depression and anxiety, and were judged to provide a more appropriately stimulating and organized home environment. However, there was not a significantly higher proportion of securely attached children in the intervention group than in the control group. Despite this finding, van IJzendoorn, Juffer, and Duyvesteyn (1995) caution against dismissing the utility of longer-term interventions that focus upon changing parents' mental representations. The authors note that it may take more time for mothers to change these mental representations than to learn new behavioral strategies. Indeed, there was a trend for the children who participated in Project STEEP to move toward a more secure relationship during their second year of life. Control children showed a tendency to move toward insecure attachments.

What are the implications for work with parents and caregivers of older children who manifest insecure attachments and have grave difficulties relating in healthy, adaptive ways to others? Although the effects of long-term interventions that focus upon changing maternal attachment representations seem very modest (but statistically significant), they still have important practical applications. Maltreated children who continue to be raised by individuals whose parenting is deleteriously influenced by their own painful and hurtful child experiences may well be at risk for further abuse and neglect. The psychotherapeutic outcome for these children will also be attenuated or even obviated by living in such a child-rearing environment. This variable must be thoroughly evaluated in the assessment phase. Appropriate interventions must be developed and offered to the parent. For many such parents, intensive psychotherapy may be the treatment of choice; we have already reviewed some basic principles of this approach. Parents must be made aware of how their mental representations, formed in early childhood, affect their parenting. A principal strategy is to use the parent's current experiences with their children to elicit and examine memories from their own childhood and to access feelings of anger, sadness, and loss. Acknowledging resentment about caring for their child because no one ever cared for them may be a first step in jettisoning those feelings that interfere with being the kind of parent they really want to be. Parents are encouraged to think about experiences they wish they had had as children and to replicate these interactions with their own offspring. An awareness of these profound feelings of sadness, loss, and anger may help parents see experiences, such as their abusive or neglectful care of their own children, from the child's perspective. The psychotherapeutic relationship is also used to change parental expectations and beliefs about the self and others. The reader would be wise to consult the classic work by Fraiberg et al. (1975); recent contributions by Crittenden (1992b), Erickson et al. (1992), and Lieberman (1991, 1992; Lieberman & Pawl, 1990; Lieberman, Weston, & Pawl, 1991); and a more recent work by West and Sheldon-Keller (1994). These works provide a comprehensive review of this approach, particularly the relevance of attachment theory to the conduct of adult psychotherapy.

Other parents or caretakers may have had a positive upbringing and therefore are not influenced by negative representations derived from childhood. Their parenting skills may be solid, but they may be caring for children who have severe deficits in establishing and maintaining secure and healthy relationships with others. How can we help caregivers form relationships with these children that will counter the children's negative internal working models of others and the self?

Forming intimate relationships with others is often a threatening experience for many maltreated children. When they become closer to others, they have even stronger feelings of vulnerability. Intimacy is equated with harm, threat, and betrayal and therefore is to be avoided. There are other reasons that inhibit maltreated children from establishing close relationships.

They believe that intimacy with a person other than their parent constitutes an act of disloyalty to the absent parent, whom they expect to reject them if they discover the child's growing affection for the substitute caregiver (James, 1994). Other youngsters may attempt to provoke rejection by the parent via defiant, negative, and oppositional behavior. This behavior allows them to gain some control over the rejection they believe is inevitable. A child may derive some measure of security and control by controlling rejection rather than passively waiting for rejection to happen.

Through small, repeated demonstrations that the parent cares, the child's negative internal working model of others and the self may begin to change. The child may well have to undergo a great many of these experiences before he or she actually begins to trust the authenticity of the parent's positive intent. As we have stated elsewhere, the child may need many other interventions to facilitate an accommodation of the internal working model in a more favorable and positive direction. The therapist can help the parent or caregiver identify opportunities to manifest this commitment and to formulate concrete ways to show this caring attitude. For instance, parents should follow through with any promises made to the child. Also, the therapist can help the parent become more attuned to the feelings and conflicts underlying the child's sometimes provocative and perplexing behavior. Exposure to sensitive adults who articulate empathy may be a novel experience for many children; it may well be the start of a reparative process by which their trust in others is restored.

Children with negative expectations of others often subject parents or caregivers to numerous tests of their commitment. When these children begin to feel a closer connection to the parent, they may engage in provocative, defiant, and oppositional behavior to determine if the adult will reject or abuse them. It is particularly important to give parents an explanation of this phenomenon. Moreover, parents must impose firm and consistent limits on this behavior at these times. It is very easy to give up when faced with a child who thwarts any attempt at closeness or intimacy and whose behavior remains refractory to typical child management strategies that were previously successful with other children. Parents should tell the child directly that they will set limits and consequences because they want to ensure the child learns how to behave appropriately. Parents should also emphasize that these measures, which may seem draconian to the child, are based upon the adult's deep commitment to the child. Parental failure to control the more negative aspects of a child's behavior not only results in a further deterioration of the child's behavior; the child may interpret this parental lack of action as meaning the parent no longer cares about the child's welfare. In the child's mind, if the parent's had cared, they would have expended the effort necessary to manage the child's behavior.

To counter the child's deep mistrust of others and fear of closeness and intimacy, the parent or caregiver must make a concerted effort to include the child in mutually positive and pleasurable experiences and activities (James, 1994). Each may begin to enjoy the other's company and have some fun together. Participating in these kinds of activities helps the child learn that interpersonal relationships can be rewarding. For the adult caregiver who derives little satisfaction from the child's negative, hostile, and sometimes even outrageous behavior, these experiences may counter the adult's growing disenchantment and reinforce efforts to engage the child. Although parents and caregivers can often readily arrange such experiences, the therapist may have to meet with some parents and children to help identify what activities would be mutually pleasurable. James (1994, p. 73) provides several good suggestions for such activities. Positive cognitive experiences may include going to a museum or carrying out a building project together. Pleasurable emotional experiences include the child and adult caring for a pet together or watching an emotional movie. Parents and child may share spiritual experiences, such as attending church together. There are many other fun activities that parents and children might share: playing simple board games at home, participating in sports together, or reading to a child. With the therapist's guidance, parents and children can usually think of something that would be fun to do with one another. In subsequent sessions with the therapist, the parent and child may be encouraged to review such an activity, emphasizing its positive aspects. The therapist may ask each to identify what they liked most about being with the other. Souvenirs of these activities or outings (e.g., a movie ticket stub or a photograph of the child and parent playing catch) should be retained and kept in a special place in the home. These souvenirs serve as concrete reminders of shared good times, especially when both the child and adult become pessimistic about the chances that their relationship will ever work.

Some parents, especially those who might have contributed to the child's maltreatment, may encounter real difficulty doing this task. They may have little motivation or expect that the child will reject their overtures to participate. The therapist may help by encouraging the parent to begin thinking of brief activities in which there is a reasonable chance the parent and child will have some fun together. Again, the therapist must consult closely with both child and parent concerning the choice of these activities. The activities might be something as simple as a game of checkers, walking a dog together, or reading together for 10 minutes. Asking that they participate in more intense and prolonged activities, such as completing a science project together, may be too threatening for the parent and child, and the activity will quickly be rejected by both participants. However, success with limited activities may start the process of instilling some hope that the participants can relate better. Parent and child may then be encouraged to try longer activities with one another in the future.

There are also some parents who do not have the skills to interact positively or play appropriately with a very young child. In some programs, attempts have been made to increase parental sensitivity to an infant's cues and to select and implement a response that meets the baby's needs (e.g., van den Boom, 1994). A meta-analysis of different intervention studies revealed that interventions are more effective in changing parental insensitivity than in changing children's attachments, although the latter were still statistically significant (van IJzendoorn et al., 1995).

The same kind of approach may be necessary with parents or caregivers of older children. The first step may be for the parent to observe the therapist and child in the playroom engaging in typical activities such as board games, painting, or playing with dolls and trucks. For a parent, these activities model some specific ways to interact with the child. Then the parent might be invited into the playroom to play with the child and the therapist. These joint sessions provide another opportunity for the parent to model healthy and appropriate interaction and to give the parent concrete tips about his or her interactional style with the child. Do not assume the parent knows how to interact in seemingly simple activities such as drawing or building with blocks. Some parents with minimal skills in this area feel threatened by the thought of having to play with their child. They feel relieved and supported by the therapist's guidance and suggestions. The therapist may serve as a mediator if things start to go wrong, leading the child and parent through a problem-solving process. When parents feel more confident, the therapist may leave the room and watch via a one-way mirror or videotape the interaction. Afterward, the therapist gives the parent some feedback, emphasizing the parent's strengths and capabilities. Watching segments of the videotape may enable parents to become more sensitive to their child's cues and better able to make appropriate interventions.

James (1994) describes other useful strategies designed to increase the child's sense of belonging to the family. These strategies include the adult making verbal references that emphasize the child's tie to the family, as well as more concrete demonstrations, such as having a new family picture taken together (for a child placed with an adoptive or foster family or a child just returned to a parent from foster care), selecting a special place for the child at the dinner table, or purchasing a gift for the child's room.

James also recommended that abused children need "positive, intimate, physical touch" (James, 1994, p. 76). To prevent an escalation in the child's anxiety, James advises that the touching behavior be explained to the child. She suggests that parents or caregivers begin with grooming behavior, such as shampooing and styling the child's hair. We also believe it is critical for the parent or caregiver to proceed slowly and gradually in this area. For children who have been physically or sexually abused, touching that seems innocuous to most people may be associated with some frightening and painful experiences. For instance, an adult who sexually abused a child might have initiated the assaults by giving the child a back rub and then progressed to sexually intrusive behavior. Other sexually abused children might find this kind of touching to be sexually exciting, thereby eliciting significant anxiety. Parents or caregivers would do well to go gradually and take their cues from the child's ability to tolerate touching. Parents must also explain to the child the distinction between the current touching and that associated with the maltreatment (e.g., "When I hug you like this, it means that I like you and care about you. It does not mean that I am going to touch your private parts.").

Many maltreated children are permanently removed from parental care, and they must have alternate supports before they can acknowledge their parents' inability or unwillingness to provide the love and care they deserve and to accept this loss (James, 1994). It is often difficult for such children to acknowledge openly that their parents cannot care for them or may not even love them. These children would be overwhelmed by feelings of abandonment if they acknowledged their parents' lack of commitment. In making this acknowledgment without support, these children would need to admit that they had no one who loved them, a truly frightening prospect for a young child. They then tend to deny the parent's ongoing difficulties, adamantly maintain the parent will change for the better, and often present an overidealized portrayal of the parent that runs counter to the painful reality of the parent's deficits and failings.

Alternate caregivers like foster parents may become somewhat frustrated with the child's use of these defensive strategies, particularly if their strenuous efforts to make the child feel wanted and cared are met with hostility, defiance, and even more negative behavior. The therapist may play a significant role in educating the caregiver about the function of defenses such as overidealization and in explaining how the child's negative behavior may be a test of the caregiver's commitment. The caregiver should not argue with a child who steadfastly maintains that his or her parents have now resolved all the problems responsible for the child's apprehension from the home. Instead, the caregiver should empathize with the underlying fear or anxiety that drives the child to make such assertions, even when confronted with clear evidence that the parents still have many difficulties. The caregiver who identifies all the parent's glaring deficits and foibles and tries to convince the child that the parent is unfit will probably engender even more resistance by the child in acknowledging these problems. The therapist should teach the foster parent how to empathize with some of the child's underlying feelings. This empathy might be communicated through statements like, "It would make you very happy if your mom was able to stop drinking and take you home again," in response to a child who claims that she will soon be going home because her mother has surmounted her longstanding problem with alcoholism. The establishment of even a limited connection with an alternate caregiver begins to attenuate the child's profound sense of abandonment. Along with the alternate caregiver's ability to convey a deep understanding of, and empathy for, the child's plight, such a connection helps the child acknowledge the significance of his or her loss and begin expressing intense feelings of rage, sadness, and grief. By normalizing these feelings, helping the child find appropriate words rather than acting out the feelings through aggressive or destructive behavior, and maintaining firm and consistent limits on any negative behavior, the caregiver helps the child through the grieving process. These strategies also strengthen the child's ability to self-regulate feelings and behavior. Some caregivers take solace from the fact that the child now can mourn the other parent's loss because the caregiver has been successful at making a connection in which the youngster feels a certain measure of safety and security.

Enlisting the cooperation of the parent whose loss the child is mourning may facilitate recovery. Specifically, both child and parent may benefit from joint sessions in which the parent gives the child explicit permission to form a close relationship with alternate caregivers. At this time, the parent assures the child that he or she will not be threatened by the child's close relationship with new parental figures. For children who believe their negative behavior in the foster home will break down the placement and result in a return home, a clear and unequivocal message from the parent may contribute to a deescalation of the negative behavior. These discussions are difficult for children; they may require some individual sessions to express their sentiments about the loss, to formulate questions for the parent (e.g., "Why did you give me up?"), and to decide how they want to say good-bye to their parents. Parents also may need some preliminary individual sessions with the therapist to express their grief and anger about losing the child and to rehearse what they will say. Of course, some parents vehemently oppose losing their parental rights. They are unwilling or unable to give their child explicit permission to become close to another individual, they may even blame the child for what has happened. Other parents who have lost parental rights are so egocentric or dependent upon their child that they cannot let go and allow the youngster to establish alternate relationships.

In Chapter 1 it was pointed out that many maltreated children do not have a solid sense of self. Again, James (1994) provides some good suggestions about how to help children establish a sense of self and identity. As well as being applicable to therapy sessions, a number of her suggestions can be used by parents and caregivers. These suggestions include sharing the caregiver's comments about the child's uniqueness and soliciting the child's opinions about his or her personal feelings, thoughts, and bodily experiences. Extensive or in-depth discussions about these opinions or the child's dislikes and likes contribute to the child's further differentiation of self.

Helping the Parent or Caregiver
Develop Child Management Skills

We have already discussed how parents or caregivers may benefit enormously from concrete suggestions and advice from the therapist concerning behavior management strategies. Sessions covering these topics may take place in an office setting or in the home in order to provide parents or caregivers with hands-on teaching and guidance. For their part, parents or caregivers must be willing to work as part of the treatment team, to openly communicate information about the child and their own struggles, and to be willing to seek out help and guidance when required (James, 1994).

Providing Ongoing Support to the Parents or Caregivers

Parenting and caring for a maltreated child with significant symptomatology can be exhausting, frustrating, and daunting. These parents and caregivers deserve enormous amounts of support and assistance. There are other ways therapists can provide this kind of support besides advice and guidance concerning behavior management and strengthening the parent–child relationship.

First, the therapist should normalize and validate some of the parent's reactions to the child. The child who responds to the parent's overtures of caring and love with increased hostility, defiance, or even rejection poses a real threat to many parents, especially for those who want a mutually reciprocal and intimate relationship with the child. These parents not only become angry with the child but begin to question their own skills and worth as parents and individuals. Consequently, they may feel like giving up and having the child removed from the home. Foster parents sometimes complain that they feel they have been "sucked dry." Compounding these feelings is the disruption of the entire family and the incessant demands by others to "do something" to bring the child's behavior under control. Therapists should encourage caregivers to respond to the needs of other children in the family. Often these children tend to receive less active parenting because of the very high demands of the maltreated child.

Having the opportunity to articulate these feelings and frustrations can alleviate a parent's distress. In particular, participating in a support group with other parents or caregivers facing similar challenges and frustrations may attenuate the parent's sense of isolation. Preparing parents for their child's possible behavioral regressions as a function of upcoming events (e.g., court appearance) and helping the parents develop plans to cope with these contingencies decrease their feelings of powerlessness. Although time consuming, regular consultation with these caregivers usually results in an improvement in the care the child receives. Parents also benefit from some respite care; for instance, having the child spend one weekend per month with another family. Again, the therapist should advocate for the provision of this service.

WORKING WITH TEACHERS

As well as working with parents and other caregivers, the therapist who involves teachers in the treatment plan has a better chance of helping the maltreated child recover. Teachers have a great deal of contact with the child and often see and experience the child's difficulties firsthand. They are in an excellent position to help remediate some of these problems.

In Chapter 4 we discussed the importance of gathering information from teachers during the assessment. The therapist should request their continued involvement in the treatment phase. An offer by the therapist to visit the school and meet with staff is often well received. Like the child's parents or caregivers, teachers may be frustrated and exhausted from dealing with some extremely difficult behavior. However, the therapist should not portray himself or herself as the "expert" who dictates how teachers should manage the child. Instead, the therapist must be willing to work cooperatively and collaboratively. The therapist must realize that school personnel probably already have valuable insights and ideas about the child and how best to help.

Given the sensitivity of information concerning the child's history and current circumstances, the therapist must be prudent when deciding how much of this information to share. The therapist should have discussed this issue with the child's parents or legal guardians and received explicit permission regarding the kinds of information that may be communicated before they talk or meet with teachers. The child, particularly an older one, should be informed that the therapist wishes to meet with his or her teachers so that everyone can work together on the child's behalf.

One of the first things a therapist might do is to provide teachers with some information regarding the reasons for the child's behavior. Appropriate reference should be made to those historical and current factors that have contributed to the child's functioning. For those who teach children with chronic and long-term difficulties resulting from maltreatment, the therapist might help them develop realistic expectations about the child's prognosis and the rate of change. Although the therapist may help the teacher understand that change will not be immediate, an overly pessimistic attitude may set up a self-fulfilling prophecy that might prove to be detrimental. Teachers with a solid understanding of the basis of the problem behavior may begin to see the child in a different perspective and are less likely to personalize the child's reactions.

Teachers should be encouraged to limit any physical aggression or sexually inappropriate behavior firmly and consistently. They should work with the therapist to develop some concrete strategies. Some teachers with whom we have worked have agreed to institute daily "check-ins" with these children. The teachers spend 5 to 10 minutes alone with the child near the beginning of the school day to review classroom expectations, identify situations that might pose problems during the day, and discuss possible coping strategies. Therapists should assist teachers who deal with extremely anxious children by reviewing the rationale and basic procedures of common techniques such as thought stopping and relaxation training. During these daily check-ins, the teacher might remind and encourage the child to use these techniques.

The teacher may intervene in other ways. Some sexually abused children indiscriminately discuss details of their victimization with schoolmates or in front of the entire class. The teacher should learn to curtail these discussions quickly and then talk privately with the child about the most appropriate times and contexts for such discussions. Teachers should encourage maltreated children to participate in school activities and follow a regular classroom routine. These activities will demonstrate to these children that they still can function and cope with the daily demands of life, despite their abuse or neglect. Excessive sympathy by the teacher often results in he or she placing few demands upon the child, which just reinforces the child's feelings of low self-esteem, helplessness, and inadequacy and the pattern of underachievement or behavioral problems.

By maintaining regular contact with the teacher, the therapist gains valuable information about the child's functioning and whether changes that might be necessary in the treatment plan to better suit the child's needs (e.g., slowing the pace of introducing abuse-related stimuli in treatment sessions). The teacher should alert the therapist to special circumstances or events in school that may be stressful to the child, such as the initiation of a sex education program in the classroom. The therapist who is alerted to such an event may raise the issue in therapy and help prepare the child. The therapist and teacher should collaboratively develop an intervention plan for use in the classroom if, for instance, the sexually abused child begins to feel anxious and distressed during sex education programs.

To maintain this high degree of cooperation, contact between the therapist and teachers should be regular and frequent (i.e., weekly). This contact is especially important for those children who present serious problems in the classroom. Many whose behavior is out of control are reassured when they know that the therapist and teacher talk with one another regularly.

For example, 10-year-old Bob (whose Rorschach responses we described in Chapter 4) was aware that his therapist would call his teacher at the same time on the same day every week. Bob derived a great deal of comfort and security from the knowledge that two significant adults were communicating openly and frequently about his welfare. He realized that they were working together to help him. This was the first time Bob had adults in his life who worked together as a team and showed enough commitment to take the time to talk with each other about him predictably and consistently. He always asked his teacher just after the scheduled phone call whether she had talked to the therapist, and he asked the same of the therapist in their weekly sessions. Bob appeared visibly relieved when assured by both that they had indeed talked with each other about him, even if part of their discussion had been devoted to some of Bob's negative behavior.

Finally, teachers often have ongoing contact with the child's parents. The therapist and teacher should ensure that they are providing the parents with consistent information and suggestions. Some parents are extremely difficult to deal with. In such cases, the therapist might be able to provide the teacher with ideas about how to best handle these interactions.

WORKING WITH CHILD WELFARE PERSONNEL AND THE LEGAL SYSTEM

Although child welfare workers and lawyers do not have the same frequent contact with a maltreated child that parents, foster parents, other caregivers, and teachers do, their involvement can have a powerful impact on the child's life. Many maltreated children and their families have contact with child protective services at some time during the children's growing years. These contacts may arise through investigation of reports of abuse and neglect, provision of support to children and families, or removal of children from their families under child protection legislation. Any therapist involved in clinical work with maltreated youngsters and their families will need to work with additional professionals to optimize the benefits to children.

An important role therapists play in the child welfare system is that of advocate for their young clients and their families. A child welfare worker will usually have to make a number of decisions that have a profound effect on a child's life. Should the child remain in care or be returned to the family? Is the child a suitable candidate for adoption? The therapist, with detailed knowledge of the child, can provide the child welfare worker with valuable information and opinions about these and other issues, especially if the therapist has known the child for a long time. For a child who has gone through multiple foster homes and seen a parade of child welfare workers come and go over the years, the therapist may be one of the most consistent figures in the child's life and can therefore play an especially important advocacy role.

There are other areas in which therapists can be advocates for their child clients. The therapist must notify the child welfare worker about any significant concerns regarding the child's safety. We mentioned earlier that participating in therapy may elicit children's anger, which in turn may place them at risk if their parents are unprepared to cope with this anger. Therapists should thoroughly familiarize themselves with their jurisdiction's legal statutes concerning abuse and neglect, as well as reporting requirements and protocols. They may also have to advocate for the provision of other services, such as in-home teaching of parenting. The therapist will soon encounter some of the broader systemic obstacles that impede children's recovery (e.g., long court delays, scattered and limited resources for parents). Although advocating on a case-by-case basis is necessary, therapists must remember that some of these larger problems will be solved only by concerted action and widespread pressure for change.

Therapists must expect that child welfare workers and lawyers will seek their opinion and should make themselves available for consultation by promptly returning phone calls and providing timely, concise reports. Excessively lengthy reports replete with technical jargon usually are not useful. Furthermore, therapists' reports in which the limitations of the report pertaining to the conclusions are openly acknowledged and a balanced perspective on a case is maintained are usually better received and more highly regarded by other professionals, as well as the courts. Although some professionals may take exception to others' opinions that do not confirm their beliefs, we encourage therapists to state their opinions honestly and remember that in many cases there are no easy or clear-cut answers. Rather than offering an unequivocal opinion that may not be supported by the data, therapists instead should describe the advantages and disadvantages of a particular course of action. Such an approach may also alleviate the anxiety of therapists who feel a sense of discomfort at becoming an agent of the courts or of the child welfare system. Therapists must realize that although they may have some specialized knowledge about a child, they do not have all the answers and that others also have useful and important information. This realization may help novice therapists who often believe they must provide an unequivocal opinion or recommendation to a court and that the entire responsibility for decision making rests with them.

The therapist's close involvement with child welfare workers and the courts may provoke considerable anxiety or resistance in some abusive and neglectful families. The latter may feel threatened by disclosing information to the therapist. This issue should be addressed before therapy begins. The therapist should inform parents clearly of the limits of confidentiality and the conditions that would compel the therapist to contact child welfare authorities without the family's permission. Parents and therapists should discuss other situations in which information will be shared and negotiate the manner in which it will be done. Child welfare workers should be included in these discussions at some point so that all relevant parties can reach an agreement. Despite this preparation, therapists must realize that some parents may refuse to bring themselves or their children back to therapy after the therapist has shared what parents consider to be damaging information with child welfare authorities or the courts. If the child involved is old enough, the therapist should discuss with her or him the fact that the therapist will be meeting with a child welfare worker. This discussion affords an opportunity for them to talk about the child's progress in therapy, the remaining issues that need to be addressed, and any recommendations to the child and family about intervention. We have found that alerting the child to these meetings often provides a greater focus for discussions between child and therapist. Sometimes children who are reluctant to speak with a child welfare worker will express their opinions in no uncertain terms to their therapists about such issues as the possibility of returning home. The child may be more motivated to express his or her opinions about these matters if the therapist expresses a willingness to act as spokesperson for the child in settings such as case conferences or court hearings where the child will not be present, even if the therapist's opinions are different from those of the child. The therapist must be honest in identifying any areas of disagreement with the child concerning these issues. Although the child may be quite upset with, for example, the therapist's decision to recommend that the child not return home, such disagreement will often provoke even more discussion that facilitates the child's active examination and consideration of these issues.

Convening regular case conferences is a good way to ensure open communication with child welfare workers and others. A case manager, typically the child welfare worker, should be appointed for particularly complex cases. One duty of the case manager is to facilitate a coordinated approach to intervention and delivery of services, including such items as scheduling and arranging case conferences.

In our work, we quickly learned that we had to devote significant time to communicating with child welfare workers and collaterals such as teachers or other therapists when we began to work with them. Our subsequent experiences have reinforced our initial impression that contact with collaterals is time consuming and often imposes many demands upon therapists. However, it is critically important. Therapists who believe they can work in total isolation from others and confine all their efforts to a weekly 50-minute session are missing the mark. Although clinicians must pay particular attention to many aspects of the actual therapy with their young clients, they must not lose sight of the fact that other individuals, such as natural parents, foster parents, teachers, and child welfare workers, often have as much or even greater influence upon a child. It is only by recognizing the significance of these people and their potential role as allies and by incorporating them into the treatment program that we can maximize the benefits of psychotherapy. This notion is well articulated by Cicchetti and Toth (1995): "Therapy with a maltreated child cannot be limited to the confines of the playroom, but must transcend the safety of the office to confront and impact the factors that may continue to assault the child in his or her daily life" (p. 557).

SEVEN

The Therapeutic Relationship

Peter was an 11-year-old boy who was referred to a therapist because he had been sexually abused by his stepfather from the ages of 7 to 9. When he was 10 years old, Peter disclosed to his mother that he and his stepfather had engaged in numerous episodes of oral sex and mutual masturbation and had viewed pornographic videos together. He was referred to therapy because of his preoccupation with sexual matters. Peter had begun to tell his mother that he was bothered by frequent sexual fantasies, including having sexual intercourse with other children and babies. There also had been several occasions when he initiated oral sex with younger children. Peter refused to complete any academic work and was in danger of failing in school that year. He was defiant and oppositional with his teacher and his mother. The latter was becoming increasingly frustrated with her inability to manage Peter's behavior. He began to associate with adolescent boys who had an unsavory reputation in the community, stayed out late at night, and began to lie and engage in petty theft.

Initially Peter was assessed by another clinician who had referred him to therapy because she did not believe she had the skills to help this youngster and his mother. When the second therapist introduced himself in the waiting room, Peter avoided all eye contact and reluctantly and weakly shook the therapist's hand. He agreed to accompany the therapist to his office but remained 10 feet behind as they walked down the hall.

For the first 30 minutes of the meeting, Peter responded to all inquiries with one- or two-word answers. For most of the time, he either looked at his watch or cradled his head in his arms and periodically shut his eyes. He explained to the therapist that he was "sleepy," since he had slept at a friend's home the night before the appointment and had not gotten much sleep. He claimed he did not know whether he had any problems to address in therapy and on several occasions asked if he could "go now." Overall, Peter conveyed an attitude of indifference to the therapist and to the possibility of actually receiving any assistance for his serious problems. After an hour with this seemingly unresponsive youngster, the therapist felt a certain degree of frustration about Peter's lack of interest in his efforts to help the boy and his own inability to form any connection with the youngster. Also, the therapist felt he had done "all the work" and was exhausted by the end of the hour. He looked forward to the next session with Peter with some anxiety and trepidation.

Unfortunately, this kind of experience is not uncommon for therapists who treat maltreated children. It occurs especially with children who have been exposed to severe and longstanding abuse and neglect and who now manifest some of the serious developmental effects described in Chapter 1. For example, a close reading of Peter's assessment report prepared by the first clinician revealed that besides sexually assaulting him, his stepfather had met none of Peter's needs for nurturance and attention from a paternal figure. His mother reported to the first clinician that Peter had "chosen" this man, an acquaintance of the family, as his father when he was 6 years old. Peter had started to call the man Dad before he and Peter's mother began to date. As a young boy and even before meeting his future stepfather, Peter had talked incessantly about wanting a dad with whom he could "do sports stuff." The only time his stepfather gave him any attention, however, was during the sexual assaults. The assessment also indicated that Peter blamed his mother for not having known about these assaults and for not protecting him. His mistrust of her was compounded when she sought employment outside their community immediately after his disclosure, leaving him for several weeks with two alcoholic caretakers. In subsequent discussions with Peter's therapist, his mother revealed she had been overwhelmed by the demands of single parenting. She had felt depressed for much of her son's infancy and toddlerhood. She described parenting in these early years as "going through the motions" and acknowledged that she frequently rejected Peter's attempts to obtain her attention and affection. On occasion she would hit him or angrily rebuff his efforts to interact. Given this history and experience with others, why would a youngster like Peter put himself in the vulnerable position of becoming close to someone, especially an adult male? Why would he want to talk to a therapist, or anyone, about embarrassing problems such as his sexual behavior and fantasies when others had been so unhelpful in the past?

Let us now consider another 11-year-old boy, Derek. He had also been referred to the therapist after assessment by another clinician.

Derek had been sexually assaulted once by an adolescent male baby sitter who lived next door. The day after he had been abused, Derek disclosed this episode to his parents, who in turn quickly notified the police. Derek provided a clear disclosure to the police. When confronted, the adolescent baby sitter quickly admitted his guilt. Throughout the whole episode, Derek had the full support of his parents.

Derek was referred to a therapist because of some anxiety-related symptoms, including nightmares and intrusive memories of the assault. Although he appeared somewhat anxious in the therapist's waiting room, Derek readily shook his hand. Derek accompanied the therapist to his office without any undue hesitation or reluctance, walking beside the therapist and chatting about how he had been to the same hospital several years before after falling off a bike.

In this initial interview, Derek readily responded to the therapist's questions, maintained good eye contact, and displayed a wide range of affects, including his sadness about having been assaulted by this older boy who, in the past, had been kind to him. He quickly identified his recurrent nightmares as the primary problem he wanted to address and was enthusiastic about returning for another appointment to begin work on this problem.

Before this isolated assault, Derek had had the good fortune of living in a family in which he was not maltreated and in which the parents consistently afforded him excellent care. Given this history, Derek entered therapy with the expectation that the therapist, like everyone else in his life, would treat him respectfully. He expected the therapist would provide the help and support he needed at this time. Although he was somewhat nervous at the beginning of the interview, his anxiety soon abated after the therapist provided a clear description of his role and of the therapeutic process. After a short course of therapy, Derek's frightening dreams and intrusive memories disappeared. Although Derek and the therapist established a positive therapeutic alliance in the first session, much of the intervention focused upon providing the boy with cognitive–behavioral strategies to cope with his symptoms. In contrast, therapy with Peter was a long and sometimes arduous process. A significant emphasis was placed upon Peter's relationship with the therapist to counteract his longstanding feelings of mistrust and betrayal by others.

These two boys and their initial presentations in therapy illustrate the two major perspectives on the relationship of child and clinician in child therapy as described by Shirk and Saiz (1992). As we reported in Chapter 5, the therapeutic relationship can be used as a medium for change with some child clients. Certain relationship qualities, such as the therapist's unconditional regard and acceptance of the child, are seen as the primary variables that promote change. We also proposed that interactions between the therapist and the maltreated child offer the therapist many opportunities to facilitate the child's growth, especially to counteract negative internal working models of the others and self. However, we posited that an exclusive focus upon the therapeutic relationship is usually insufficient and a number of other intervention strategies must be implemented.

In the other perspective on the relationship in child therapy, the use of the relationship as a means to an end is emphasized (Shirk & Saiz, 1992). In this conceptualization, the child's positive feelings for the therapist allow the child to accept the therapist as someone who will assist in resolving emotional or behavioral difficulties. The relationship itself is not a curative agent; instead, it promotes the child's participation and collaboration in specific therapeutic tasks or interventions. Derek's progress in therapy exemplifies the establishment of such a therapeutic alliance. His positive feelings toward the therapist and the therapeutic process enabled him to quickly and actively learn and adopt some cognitive–behavioral strategies that ultimately reduced his anxiety and alleviated his distress. The therapist did not have to use different facets of the therapeutic relationship to help this young boy, as he did with Peter.

This chapter is divided into two major sections. In the first, we review and describe different strategies that may be used to engage children in the psychotherapeutic process, including those who form a therapeutic relationship with relative ease. We also discuss engagement strategies for children whose abilities to establish and maintain relationships have been deleteriously and significantly affected by maltreatment. In the second section, we describe aspects of the therapeutic relationship for use in the middle phase of therapy, especially in remediating the effects of insecure attachments and negative internal working models.

ENGAGEMENT PHASE OF THERAPY

Orienting the Child to the Purpose, Process, and Structure of Therapy Sessions

The therapist must orient every child to the therapeutic environment and to the purposes and process of therapy. This orientation is necessary to help the child form a therapeutic alliance with the therapist so that the work of therapy can proceed: the child and therapist must reach some agreement or consensus about the reasons for therapy sessions and how they will be conducted.

In Chapter 4 we described strategies to orient the child to the assessment process. The clinician may have already done an evaluation of a particular child who is now beginning treatment and may have reviewed the assessment results with the child and family. In the first therapy session, the therapist should briefly review this information. The therapist should reiterate the consensus reached in the feedback session regarding the youngster's participation in treatment and the goals to be addressed in this process.

When a therapist is beginning therapy with children who have been assessed by other clinicians and whom they are meeting for the first time, the therapist should ask the child why he or she was brought to see the therapist, who should show empathy with the child's fear or anger about attending therapy. The therapist should explore and clarify any of the child's fantasies about participating in therapy and quickly correct them to alleviate anxiety. It is well worth the time involved to review the initial assessment results with the child to establish an agreement about the child's participation in treatment. As we advocated in Chapter 4, the therapist should clearly and directly inform the child that he or she knows the child has been maltreated and that the maltreatment is one of the primary reasons for the child's participation in therapy. Besides setting expectations for the work of therapy, the therapist who talks directly about the child's victimization conveys an expectation that the child will eventually be able to handle this topic and begins to desensitize the youngster. This direct account of why the child was referred to therapy serves to counter his or her expectation that adults will be dishonest.

What might the therapist say to the child about the purpose of therapy? We believe the child requires a clear and simple explanation of why he or she has been brought to see the therapist. The explanation might be something like "I help kids figure out how they feel about being beaten up by their dad [or whatever expression may be appropriate to the specific form of maltreatment] and what they think about it. Sometimes kids feel really upset or mixed up about what had happened to them. I try to help them think of other ways of letting out their feelings about what happened." Of course, the language must be appropriate to the child's developmental age. The therapist might refer to some of the child's specific difficulties as potential targets of intervention. The therapist must be prudent not to give any false reassurances, such as saying that therapy will make the youngster "forget" the maltreatment. Children should be reassured that talking about these matters is often difficult, even for adults, and that the therapist understands this anxiety and will not force the child to deal with material before he or she feels ready. The therapist should inform the child that he or she has many different ways of helping children "get out" their feelings and thoughts about their experiences in safe ways. Ultimately, the child has control over what is shared with the therapist. Such statements convey respect for the child's need to get to know the therapist better and to feel a measure of safety in the therapist's presence, thereby reassuring an anxious or frightened child. Telling a child that the therapist sees other children who have gone through similar experiences also reduces the sense of isolation and stigmatization many maltreated children feel.

Besides orienting the child to therapy's purpose, the therapist must talk with the child about the process and structure of therapy. Even young children can benefit from brief and simple explanations of what therapy is about; that is, about the process. For those who will be participating in therapy in which a heavy emphasis is placed upon direct verbalization, a brief rationale of the benefits of talking about the maltreatment should be given. A child might be told that talking provides alternate means to expressing feelings than acting them out in ways that cause the child and others trouble. Talking about the maltreatment gives children the opportunity to think differently about what has happened to them, such as reformulating the belief that they were responsible for their victimization. The therapist should tell the child he or she may use whatever words or terminology the child prefers in therapy and also give the child permission to tell the therapist he or she is not yet ready to talk about or deal with certain topics. Children who will be participating in more indirect methods of intervention, such as play therapy, deserve a simple explanation of this approach. For example, they might be told, "Sometimes the way kids play tells us what's bothering them. Playing also helps us think of some new ways you can use to feel better about what happened to you."

Besides setting the expectation that there is work to be done in therapy, these brief descriptions alleviate a child's anxiety about the therapeutic process. In Chapter 4 we described how some sexually or physically abused children expect similar treatment from a therapist. They deserve and require honest explanations of the treatment process, in particular that the therapist will treat them with the respect and dignity they and all children deserve. The therapist must be especially sensitive to situations or interventions that may replicate some aspects of the original maltreatment, being sure to draw the distinction for the child. For example, the therapist may need to reassure the child that talking about sexual matters behind closed doors with an adult will not be the initial stage of a process in which the child will be sexually abused. Drawing this distinction not only attenuates the child's anxiety but starts modifying his or her internal working models of others in a more positive direction, that is, "Not everyone is going to hurt me."

The therapist must also educate the child about the structure of the sessions. Again, these discussions serve to allay the child's anticipatory anxiety and fears about treatment by providing a sense of predictability about what will happen from session to session. This approach may be particularly reassuring for those anxious children who have lived in unpredictable, chaotic environments, where they developed the belief that adults are untrustworthy, unreliable figures. Although the therapist's actual actions and behavior are critical in establishing and maintaining predictability, the therapist should begin the process in the first session by explaining the structure of therapy (e.g., locale, duration of sessions), as already discussed in Chapter 4.

The child must be informed about the therapist's contact with parents or caregivers. The child should be told that the therapist will meet regularly with these individuals to assist them in helping the child and to inform them of the child's therapy progress. Also, the therapist might say that although he or she will not disclose information without notifying the child first, there will be limits on confidentiality. For example, the therapist will not keep secrets about someone hurting the child. Besides talking with them privately, the therapist might have the child present during discussions with parents about the youngster's progress.

Regularity, Consistency, and Safety in the Therapy Sessions and Therapeutic Relationship

Many maltreated children have internal working models of other people as inconsistent, unreliable, and dangerous individuals. These models may prove to be detriments to the child's participation in therapy. Furthermore, the child who believes the therapist cannot keep him or her safe from acting out overwhelming feelings will be reluctant to address salient aspects of the maltreatment. "Opening up" may overwhelm a child's fragile defenses and threaten his or her precarious ego controls, placing the child at higher risk for expressing feelings maladaptively. There might be some regression in the child's behavior (e.g., enuresis, physical aggression), or the child might begin complaining of being bothered by intrusive thoughts or nightmares as he or she is flooded with feelings and memories associated with the victimization. It will be safer to avoid these issues and not deal with them if the child has little confidence in the adult's ability to limit this acting out.

Promoting Predictability and Safety

The therapist can begin developing an atmosphere of predictability and safety in many different ways. Sessions should be scheduled at the same time and day(s) during the week and should use the same therapy room or playroom, along with the same toys and/or equipment. Switching from one office to another or having different toys available from week to week may erode any trust that the child is beginning to develop in the therapist. The clinician might set up a special box or folder to hold the child's art or other therapy productions. Taking the holder out at approximately the same time in each session and then putting it in its special place at the end of the session reinforces constancy and predictability. The therapy session may include other rituals that serve the same purpose. Some children enjoy and experience reassurance from the same ritual greeting every week, such as a special handshake (Friedrich, 1990). Others hide under a table in the waiting room while the therapist feigns ignorance about their whereabouts and then expresses happiness and pleasure when "finding" the child. Yet other children may have to play the same game or engage in the same activity at the beginning or end of each session. These opening and closing rituals provide predictability and regularity and also serve as concrete markers or cues for different aspects of the child and therapist's participation in the therapy session. For example, playing a simple board game like checkers may serve as the stimulus to discuss the past week. Closing rituals may include putting away the toys and equipment, shutting off the lights, and closing the door. These actions may come to symbolize the child's attempt to contain the material elicited and processed in that particular therapy session; they also allow the child to move on to the routine demands and tasks of everyday life.

The therapist may impose similar regularity and predictability on other aspects of the relationship with the child. Cancellations or changes in appointment times should be avoided as much as possible. Such changes may elicit feelings of disappointment or rage in the child. These extreme reactions are the result of the child's perception that people are again treating him or her unreliably. Since some changes or cancellations are unavoidable, the therapist should clearly explain the reasons and emphasize that they have nothing to do with the therapist's feelings for the youngster. A therapist's extended vacation may prove to be a particularly difficult problem for children who require preparation for any scheduling change. To alleviate a child's anxiety stemming from the belief that he or she will never see the therapist again, the therapist might give the child a copy of a calendar on which the date of the next therapy session is clearly identified. Showing the child maps of the therapist's intended destination also may attenuate the child's distress and confusion about the therapist's whereabouts. These strategies begin to alleviate the child's fear that the therapist might reject or forget the youngster. They also promote the internalization of the mental representation of the therapist as a reliable and consistent figure.

Promoting Object Constancy

Frequently, maltreated children have great difficulty in maintaining an image of the therapist or even the therapy room in their minds (i.e., "object constancy"). They believe they will never see the therapist again or that the therapist will change significantly in personality or behavior from one session to another. There are several concrete strategies a therapist can employ to help children cope with this kind of anxiety generated between weekly sessions. A calendar may be used to show the child not only the date of therapist's return from an extended vacation but also the date of the next weekly session. An appointment slip with the therapist's and child's names on it will serve the same purpose; the child takes the slip home as a reminder that another appointment is scheduled. Some children benefit by taking home a small object as a "souvenir" of the therapist and the therapy sessions. They might then bring back the object, such as a pencil, to the next session and exchange it for another small token. It is unwise to allow the child to take home toys from the therapy room, particularly if the toy is used by other child clients regularly or if the toy is associated with significant issues or feelings for the child. In the latter situation, bringing the toy home may result in an escalation of anxiety or acting out at home. The toy should be left in the therapy room so that these feelings will be contained. Another strategy we have used is to have photographs taken of ourselves and the child together. The child may take the photograph home as a concrete reminder of the relationship and its importance to each participant. Some children are reassured by receiving pictures of their name drawn in fancy letters by the therapist. Others may be reassured by doing a drawing that they put on the therapist's wall so the therapist will be reminded of the child during the week.

The therapist might help parents or caregivers use similar techniques with children who have problems with object constancy. Joan, an 8-year-old girl, had been removed from her mother's care because of psychological maltreatment, especially verbal abuse, neglect, and frequent episodes during which she was abandoned for prolonged periods and left to fend for herself. After being placed in foster care and beginning school, Joan's behavior in the classroom began to undergo a notable deterioration near the end of each school day: she would become defiant and oppositional and would have great difficulty in concentrating on academic tasks. She subsequently revealed to her therapist that she was afraid her foster mother would not pick her up at the end of the school day as she had promised. The child worried even though the foster mother had never failed to do so and in fact usually arrived a few minutes before dismissal. Joan believed that her foster mother might "forget about me." She also thought her foster mother's personality might change drastically between the morning and the end of the school day, so that she would abuse Joan later, in the school yard. To promote and consolidate Joan's belief that her foster mother would be reliable, predictable, and caring, the therapist suggested she have a picture taken of the two of them engaged in a positive activity. The foster mother subsequently arranged for such a photograph, and Joan's teacher permitted her to tape it prominently on her desk. The therapist instructed Joan to look at the picture each time she began to feel worried about her foster mother's commitment. This strategy resulted in a significant decrease in Joan's anxiety. Young children require such concrete cues and reminders so that these more abstract concepts will become relevant and meaningful.

Dealing with Provocative Behavior

Early in therapy, some maltreated children may begin to test whether the sessions and the therapist will provide them with a measure of safety and protection. Is the therapist someone who will protect the child from acting out strong feelings in provocative, dangerous, and unhealthy ways? Is the therapist someone who will react to provocations with firm yet appropriate responses? Sometimes telling children about basic rules (e.g., "We aren't allowed to hurt each other or break anything in the room") diminishes their anxiety about being permitted to act out strong feelings and urges in whatever way they desire. However, providing children with an elaborate set of rules may constitute a challenge to those who need to test the therapist. Interactions characterized primarily by contention and conflict in the engagement phase detract from the therapist's efforts to form a therapeutic alliance. It is usually more beneficial to lay down a minimum of rules and then deal with further incidents and infractions as they arise.

Children use varied and often creative ways to address these questions. Some children engage in daredevil and reckless behavior, such as climbing up the shelves of the play therapy room. When confronted with this behavior, the therapist should quickly and firmly insist that the child stop it, pointing out the potential dangers to the child's safety and emphasizing that the therapist does not want the child to be hurt. The therapist should show a willingness to take the steps necessary to ensure the child's safety. Alternate behavior can then be suggested, such as helping the child stand on a chair to reach for a toy on an upper shelf. Many of these children have never had parents or caregivers who were this solicitous about their welfare. The therapist's actions are concrete demonstrations of caring and commitment. Still other children become physically aggressive or try to engage therapists in sexual behavior to determine whether the therapist will physically or sexually abuse them. Although we discuss this issue in more depth in the second half of this chapter, it is important to note here that the therapist should curtail any such behavior quickly and in a straightforward and matter-of-fact way.

Physical Contact with Abused and Neglected Children

The therapist should exercise considerable caution in touching an abused or maltreated child. Such a gesture, although well intended, might be misinterpreted by the child as a sexual advance or physical threat. Many maltreated children are extraordinarily sensitive to any form of touching by an adult because of their past histories. Young sexual-abuse victims who have experienced longstanding sexual molestation may not be able to discriminate between sexual and nonsexual touching. On the other hand, some children crave physical contact with the therapist because of their chronic histories of psychological and emotional neglect. In the case of the child deprived of physical affection, the therapist must introduce other forms of positive interaction. The child's indiscriminate physical contact must be limited, but a hug at the beginning and closing of the therapy session may be allowed. By failing to curtail this interpersonal style, the therapist places the child at risk for exploitation from adults who prey upon children who crave a great deal of attention from others.

Some sexually abused children may have learned to gain attention and affection from others primarily through sexual means, and they may make direct sexual advances to the therapist. These advances must be quickly curtailed. They may also be a test of the therapist's boundaries and whether he or she would respond sexually to the child (Van de Putte, 1995). Furthermore, allowing this behavior will just escalate the child's anxiety and may place the therapist in jeopardy; he or she may be accused of improper conduct. The therapist should explain that he or she knows the child had a relationship with an adult involving sexual activity and also that sexual feelings in general are normal. However, the therapist must be emphatic in asserting that the relationship between the child and the therapist will not include this kind of contact. In this new relationship, they are to communicate by means of talking and playing; the child should understand the he or she has no need to use sexual behavior to establish a nurturing relationship with an adult. The sexualized child should be taught more appropriate ways of physical contact, such as a handshake. It is also well to be aware that the child's sexualized behavior often generates intense feelings and reactions in the therapist. Chapter 12 contains a review of the strategies available to therapists in coping with their own emotions and issues elicited by this demanding and difficult clinical work.

Countering Regressive Behavior

During the engagement phase, some maltreated children begin to recount many details of their victimization. For some children, talking about their victimization may be intensely frightening; they are flooded with painful memories and feelings that threaten to overwhelm their fragile defenses. Also, their symptoms may increase or they may begin to show even more regressive behavior. Although we discuss this issue in more detail in Chapter 8, it is important to state here that the therapist must structure sessions tightly and control their pace to ensure that the child is not overwhelmed. For example, the therapist should restrict these discussions to a limited amount of time in each session and request that the child deal with only one memory or issue per discussion. The remainder of the session should be devoted to less intense activities such as nondirective play (James, 1994).

Ten minutes or so should be reserved before the session's end to ensure the child is behaving more maturely. It is not desirable, for instance, to have a child who has been acting like an infant and demanding feedings from a baby bottle to leave the session in that state and then have to cope with classroom demands. The therapist might tell the child that that part of the session is over and that the play must now stop. At the same time, more mature behavior can be encouraged, such as having the child help clean up the playroom. The therapist and child might discuss the demands to be faced in the next several hours and how these demands can be best met. Allowing a child to leave a session in a highly regressed or distressed state does that child a real disservice. There must be some closure on each therapy session to promote the child's adaptive functioning in the everyday world. Again, closing rituals help by symbolically containing the sensitive and painful therapeutic material elicited in the session. For example, as described earlier, the child might place his or her art productions in a special folder and "pack it away" until the next session.

Being Empathic about the Child's Affective Expression

By articulating an understanding of the child's feelings, the therapist begins modifying the child's expectation that others will be insensitive and unaware of his or her internal states. The therapist might start this process in the first session. Because of various factors, including the child's fears and expectations of being maltreated by the therapist, the child may seem highly anxious during the first several sessions. By commenting simply and directly about the child's anxiety (e.g., "It's scary when you think that you might have to talk about what happened to you") and explaining the reasons for therapy and what will transpire during sessions, the therapist not only clarifies what might be expected of therapy; he or she also demonstrates sensitivity to the child's fears and anxiety. Other types of therapist behavior reinforce an understanding and appreciation of the child's plight. With a highly anxious, maltreated child, the therapist might leave the office or playroom door ajar so that the child feels a sense of safety (i.e., the child feels he or she can readily escape or that others outside will be able to monitor therapist and child interaction to ensure the child's safety). We have already talked about maintaining appropriate physical distance from the child so as not to elicit even more anxiety about possible further physical or sexual abuse. Care should be taken to ensure that the therapist does not "corner" or tower over the youngster. Such actions merely reinforce the child's sense of vulnerability and powerlessness. Having a supportive adult or parent present for the initial therapy sessions also allows the child to relax. The other adult may then be gradually permitted to leave the room, as the child begins to feel more comfortable in the therapist's presence.

Even while setting limits on a child's physically aggressive or sexually inappropriate behavior, the therapist may still convey an understanding of the child's internal world. The key is to validate the child's underlying affects while assisting him or her to develop more appropriate ways of expressing these feelings. For example, the therapist might comment about the normalcy of the intense rage and anger in the maltreated child who attempts to break toys while talking about his or her physical abuse. At the same time, the therapist must quickly intervene to stop this destructive behavior and propose other ways to ventilate the rage. Likewise, with a sexually abused child, the therapist should convey the notion that sexual feelings are normal and that the child is not perverted or depraved. Concurrently, firm and consistent limits should be placed upon the inappropriate expression of the sexual feelings. The child can then begin to think of the therapist as someone who not only accepts his or her feelings but also cares enough to ensure that the child will not act them out harmfully or inappropriately. As well, the therapist begins to introduce coping mechanisms that promote the child's self-regulation of behavior and emotion.

The Role of Play in the Engagement Phase

For children who are particularly frightened of therapy or the therapeutic relationship, play often provides a medium through which they can begin to communicate with and relate to the therapist. The second half of this chapter is devoted to a more detailed discussion of the use of the therapeutic relationship with these avoidant children. However, we think it is appropriate to make several comments here about the use of play in the engagement phase.

Nonverbal interactions may help the child become more comfortable with the therapist. Rather than subjecting the child to countless questions and inquiries, the therapist should follow the child's lead and pace during these play activities. By mirroring the child's body language and/or vocal quality, the therapist conveys his or her sensitivity to the child's feelings. The therapist demonstrates interest in the child and encourages the development of verbal expression by reflecting or paraphrasing the child's statements (Brady & Friedrich, 1982). Being allowed the choice of play activities or materials gives the child a sense of control over what happens during therapy sessions, thereby increasing the child's sense of safety. Initially, children may choose activities in which they are confident they will meet with some success. Sometimes these activities may be characteristic of a much younger child's play; the youngster may expect that success is possible only with simple and unsophisticated materials and that failure is inevitable with anything more difficult. Although the therapist should allow this activity for a time, the child should gently be encouraged to move on to an activity that will challenge the child's abilities. However, the activity must be one that will bring the child some success. Also, there is a fine line between pushing a child too strenuously to the point of eliciting overwhelming anxiety and allowing a child to repeat endless activity. The latter does nothing to raise the child's self-esteem or make therapy a profitable or positive experience.

Let us return now to 11-year-old Peter, whom we mentioned at the beginning of this chapter.

> By the second session, the therapist and Peter agreed that he needed to come to therapy to work on some of his problems but that he needed the opportunity to get to know the therapist better before he would discuss or address these issues. Peter quite readily agreed to spend several sessions with the therapist in the playroom in order to "check out" what therapy would be like. During the first play therapy session, Peter played with large building blocks that much younger children typically use. He built extremely simple constructions and resisted suggestions to build anything more complicated. He eventually found a checkers game and commented that he was quite a good player. However, he refused the therapist's invitation to play the game but reluctantly agreed to do so in the next play therapy session. In fact, Peter was quite an astute player, but he made several comments about making "dumb moves" and stated several times that he knew he was going to lose. The therapist empathized with his fears of losing and feelings of inadequacy, which resulted in a more extended discussion of Peter's concerns that everyone thought he was "stupid." He felt that his poor school performance was incontrovertible proof of his low intelligence.
>
> In the third play therapy session, the therapist suggested they play Chinese checkers, a game with which Peter was unfamiliar. However, Peter immediately insisted that he would never be able to learn the game. He agreed that, at a minimum, he would listen to the therapist's explanations and then decide whether he wanted to play. Although still anxious, he finally agreed to play a game. Despite losing, Peter made a number of good moves. The therapist provided Peter with a great deal of reinforcement about how quickly Peter caught on to the game and cited some of these moves as concrete evidence of his ability. Peter agreed to play a second game and in fact won, which left him obviously pleased.

These initial play sessions allowed Peter to begin establishing a therapeutic alliance in which he felt safe, accepted, and validated. Rather than laughing at his initial attempts to play the new game, the therapist gave gentle encouragement and instruction that resulted in some success. Peter encountered his first successes in the playroom, which made his participation in therapy more appealing. Furthermore, Peter actually had some fun with this adult, which reinforced the attraction of the therapist and the therapy process for this young boy. The therapist's sensitivity to Peter's deep sense of insecurity and inadequacy and his permitting Peter some control over the play activities began to diminish Peter's expectation that adults, particularly men, would subject him to further abuse, humiliation, and degradation.

Teaching Neglected Children How to Play

As we have just mentioned, these initial play therapy sessions should be fun so as to encourage the child's interest in participating in therapy. Similarly, the child must experience some degree of success, even if it is with such simple activities as board games. Such successes counter feelings of stigmatization and personal failure that often accompany the beginning of the therapeutic process. However, we must note that some maltreated children encounter grave difficulty in succeeding with even simple play activities. Typically, these are children who have been subjected to great deprivation and neglect and have never learned how to play. When brought into the playroom, they are unimaginative, inhibited, confused, and unable to use toys or equipment purposefully. Rather than allowing the child to stand immobilized, thereby compounding his or her feelings of failure and inadequacy, the therapist must take the initiative and teach the child how to play. For example, the therapist may have to teach the child how to use paints, building blocks, or other simple materials. The therapist might model the activity and then gently encourage the child to begin participating in the activity along with the therapist. The therapist should reinforce the child's attempts to take some initiative in the play.

Over the years, we have formed the clinical impression that children who have been severely physically or psychologically neglected are often preoccupied with food. They frequently worry that they will not get sufficient food and engage in behavior like hyperphagia (increased food intake) and stealing and hoarding food. There is some support for this observation in the literature. Demb (1991) has identified a subsample of children in foster care because of parental substance abuse. Their foster mothers reported they had an excessive appetite for food. Furthermore, the consumption had a driven quality, and there was an apparent lack of satiety, as well as frequent eating to the point of gastric pain or vomiting if food intake was not externally limited. We wonder if food is equated with psychological nurturance for some children raised in environments characterized by emotional and physical deprivation. Food may be profitably incorporated into the treatment plan of severely deprived children. Small snacks at the beginning or end of each session in the early phase of treatment are often well received. Food serves as evidence that the therapist is sensitive to the child's needs and demonstrates the therapist's commitment to the youngster. Food may also bring clinical issues into prominence during sessions. For example, the child may devour the snack voraciously and angrily demand more. This behavior may be an opportunity for the therapist to articulate the child's anger, which is elicited when the youngster is "not getting enough" and his or her disappointment when the therapist cannot meet all of the child's massive needs.

Therapist as a "Secure Base"

Bowlby (1988a) argues that in psychotherapy, the therapist assumes the role of a secure attachment figure as the client begins to sense safety and predictability with the therapist and the therapeutic process. By inspiring trust in his or her availability and responsivity to clients, the therapist provides a secure base from which children can confidently explore their internal world, including their working models of others and the self. Sensing safety and feeling increasing confidence that the therapist will meet his or her needs for comfort and empathy, the maltreated child may now more readily raise and confront some more challenging and distressing issues. These issues include the child's distorted conceptions of the therapist, based upon the child's negative internal working models and other aspects of his or her victimization. The establishment of this secure base is similar to the notion of the therapeutic alliance. In each conceptualization, qualities of the relationship between child and therapist facilitate the child's active participation in treatment.

This task of promoting the therapist as a secure base often runs throughout the course of therapy. However, the therapist must pay particular attention to it in the first stage, using some of the strategies described above to begin engaging the child in the therapeutic relationship. The therapist must be aware that forming a relationship wherein the child can begin to feel a sense of safety, regularity, and commitment is often a slow and gradual process. There is no one intervention or therapeutic technique that suddenly turns these children around and dissolves the strong barriers of mistrust and avoidance they had developed over numerous years to protect themselves. James (1994) eloquently articulates this sentiment:

> Children who have learned not to trust adults and who are intimacy-avoidant may not show signs of relationship development with the therapist for many months. It is a fairly common occurrence in work with attachment disturbance that the clinician becomes suddenly, rather than gradually, aware that the child experiences sufficient relational support to begin deeper work. This sudden "opening up" may be understood as the child responding to specific clinical intervention or technique, rather than as the child having developed emotional readiness.

It is an error, though tempting, to consider such a clinical occurrence a "breakthrough." The phenomenon may appear to be an instant shift caused by a specific action or event: a wall of "resistance" that the child or therapist shatters, splits apart, or bursts through. The process leading to children being able to trust their therapist, allowing themselves to be vulnerable and revealing tender feelings can be likened to the slow, complex development of a critical mass of emotional safety, not a sudden breakthrough. (pp. 61–62)

If the child feels somewhat secure and safe with the therapist, the therapeutic relationship may deepen. It will then provide more examples of the child's maladaptive internal working models, other feelings and cognitions related to the maltreatment, and further opportunities for intervention.

MIDDLE PHASE OF THERAPY

This phase offers the therapist more opportunities to modify the child's internal working models of others and self. Here we discuss the use of the therapeutic relationship as a tool to help children who display a number of features of different attachment organizations. Our ideas and thoughts build upon an earlier paper (Pearce & Pezzot-Pearce, 1994) and are derived from some of the basic tenets and ideas of attachment theory.

We begin with a review of strategies that may be applied within the context of the therapeutic relationship to characteristics of an avoidant attachment organization. Then we discuss strategies to assist those youngsters with an ambivalent–resistant attachment organization. However, this distinction may be somewhat arbitrary, since there is considerable overlap in the characteristics of different attachment organizations. It is our impression that some older children manifest a mixture of characteristics, although much work is needed to determine the extent of such overlap. As well, strategies may have broad applicability to features of different attachment organizations that present problems. Because many strategies for avoidant or ambivalent–resistant children can be applied to youngsters with a controlling–disorganized classification, they will be integrated and identified in the discussions concerning avoidant and ambivalent–resistant children.

Children with an Avoidant Attachment Organization

These children fear further rejection or maltreatment from attachment figures and block information about their own feelings and emotions. We have seen children display elements of this avoidance in the therapeutic relationship. For example, a child may play quite independently, rarely inviting the therapist to join in the play. The therapist is on the sidelines, watching rather than participating. The child makes little eye contact and maintains considerable psychological distance. The child, expecting that the therapist will hurt, reject, or disappoint him or her as others have previously, will avoid interactions with the therapist as a protection from the consequences of a close relationship. Peter's indifference to the therapist in the initial sessions probably reflects this strategy. He did not want to become involved because his previous experiences with other people, especially his mother and stepfather, generated expectations that he would be hurt again and that others would not recognize or alleviate his distress. Peter also avoided acknowledging and expressing his intense and sometimes conflicting feelings, another primary characteristic of children with an avoidant pattern of attachment. In Chapter 8 we discuss in detail ways to help children identify and express their feelings.

The child may engage in other interactional patterns to avoid a truly reciprocal or close relationship with the therapist. By behaving in a very controlling, omnipotent fashion in therapy sessions, the child feels mastery and control over the interaction that is expected to result in even more maltreatment. This behavior and expectation are reflected in the process of therapy sessions wherein the child chooses the play materials and activities and the therapist is relegated to a minor role. Let us return to a description of some other early sessions in Peter's therapy that illustrate these patterns.

> After participating in several sessions, during which he insisted playing Chinese checkers (and winning many games, which probably facilitated engagement), Peter began to engage in dramatic play for several months. Peter's relationship with the therapist during these sessions reflected his reluctance to become engaged in a relationship marked by reciprocal interaction. Despite the therapist's request to become more involved in the play, Peter adamantly told the therapist that his role was to be the "audience." He was to sit quietly while Peter pretended he was "Superman" and provide him, on cue, with praise and approval for his strength and power. As Superman, Peter portrayed himself as a powerful figure who could fend off any kind of attacker. He placed much emphasis upon his physical prowess, rolling up his shirt sleeves, flexing his muscles, and pretending to pick up objects such as cars and buildings.
>
> Peter insisted upon enacting this play scenario and rigidly enforced the therapist's minimal involvement for many weeks. The therapeutic relationship underwent a significant change when Peter asked the therapist to play the role of the "bad guy." This play, which lasted for approximately 2 months, invariably began in each session with Peter telling the therapist to think of increasingly devious ways of abducting or hurting small, plastic animal figures. These figures were usually defenseless creatures like puppies or birds. As Superman, Peter "rescued" the animals from the therapist, who

always had to portray a menacing and dangerous figure. This play culminated in a session during which Peter introduced interpersonal disputes in the play as targets worthy of Superman's intervention. Once, Peter used small dolls and a doll house to enact a quarrel between a boy and his mother. As Superman, Peter intervened and essentially acted like a referee to help these two individuals resolve their dispute.

There are several important and salient aspects of Peter's play. The interaction with the therapist at the beginning of the play was minimal. As well, Peter placed the therapist on the periphery by maintaining strict control over what the therapist could do and say. Peter tried to control the interaction that he expected might lead to aversive or harmful consequences, which reflected elements of the controlling–punitive pattern displayed by some controlling–disorganized children. After engaging in this kind of play where he gained some control and mastery, Peter seemed to feel a greater sense of safety and security in the therapist's presence. He then began to involve the therapist more actively in the play, although Peter was still in charge and continued to protect himself from the therapist, who was the "bad guy." Finally, the play revealed Peter's need to master traumatic experiences. Rather than being the passive victim, he now saved others from physical dangers and, ultimately, took the initiative and solved difficult interpersonal problems. Typical play themes include the child's self-portrayal as a strong, powerful figure who can defeat all sorts of enemies and adversaries. In this play, which relies heavily upon defenses such as identification of the aggressor, the child does not have to worry about being hurt or rejected again. The youngster achieves a sense of mastery over environmental contingencies that are believed to lead to more hurt and pain.

To counteract the child's fear of establishing and maintaining a close therapeutic relationship, the therapist might use several strategies. First, the therapist must respect the child's reliance upon the defensive use of avoidance. Insisting prematurely that the child relate in an intimate way may lead to a rapid escalation of anxiety to the point where the child will engage in even more avoidance. Confronting the child too quickly with demands for intimacy also may result in a deterioration of his behavior. Feeling so threatened, the child may begin to be even more oppositional, defiant, or outrageous so as to alienate the therapist. In these initial sessions, the therapist must allow the child a large measure of choice over play materials and activities. If the therapist had insisted upon directing or controlling the play at this early stage, Peter probably would have felt threatened by this premature attempt to become close. In the past, closeness with another male, his stepfather, was associated with some disastrous consequences. By having a sense of control and safety, the youngster may begin to regard the therapist in a more positive light. Here is someone who understands the child's fear of intimacy and closeness. This person is willing to gradually establish a relationship in a manner that does not threaten to overwhelm the youngster with anxiety and fear. This may well be the start of the process whereby negative internal working models of others are modified.

As in the engagement stage, it is critically important for the therapist to follow through with any promises made to the child. This consistency demonstrates the therapist can be trusted. For example, in one early play session in which he pretended to be Superman, Peter wished aloud that he had a red cape. To show his trustworthiness and commitment, the therapist told Peter that he would bring some red cloth for a cape to the next session. When Peter entered the playroom the next week and found the cloth, he looked at the therapist and exclaimed, "You really did it!" Besides being a concrete demonstration of the therapist's commitment, this incident provided the therapist with an opportunity to comment to Peter that he seemed surprised that somebody would follow through with a promise. Peter agreed that he was indeed surprised. In response to inquiries about who had disappointed him in the past, Peter named his stepfather. Although unwilling to talk about the sexual assaults in this session, Peter told the therapist that before his stepfather and mother married, he had promised to participate in sports activities with Peter. However, his stepfather reneged on this promise. While recounting this incident, Peter looked and sounded sad. Although he would not pursue the matter any further, Peter quietly agreed with the therapist's statement about how sad and disappointed Peter must have felt. This was the first occasion when Peter could acknowledge his feelings of loss. It was followed in the months ahead with more direct discussions of these and other feelings. This episode started the process wherein the therapist began to help Peter develop more appropriate ways of expressing feelings (i.e., using words to communicate feelings of loss rather than other, more maladaptive strategies). The therapist's empathic response to these concerns was another demonstration that he was listening keenly to Peter and making a concentrated effort to understand what Peter was trying to say. The therapist's sensitivity and his follow-through with the promise to Peter the week before were two examples of many actions the therapist had to repeat to help this boy reformulate his expectations of others.

At this point, the child may be more tolerant of the therapist's participation in sessions and of his or her attempts to form some kind of relationship. Rather than taking the very nonintrusive and nondirective approach that characterized initial sessions, the therapist should try to become more involved and interactive, albeit gradually. The intent is to expose the child to increasingly larger doses of positive interaction to alleviate his or her fear of close relationships and subsequent avoidance of interaction. Becoming a more desirable person to the child may also restimulate the child's need for other relationships of a similar nature.

Some common play themes emerge that will offer further opportunities to reinforce the therapist's representation in the child's inner world as positive and helpful. The child may begin to nurture himself or herself: nursing on a baby bottle, feeding baby dolls, and taking care of sick or wounded animals or protecting them as Peter did from abusive and menacing adversaries are common play themes of maltreated children (Frazier & Levine, 1983; Mills & Allan, 1992). One notable aspect of this play is that the child is in control. The youngster assumes the role of the protector in the play, thereby gaining a vicarious sense of nurturance and gratification. The child cannot let the therapist nurture yet because of beliefs and expectations that adults are unresponsive, unreliable, and unwilling to care for children in this manner. This pattern may characterize the controlling–caregiving pattern of some controlling–disorganized children.

> After reenacting many episodes of protecting small animals from physical danger and solving interpersonal disputes, Peter began to have Superman care for and nurture individuals in other ways. As Superman, he hosted a birthday party for his "100-year-old grandma" to which the therapist was invited. Using toy food, Peter prepared a banquet for everyone. However, Peter made it clear that he still regarded the world as dangerous, and he could not relinquish his omnipotence. He pretended there were "wild animals" outside the house in which the birthday party was held and instructed the therapist to "act scared." He went out of the house on several occasions and calmed these animals with a mere glance and a few brief words of warning.

Peter was beginning to allow himself to relate more closely to others (exemplified by inviting the therapist and imaginary grandmother to the birthday party and feeding them). However, he still needed to control this interaction because he still regarded the world as dangerous and threatening. For children like Peter, relationships are characterized by ambivalence: the child longs for nurturance and attention but remains frightened about becoming too close and therefore more vulnerable.

The therapist began to give voice to these conflicting sentiments. In his role as a guest, the therapist stated he felt "really good" when people cooked wonderful foods for him (validating Peter's desire for nurturance). The therapist added that he felt "scared" by the presence of wild animals outside the home and wondered aloud whether he would be safe. He said that having someone like Superman to "take care of him" made him feel better. These comments empathized with Peter's fear of being hurt again and his desire for a strong, powerful figure who would protect him from harm. Verbally articulating or somehow identifying and expressing these feelings is an important component of treatment for the avoidant child who routinely disconnects from these affective states. By articulating them in the play, the therapist brings them into consciousness and provides an opportunity for the child to ultimately gain some control over their influence. Furthermore, talking about these conflicted feelings as if they belonged to someone else (i.e., the therapist's role as guest at the birthday party) was more tolerable to Peter. If the therapist had brought this material out of the metaphor in this early stage, he would have elicited too much pain and distress. Peter might have then avoided this play to protect himself from the anxiety generated by the therapist's direct interpretations. The therapist who expresses these conflicting feelings, either directly or via indirect metaphorical methods, is again modeling a more adaptive way of expressing them. This in turn promotes the child's growing ability to regulate his or her behavior and affects.

The therapist should not allow the child to continue to play the role of exclusive nurturer indefinitely. The therapist must initiate interaction that demonstrates goodwill and a willingness to meet some of the child's emotional and psychological needs. For example, the therapist might offer to prepare some food for the child who is feeding a baby doll. If the child seems comfortable with these relatively nonintrusive attempts to be more nurturing, the therapist may eventually offer to feed the baby. As we have commented, children may prepare elaborate meals for themselves and the therapist. Initially the child is in charge of providing this nurturance because of his or her minimal trust in the therapist's ability or willingness to care for the child this way. The therapist might begin taking a more active role by first offering a few menu suggestions; offering to prepare one or two dishes; and then preparing most, if not all, of the meal. It is served to the child, who is treated like an honored and valued guest. These strategies may be beneficially applied to children displaying a controlling–caregiving pattern. Their sense of responsibility for the therapist's welfare may be reflected in this symbolic play, wherein they nurture, feed, and generally take care of the therapist.

> Peter continued to host these birthday parties, for which he made all the preparations. After Peter assumed this exclusive role in several parties, the therapist suggested that he, as a guest, be allowed to bring one dish to the party in order to "help out," since Peter had so much work to do. Peter agreed with this plan and seemed pleased when the therapist prepared his own pretend food. Each week the therapist suggested that he prepare more food and Peter agreed.
>
> As the therapist began to play a greater role in the play, Peter began to invite other guests to these parties, including some small animals (the weak, defenseless creatures whom he had previously protected from all sorts of danger and harm). Peter pretended that these animals had a great deal of fun at the parties and had them become increasingly interactive with

the therapist. Initially, he had each animal physically approach the therapist and then put each of the small animal figures on the therapist's arms and shoulders. While doing so, Peter portrayed them as very shy. He agreed with the therapist's remark that some of them had difficulty "trusting" the therapist because they were uncertain of whether he would hurt them. Immediately after this comment from the therapist, Peter stuffed a small bunny into the sleeve of the therapist's shirt. He stated that the bunny did this because she wanted to "smell him [the therapist] to get to know him better."

After several more weeks of this play, Peter began to enact a series of vignettes that were more direct reflections of his ambivalence about trusting others, particularly paternal figures. Peter called this play "father and son." He assumed the role of the son and the therapist was the father. The "son" demanded lots of toys from the father, who met these symbolic demands for attention, love, and nurturance. Besides the "father" giving the "son" these gifts, the father and son had fun together on the beach, building sand castles in the sandbox. This play was an expression of Peter's longing for the idealized parent who would provide the nurturance, caring, and protection he had so sorely lacked in his early years. It was accompanied by more direct expressions of Peter's growing affection for the therapist. He began to initiate some physical contact, such as putting his hand on the therapist's shoulder. He expressed a desire to prolong the weekly sessions, and once he left a note in the therapy room to the therapist that stated, "I like you."

However, Peter's fear and anxiety about closeness with the therapist reemerged in subsequent sessions. He began to test the therapist's commitment. He knocked the therapist's marker off a board game so forcefully that it flew across the room, refused to leave sessions, and was somewhat rude. Unfortunately, this behavior coincided with the beginning of the therapist's summer vacation. When the therapist explained that he would see Peter one more time before a 4-week holiday break, Peter immediately and angrily responded that he never wanted to return for another session. He could not provide any specific reasons for this statement. The therapist empathized with Peter's anger regarding the therapist's absence. He normalized it and told Peter that he understood why Peter was so angry about not being able to see someone he liked. When the therapist firmly told Peter that he would be returning, the boy seemed relieved but needed to take home a small souvenir to reassure himself of their relationship.

At this point, the therapist could talk directly with Peter about his fears of becoming too close to the therapist. Although intellectually aware that the reason for the 4-week break was the therapist's vacation plans, Peter expressed his fear that the therapist might forget about him or no longer want to see him. Although he enjoyed his closer relationship with the therapist, it filled him with anxiety. He and the therapist talked about the differences between the ways Peter was treated by his stepfather and the therapist. Peter and the therapist were able to identify many previous occasions when the therapist had proven his commitment to Peter. This was the first discussion of many that enabled Peter to think about and critically identify his unconscious assumption (i.e., internal working model) that the therapist and others would mistreat him as his stepfather had.

When therapy resumed after the vacation, Peter was able to tolerate more direct discussions of his relationship with the therapist. In particular, he discussed how his fear of closeness was sometimes associated with his behavior in therapy sessions that was designed to push away the therapist and test his ongoing commitment. They identified similar behavior he used in other relationships when he expected people to reject or abuse him. The frequency of this provocative behavior declined as Peter became more cognizant of his unconscious reliance upon this strategy and the internal working model upon which it was based.

As we have already noted, the child may be uncertain about his or her nascent belief and expectation about the reliability and trustworthiness of others. For example, the child may introduce calamities (e.g., the therapist and child are attacked by monsters) during a play episode in which the therapist is symbolically nurturing the child. For several weeks, Peter pretended the father and son playing on the beach were attacked by pirates. As the son, he took the lead in protecting them, but the pirates would abruptly and unexpectedly attack again after Peter had defeated them. This is reminiscent of the "chaotic" play of controlling–disorganized children. Catastrophes and dangers arise and, although vanquished each time emerge repeatedly. This pattern and in particular the abrupt shifts suggest that Peter was still having difficulty in successfully defending himself or resolving anxiety. Although he showed many features of an avoidant attachment organization, his play reflected disorganization and dysregulation of defensive strategies. Peter had to fight these adversaries to restore a sense of control and power over interactions that he still regarded skeptically.

Although the therapist attempted to create a warm, positive, and accepting therapeutic environment from the beginning of therapy with Peter, he also intervened with specific strategies. As we have seen, the therapist began taking more initiative to increase their positive interaction, demonstrating to Peter that others could be trusted to meet his needs. The therapist helped Peter identify some reasons for his avoidant pattern and the conditions in which he used it to cope with anxiety and fear about intimacy. Peter was encouraged to critically question his assumption that others were going to hurt him as his stepfather had. To help Peter identify and develop more appropriate ways to express his conflicting feelings about relationships, the therapist began to articulate these affective states. For Peter, talking about his fear that the therapist would forget him during the 4-week vacation and ultimately reject him was a more adaptive coping mechanism than acting out to create much-needed distance in the relationship. Fortunately, Peter's mother was able to effect some changes in the way she parented Peter. She became more consistently available to him, set firmer and more consistent limits on his defiant and oppositional behavior, and became more empathic and sensitive to his anxiety and fear. Although Peter's therapy included many other important components, we believe the therapeutic relationship helped this young boy overcome some of the more serious developmental effects associated with his maltreatment history. The therapeutic relationship, in both its direct and indirect forms, introduced an element of discontinuity into Peter's life and helped him modify these negative internal working models. Therapy was ultimately supported and complemented by other favorable and positive experiences in his environment.

Children with an Ambivalent–Resistant Attachment Organization

There is considerable support for the notion that relatively low maternal availability is associated with the ambivalent–resistant pattern of attachment (Cassidy & Berlin, 1994). In response to a parent who is minimally or inconsistently responsive, the infant heightens his or her emotional arousal to gain parental attention. As well, the extreme dependence of these infants can be regarded as another strategy to gain the mother's response. Goldberg (1991) describes the characteristics of older children who are classified as dependent–preoccupied (ambivalent–resistant). Like infants, they are preoccupied with the parent–child relationship at the expense of other activities, notably that of exploring the environment. The child and parent seem engaged in a constant struggle for control, and the child may appear as whiny and contentious. Alternatively, the child may emphasize his or her dependency with extreme coyness (e.g., whispering) or feigned helplessness.

Similar interactional qualities emerge in the therapeutic relationship. Initially, the child may become overly dependent upon the therapist. This dependency is manifested in behavior such as asking to return the next day for another session, requesting the therapist's phone number or address, and having great difficulty in leaving the session. The child may engage in quite regressive play; for instance, demanding to be fed by in the therapist's lap by a baby bottle (Mills & Allan, 1992). However, there usually comes a point in therapy when the child realizes that the therapist cannot meet all these massive dependency needs. At this point, the rage and anger that originally developed toward the unresponsive and inconsistent attachment figure are projected onto the therapist. The child may interpret the therapist's inability to meet these needs as yet another manifestation of the basic untrustworthiness of people, proving that he or she is unlovable and unworthy. Sometimes this anger becomes clearly apparent the first time the therapist has to cancel a session.

Jodi was an 8-year-old girl who had been exposed to serious physical and psychological neglect by her young mother from infancy to 5 years of age. When she began kindergarten, the neglect was discovered by school staff, and child welfare authorities were notified. Jodi was removed from her mother's care, eventually was made a permanent ward of the state, and was placed in a residential treatment program where she was referred for individual psychotherapy.

In her first encounters with her female therapist, she wanted to sit in the therapist's lap and asked to come home with her. Jodi demanded an appointment for the following day and became angry when told that this was impossible because of the therapist's schedule. Because she became ill, the therapist had to cancel Jodi's sixth session. When therapy was resumed the next week, Jodi was hostile, answering the therapist's questions in a brusque and offhand manner. When the therapist told her that she had missed Jodi the week before because of the canceled appointment, Jodi immediately shot back, "Well, I didn't miss you!" She then ordered the therapist to do certain things for her, such as getting her different toys in the playroom. When the therapist remarked that perhaps Jodi was feeling angry because she did not see the therapist the week before, Jodi denied it. However, the frequency of her hostile and angry behavior in the session began to decrease after this comment.

Several weeks later, a case conference was held in the cottage of the treatment facility where Jodi resided. The therapist greeted Jodi when she met her in the living area. Jodi did not want the therapist to leave the cottage. In fact, she again asked to go home with the therapist. She became quite angry at the therapist's refusal. At one point, Jodi physically tried to restrain the therapist from leaving and, at another, gave her some play money as a way of buying her acceptance and affection.

What can the therapist do to help these children? In the engagement section at the beginning of this chapter, we talked about giving them a small token or "souvenir" of the therapist and therapy sessions. This souvenir provides them with some reassurance that the therapist still thinks about them when sessions are not being held. It also promotes object constancy. Anxiety about the therapist's availability may be reduced by adhering to a predictable appointment schedule and routine and by avoiding cancellations and scheduling changes as much as possible.

The play of many of these children is quite regressive, but the therapist may have to allow the child to engage in this behavior to compensate, at least symbolically, for early experiences of deprivation and inconsistent caregiving. Although she was 8 years old, Jodi insisted on enacting scenarios in which she was an infant. Her therapist had to care for her, "preparing" baby food and pretending to feed her with a spoon. The therapist's efforts to nurture the child symbolically may begin to change the child's expectations that others will be unresponsive. Furthermore, the therapist's attempts to verbalize these underlying issues may promote, in the child, the emergence of more adaptive ways of expressing his or her needs rather than the child continuing to rely on regressive or provocative behavior to gain adult attention. Simple statements like "It feels really good to pretend that you are a baby and someone is always there to look after you" may be useful in promoting this kind of self-regulation.

Although the therapist wants to nurture the child to change these negative internal working models, too much regression provides no benefit. The child does not need to act like a baby after therapy is over and he or she is about to return to an elementary school classroom. As we have already discussed, the therapist should insist that the child stop this regressive behavior 5 to 10 minutes before the end of the session. The therapist should then engage the child in more age-appropriate conversations or play activities. These activities convey the notion that although the child may regress in the playroom, it is not beneficial to continue this behavior outside therapy sessions; especially if the child has many academic and social tasks to master. Jodi's therapist always informed her that they would have to stop their "play" 10 minutes before the end of the session. The last few minutes were spent putting the doll and baby toys away while the therapist asked Jodi about the age-appropriate activities or tasks she would confront later that day (e.g., participating in Brownies activities). During this time they would talk informally about how Jodi would meet some of these challenges.

Urquiza and Winn (1994) identify other characteristics of a dependent pattern of behavior. Children who show this kind of behavior are unassertive and overly compliant, and they allow other people to make important decisions for them. In therapy, these children offer little resistance to developing a relationship with the therapist and have few opinions or issues to discuss. According to these authors, "The challenge in working with a dependent child is to generate separation and individuation, to elicit a strong and determined response from the child, and [to] help the child integrate a sense of self that is based on worth, ability, and individuality" (Urquiza & Winn, 1994, p. 83).

The therapist can help children who show such characteristics by encouraging them to provide opinions about different subjects, even such trivial ones as favorite television shows. The therapist might identify an area or issue about which he or she may disagree with the child and then inform the child of the difference of opinion. Some children, upon hearing the therapist's opinion, will immediately change their minds and try to retract their opinions. The therapist should actively intervene by informing the child that it is perfectly acceptable for the child to have his or her own opinion. The therapist should then further state that his or her regard and commitment are not contingent upon the child holding identical views. Many interventions of this nature may be required. When these interventions are combined with the therapist's active attempts to demonstrate commitment, the child may begin to change his or her belief that any attempt to assert a sense of self or individuality will be met with rejection or abandonment. The therapist may consolidate the child's developing individuality and assertiveness by frequently requesting the child's choice of activities in which the youngster would like to participate. Having the opportunity to make such decisions may be quite threatening for children who fear they will evoke the displeasure or anger from the therapist if they make a wrong choice, but ultimately it may help them develop a more integrated sense of self.

Limit Setting

As we noted above, a time usually comes in therapy with youngsters who have this ambivalent–resistant attachment organization when they begin to realize the therapist cannot meet all their massive dependency needs. This realization in turn provokes considerable anger in such a child, which may be reflected in the child swearing at and insulting the therapist or even making physical attacks upon the therapist. The child may be stubbornly noncompliant and refuse to talk, play, or follow the therapist's directions (e.g., refuse to enter or leave the office or playroom). Provocative behavior may take a more disguised form in symbolic play: the therapist may be cast in the role of the helpless victim of the child's physical and psychological assaults.

Emergence of this anger in therapy offers the therapist a wonderful opportunity to relate to that child in ways different from those of the original attachment figure, thereby introducing a much-needed element of discontinuity. Rather than rejecting or abusing the angry child, the therapist places appropriate limits upon unacceptable aggressive behavior (e.g., attempts to hurt the therapist or destroy the office or playroom equipment). At the same time, the therapist acknowledges and empathizes with the underlying anger. Placing appropriate limits on children demonstrates to them in practical and concrete ways that there are adults who care enough to help them control these troublesome feelings and urges.

Limit setting also introduces the child to the notion of a reciprocal, or "goal-corrected," partnership. The therapist who stops this destructive behavior and then engages in a dialogue wherein both participants discuss and negotiate their needs exposes the child to a novel experience. The therapist is teaching the child to identify and articulate these needs for attention. For example, a child may become more oppositional near the end of each session. Rather than allowing this behavior to escalate, the therapist should help the child identify the feelings elicited by the termination of the session, encourage the child to express what he or she might need (e.g., "I want to stay here longer"), and reach a compromise solution (e.g., taking home a small souvenir). The child learns he or she no longer has to rely upon extreme displays of anger to obtain the therapist's attention or response.

There are other benefits to limit setting. Limits teach the child more adaptive ways of handling anger, such as verbalizing feelings. The child learns to have a feeling and express it verbally but also that the youngster cannot always act as he or she pleases. Limit setting ultimately facilitates better relationships with others. Finally, limits on children's aggressive or destructive behavior are necessary to enable the therapist to maintain attitudes of acceptance, empathy, and warmth, as well as to ensure the child's and therapist's personal safety.

There are several general steps in setting limits with children (Ginott, 1965). First, the therapist should recognize the child's feelings or wishes and help the child express them verbally: "You're really mad at me because you wish you could stay here for another hour." Second, the therapist clearly states the limit on a specific act: "But therapists and kids have to leave the playroom when their time is over." Third, the therapist points out alternatives: "If you're really angry about having to leave, you can say to me, 'I'm mad!' " Finally, the therapist helps the child bring out the feelings of resentment that arise when restrictions are invoked: "You sure don't like having to leave and wish you could stay longer. It makes you really angry when you have to leave." Ginott (1965) recommends that limits be phrased in language that does not constitute a challenge to the child's self-respect. Limits are better heeded when stated succinctly and impersonally, such as, "Time is up for today," versus "Your time is up and you must leave now!"

Of course, some children persist in negative behavior despite the therapist's attempts to limit it. If the limit setting described above proves ineffective, the therapist may have to stop the session. However, it is important to clarify the reasons for this step. The child may be told that the session is being stopped early because the therapist does not want the child to engage in any more negative behavior that will make the child feel worse about himself or herself. Additionally, the therapist says that he or she will not tolerate this kind of inappropriate behavior. The child must be reassured that the therapist has not "given up" and that they will see each other at their next regularly scheduled appointment. Sometimes shortening the session is effective in helping a child behave more appropriately.

The therapist will probably become angry with the child's provocative behavior. The therapist may acknowledge the anger verbally and then emphasize that he or she will not reject or abuse the youngster. The sources of the anger should be identified and connected to specific aspects of the child's behavior (e.g., "When you throw paint on me, I feel really angry") rather than to aspects of the child's self or personality (e.g., "You make me really angry"). To disrupt the stability of the internal working model and create change, the therapist should distinguish between his or her response to the child's provocation (i.e., verbalizing the anger in a nonderogatory, nonabusive manner) and those of others who have reacted in ways that reinforced the child's concept of the untrustworthiness of people.

Although the therapeutic relationship is a significant agent of change for many maltreated children, especially those who have incurred developmental effects because of their abuse or neglect, it is not the only one worthy of consideration. We now turn in the next three chapters to other ways of helping children recover from maltreatment.

EIGHT

Helping Children Express Their Feelings and Thoughts about Maltreatment

HELPING CHILDREN identify and acknowledge feelings related to a history of abuse and neglect is an especially important task. Uncovering the maltreatment is necessary to extinguish anxiety and reduce the child's reliance upon maladaptive defense mechanisms such as overidealization or dissociation. Uncovering the maltreatment and bringing it into the open offers an opportunity to explore and possibly reformulate the meaning and implications of these experiences.

In this chapter we describe specific techniques therapists may use to help children uncover and express their feelings and thoughts about having been abused or neglected. Although we describe some of our own techniques that we believe are useful, we also draw upon the work of others. In particular, clinicians such as Beverly James (1989, 1994) and others (e.g., Berliner & Wheeler, 1987; Cunningham & MacFarlane, 1991; Friedrich, 1990; Gil, 1991; Gil & Johnson, 1993; Mandell & Damon, 1989; Mann & McDermott, 1983; Urquiza & Winn, 1994) have furnished therapists with many innovative and creative strategies.

Although helping children uncover and express their feelings about victimization is a prerequisite for successful treatment, by itself it is insufficient. Therapy may often create even more difficulties if unaccompanied by interventions to help the child develop successful coping mechanisms. In their zeal and enthusiasm to help survivors of abuse and neglect, inexperienced or novice therapists sometimes believe their primary job is to "open up" clients. They encourage their clients to abreact or ventilate all their feelings about the victimization experiences. Unfortunately, these therapists pay little attention to the pacing of this process or the notion that defense mechanisms, although maladaptive in the long term, are there for a reason: they protect the individual from intense pain and anxiety. Conducting therapy in a way that overwhelms clients with their pain and provides them with no alternate coping mechanisms usually results in a deterioration in their functioning. This kind of therapy does little to encourage the client's trust in the therapist or the therapeutic process. Therapists must actively assist their young clients to develop more appropriate ways of coping with the pain, hurt, and anxiety that emerge over the course of therapy. This issue is addressed in Chapter 9.

The literature review in Chapter 1 revealed there is no homogeneous set of sequelae that discriminate among children exposed to different types of maltreatment; there seems to be more commonalities than differences. For example, a number of sexually and physically abused children present with a posttraumatic stress disorder. Although the proportion of sexually abused youngsters with this problem is higher than that for physically abused children, therapists who see physically abused children must be prepared to treat these symptoms just as they would in sexually abused youngsters. Even though the content may be somewhat different (e.g., dreams of being raped versus dreams of being physically assaulted), the treatment techniques and the underlying rationale are the same. Given these similarities and overlap, we have therefore decided to present an integrated approach rather than separate chapters on the treatment of different types of maltreatment. Chapters 8, 9, and 10 contain discussions of the three major treatment themes that confront every therapist who works with maltreated children—expressing thoughts and feelings about the abuse or neglect; developing adaptive coping mechanisms; and reformulating the meaning of the experiences. As well as describing specific techniques that have broad applicability to the sequelae of the major types of maltreatment, we review intervention strategies for the more idiosyncratic problems associated with particular types of abuse and neglect, such as the sexual behavior of sexually victimized children.

DIRECT DISCUSSIONS OF THE MALTREATMENT

Getting Started: Orienting the Child and Instilling a Sense of Safety and Control

Some maltreated children are able to talk in a straightforward and forthright manner about their victimization. To begin this process with these children, the therapist should describe the benefits of talking about the maltreatment. The therapist should reiterate that the purpose of therapy is not to forget the victimization; it is to learn to master the feelings associated with it and to think differently about what happened. Children might be told that although talking about these events is initially frightening and some-times painful, the intensity of these feelings usually will diminish.

According to the conditioning paradigm described in Chapter 2, talk-ing about the abuse may serve as a potent stimulus for the emergence of anxiety. The therapist should emphasize that he or she understands and appreciates the child's anxiety and that they will proceed at a pace tolerable to the child. As we have already advocated, the child should be given ex-plicit permission and guidance about controlling the pace of the discussion, and the therapist should structure the session in ways that will not over-whelm the child (to be discussed below). The child and therapist should devise some ways for the child to signal that he or she is feeling particularly anxious and would like a break. For instance, a simple verbal statement like "This is too fast" or "I'm getting too scared now" may be adequate. The child might instead give the therapist a nonverbal signal, such as holding up a hand with the palm toward the therapist. In order to make the child feel more comfortable, the therapist should have the child rehearse these statements or nonverbal signals beforehand.

We have maintained throughout this book that children must feel a sense of safety both outside and within therapy sessions to process the maltreatment-related material. In Chapter 7 we reviewed various ways to ensure safety, regularity, and predictability. These precautions are particu-larly important during times when the child actively verbalizes or expresses material related to the victimization. Although the therapist wants to facili-tate the child's exposure to this sensitive material, too hurried a pace will overwhelm the child with anxiety and result in the reemergence of maladap-tive defense mechanisms or regressive behaviors. The child may even be reluc-tant to attend or participate in subsequent sessions, claiming the sessions are "boring," or will adamantly refuse to discuss topics related to the maltreat-ment. The child's previous claims of being bothered by his or her abusive experiences may now be denied, and the child may say that "everything is fine." When the therapist attempts to discuss the maltreatment, the child may change the topic or engage in provocative or oppositional behavior to deflect the attention from the maltreatment.

There are various ways a therapist can structure and plan the therapy sessions to contain this kind of anxiety. For each session, the therapist and child might agree to allot a specific length of time to direct discussion of the maltreatment. It is usually best to begin with short intervals (10 to 15 minutes) so the child will not be overwhelmed by the the anxiety that might be associated with more prolonged discussions. In this way the child is ex-posed to tolerable doses of the anxiety-related material. For example, ask-ing most school-aged children to engage in a continuous 45-minute discussion of their victimization is unrealistic, given the material's intensity and their short attention spans. As the child succeeds with brief discussions and the anxiety begins to abate, the youngster and therapist should decide together how to lengthen the discussions by small increments (Urquiza & Winn, 1994). This strategy gives the child a sense of accomplishment. It also reinforces for the child that he or she is dealing with an adult who is sensitive to the youngster's feelings and needs and is willing to negotiate important issues and topics. Urquiza and Winn (1994) and James (1989, 1994) advocate interspersing these direct discussions of the maltreatment with periods of play. These play periods provide the child with some relief from the anxiety associated with verbal explorations of the maltreatment. It also provides the child with opportunities to express feelings or thoughts about the victimization in other ways (to be discussed below).

As well as negotiating the duration of direct discussion, the therapist should provide the youngster with significant control over the choice of topics related to the victimization. This approach is particularly important at the beginning of this phase of therapy, when children are especially anxious because they feel they might have no control over the conduct of the sessions. The therapist should suggest that the child begin by choosing which topic or incident related to the maltreatment they will talk about ("Why don't you choose what you'd like to talk about first?"). Talking about only one incident or aspect of the victimization in each session serves a similar purpose. Sometimes, talking while both are engaged in a parallel play activity such as drawing or playing with plasticine is helpful. In these situations, the child does not have to make eye contact with the therapist and can always fall back on the play activity when he or she does not want to say anything more. Discussions about the play activity also provide the child with a much-needed break from these intense conversations.

Facilitating and Encouraging the Child's Account

The therapist should sit quietly and listen attentively as the child begins to recount his or her experiences. Interrupting the description of what happened with a barrage of questions may discourage the child from continuing. If the child hesitates while recounting these experiences, the therapist might provide gentle encouragement by making simple statements such as "Go on" or "Can you tell me more about that?"

The therapist has several tasks during this phase of therapy. First, the therapist must help the child recall the details of the maltreatment to uncover previously denied, suppressed, or dissociated memories. The therapist might facilitate recall by asking the child to describe the maltreatment in more detail after the child has given an open-ended account of his or her experiences. For example, the therapist might begin with more neutral questions regarding the maltreatment's locale (e.g., "What room did it happen in?"), the time of day (e.g., "Did it happen at night or during the day?"), and what the child or family did earlier that day. The therapist should then proceed to ask about more sensitive aspects of the maltreatment, including the actual behavior of the perpetrator. The child should be encouraged to describe his or her experiences before, during, and after the maltreatment, including his or her feelings, odors, sights, body sensations, and reactions (James, 1994). Of course, many maltreated children do not have this verbal facility and cannot articulate their experiences and feelings in this manner. Other sections of this chapter are devoted to techniques designed to facilitate the child's ability to communicate experiences and feelings.

Second, the therapist must begin assisting the child in expressing the associated feelings and cognitions. Simple questions like, "How did you feel when he hit you like that?" may be sufficient to enable a child to express his or her sentiments. These questions give the child the opportunity to put into words the often intense and confusing feelings that were elicited by the victimization, thereby increasing the child's self-regulatory skills. Also, the child's responses to these questions allow the therapist to understand and then empathize with and legitimize the child's feelings. For example, the child may talk about his or her fear of being sexually abused in the future, which may be accompanied by nonverbal symptoms of anxiety (e.g., fidgeting, increased pressure of speech, decreased eye contact with the therapist). The therapist might convey his or her understanding with simple statements like "You're still really scared that he might do those things again to you." Subsequent statements that normalize these feelings (e.g., "Most kids would feel really scared about that") contribute to the child's understanding that his or her reactions are normal and not indicative of deviancy. In Chapter 7, we reviewed how empathic statements convey the therapist's sensitivity to the child and help modify the child's negative internal working model of others.

Phenomenological Orientation of the Therapist

It is critically important for the therapist to ensure that his or her own preconceptions are not imposed upon the child's account of the maltreatment, for instance by assuming there were no positive aspects to the relationship between the child and perpetrator. Rather than telling a child how he or she thinks or feels about the experiences, the therapist must adopt the phenomenological perspective described in Chapter 2 to understand as fully as possible the child's experience and perceptions of the maltreatment. It is important to help the child express the wide range of feelings harbored toward the perpetrator, including positive ones. If this approach not used during the assessment phase, the therapist should begin the current inquiry by requesting that the child describe the "nice things" the perpetrator did for the youngster. Some therapists may find it difficult to acknowledge that the perpetrator treated the child well in certain ways or to empathize with the child's positive feelings and possibly love for the individual. However, this attitude is critically important in helping children become aware of their ambivalent and conflicting feelings so they can ultimately express their feelings of betrayal and loss. If the therapist severly criticizes the perpetrator on a personal level by calling the individual names, even stronger feelings of loyalty from the child, are often elicited, especially if the perpetrator is a parent. In the face of the therapist attacks, the child may defend the perpetrator even more strenuously and ultimately minimize or deny the individuals's actions. A more useful strategy is to talk about the perpetrator's behavior that hurt or angered the child rather than making more personalized comments.

Anxiety-Reduction Strategies

Even though the therapist has attempted to instill in a child a sense of safety and control prior to the initiation of this kind of discussion, children frequently become anxious while recounting their experiences. Here we review some strategies clinicians might use in sessions to decrease this discomfort. A failure to do so exacerbates the child's suffering, and the youngster will quickly terminate the account.

Close Monitoring of the Child's Anxiety

If the child appears highly distressed and does not ask or signal the therapist for a break, the therapist should comment directly about the child's distress ("You look pretty upset right now"). The therapist might then ask if the child wants a break from the discussion and also inquire about the reasons for the distress. Are some intrusive memories (flashbacks) occurring during the discussion, or are there other reasons, such as fear of the therapist's reaction to a particularly embarrassing or sensitive detail or incident? The therapist should reassure the child that he or she understands the basis of the anxiety and does not think negatively of the youngster. For example, Peter's anxiety was alleviated to a certain degree when the therapist told him he did not think Peter was a "pervert" for having a sexual response while being molested. Children should be instructed to observe the therapist's reactions to their accounts closely, paying particular attention to the therapist's facial expressions or body language that might reveal those reactions. The child might then be encouraged to recount more of the distressing episode or incident. After a minute or so of this recital, the therapist should ask the child to report his or her observations of the therapist's demeanor and whether it confirmed the child's expectation that the therapist would be "grossed out." This is a variant of the "trust meter" we described in Chapter 4.

Identifying the "Worst Thing" about Talking

Youngsters may be assisted in overcoming their anxiety by identifying "the worst thing that could happen" if they told their story. A variation of James's "Worry Wall" (James, 1989, pp. 130-131) is an especially useful technique to use in identifying a child's fears of talking. The child is invited to identify his or her "biggest worry" concerning talking about the abuse and to write it down on a small card. Then the child is asked, "How big is your worry today?" If it is a little worry, the child is instructed to tack the card on the wall near the floor; conversely, if it is a significant, overwhelming worry, the card should be tacked near the ceiling. Each week the therapist invites the child to check the card and to move it appropriately to reflect changes in the child's anxiety level about talking, while encouraging the child to provide more details of the account as his or her anxiety diminishes. The card's placement on the wall serves as a concrete reminder of the therapy's progress.

Drawing the Distinction between the Verbal Expression of Feelings and Behavioral Acting Out

Some children believe that if they talk about their maltreatment they will be so overwhelmed with anger they will lose control and become aggressive or destructive during the session. It is important to reassure the child that the therapist will ensure the safety of them both and will not allow the youngster to show such behavior. The child should be encouraged to tell "a bit" of the episode or experience at a time. At the end of each of these segments, the therapist should point out that the child did not get out of control. This reminder reinforces the child's growing confidence not only in the therapist but in his or her own ability to regulate strong feelings and behavior.

Another introductory exercise that is useful in drawing the distinction between the verbal expression of emotions and behavioral acting out is "Feelings: Where Are They in My Body?" (James, 1989, pp. 93–94). The child draws an outline of his or her body and adds a legend beside the picture that describes some of the child's feelings. The child chooses colors to represent various feelings and marks their locations on the body outline using the appropriate colors. This exercise does more than help distinguish among different feelings. It also serves as a springboard for discussions about the difference between talking about feelings and acting them out, for example, using a fist to express anger. It also helps the child identify body sensations that serve as precipitants to inappropriate behavior, such as physical aggression or sexualized behavior.

Normalizing Affective Displays

Appropriate displays of affect such as crying should be normalized for the child, and the therapist should point out that he or she does not think less of the child because of such displays. In fact, the child should be congratulated for having the strength to show these feelings. The therapist should facilitate the child's general understanding of the normalcy of his or her distress and its connection to the maltreatment. This is the start of the process by which the child begins reformulating the meaning of the maltreatment experience. For example, in previous discussions the child's reactions to truly frightening aspects of the maltreatment may have been identified. Using simple language, the therapist should explain the basis of the symptoms associated with posttraumatic stress disorder or other reactions. Cunningham and MacFarlane (1991, pp. 149–164) describe the symptomatology of posttraumatic stress disorder in developmentally appropriate language. Providing children with a simple explanation for some of their reactions diminishes their fear that they are "crazy" and reduces their anxiety, isolation, and stigmatization. This is an especially effective strategy if, because of it, they begin to understand that their current difficulties, including the distress manifested in the therapy sessions, are associated with previous maltreatment experiences.

Some children who talk about their abuse or neglect experience such intense affects that they feel as if they are being revictimized during these discussions. The therapist can take several approaches to help them overcome these feelings. First, the therapist should identify the concrete and observable differences between the situation in which the child was abused and the therapy session in which the child recounts these episodes. For example, the therapist might point out that the perpetrator is not present; no one is hurting or even touching the child; and the child is reacting to feelings, not the actual perpetration. Second, the therapist should remind the child of other differences between the experience and the therapy session. The child should be reminded that he or she is now bigger, older, and more capable of asking for help and receiving protection than he or she was at the time of the maltreatment (Urquiza & Winn, 1994). This strategy may diminish the child's anxiety about discussing the abuse or neglect. It may also start the process by which the child discards the status of a victim who is powerless to protect himself or herself against future assaults.

Relaxation Exercises

Some highly distressed and anxious children need to learn specific ways of calming themselves. Deep breathing, relaxation techniques, and visualization are strategies children might learn to apply during these discussions or symbolic play reenactments of the maltreatment when they become especially anxious and distraught. Although not all children may need to use such strategies, those who have strong physiological reactions may greatly benefit from them. Often such children's physiological responses make them feel powerless and out of control, much as they felt during their victimization. Gaining control of these physiological reactions helps them regain a sense of competence and control. Before teaching children these techniques, the therapist should explain that they take time and some practice to learn. The child should not give up after only one or two tries.

We have found that various relaxation techniques may be employed successfully during sessions to extinguish the anxiety associated with these memories. The therapist should cue the child to intersperse direct discussions of the maltreatment or episodes of symbolic play with these techniques. Techniques must be adapted specifically to each child, with particular attention to the child's age, cognitive capacity, and interests. Perhaps the simplest technique is to have a child focus on breathing and slow it down; the basic technique is to count breaths in and out or to simply say, "Breathe in, breathe out" slowly. Initially, the therapist should do this prompting aloud. Once children can slow their breathing down, they should be shown how to use imagery to increase their relaxation and sense of calmness. Some children respond well to imagining they are going down a flight of stairs. With each slow breath exhaled, they take a step down and feel more comfortable and more relaxed. Others respond well to imagining they are a big balloon; with each breath out, they deflate and become softer and more relaxed. Imagining they are a limp rag doll is also useful. With each breath out, the doll relaxes further and slumps over. Still other children respond to developing an imaginary scene in which they feel safe, comfortable, and calm. During relaxation, the child breathes slowly and imagines all the details and sensations described by the therapist or on a tape. For example, some children like to imagine they are on a beach on a hot day. They are lying on a thick, comfortable towel under a large shade tree. A slight breeze is blowing, so they do not feel too hot. Gulls and children can be heard in the distance, but the child prefers to lie comfortably under the tree. The child focuses on his or her bodily sensations in this scene and feels comfortable and safe.

Hypnotherapy

Friedrich (1990) describes the use of hypnotherapy in assisting sexually abused children when they are discussing details of their victimization. He contends that hypnotherapy is rarely required to help children recall the actual details of their experiences. They are closer to the event, and other techniques such as drawing or storytelling can facilitate this process. Instead, hypnotherapy may be used to help children master and control the feelings evoked by memories of abuse. Friedrich (1990) describes a 9-year-old sexually abused girl who was behaving in a sexually aggressive manner with younger children. After a deep trance was induced, he suggested that she contain the feelings about her own victimization history in boxes. He combined this hypnotic suggestion with others that would make her feel she had contained those feelings and was now in a safe and favorite place. The girl stopped her sexual behavior with the other children after this initial intervention. Once she had mastered these feelings, she was able to focus more attentively on the therapy process. We strongly advise the reader to review the original source of this interesting and useful case vignette.

Structured Activities to Help Children
Talk about the Maltreatment

So far we have described therapy from an ideal perspective. The client is a child who can talk readily and easily about the maltreatment and its associated feelings, cognitions, worries, and concerns. Many maltreated children do not have these verbal skills or are inhibited from talking directly about their experiences for the reasons described in earlier chapters. Such children may require the psychological distance inherent in play therapy techniques that are described later in this chapter. However, even verbal children who can talk about their experiences may require specific strategies to be able to provide a more comprehensive verbal account of their feelings and experiences.

James (1989, 1994) has developed many innovative and creative techniques to help traumatized children. We have found the following particularly useful. The "Garbage Bag" technique begins with the therapist drawing a parallel between concrete pieces of garbage and the overpowering, aversive feelings associated with trauma (James, 1989, pp. 166–170). The therapist continues by explaining that keeping these feelings and thoughts secret is like carrying a bag of garbage around. The child is to get rid of each piece of "garbage" (i.e., distressing feelings and ideas about the abuse) gradually. To accomplish this task, the therapist asks the child to identify each aversive or distressing event or episode related to the trauma, which the therapist quickly writes on a piece of paper. The child is not given a chance to elaborate upon these events but is permitted to identify aversive events other than the trauma. The purpose of writing each episode or incident on a separate piece of paper is to divide the maltreatment into more manageable bits. The pieces of paper are put in a paper grocery bag that symbolically contains the memories and feelings associated with the maltreatment. Each week the child is invited to reach into the bag and pick out one piece of paper and discuss that particular episode or incident. Applying the conditioning paradigm, the child's anxiety is extinguished as the youngster is exposed to particular aspects or episodes of the trauma. The child is allowed to throw the paper back into the bag and choose another if he or she is not ready to address the first topic, thereby gaining a sense of control. If the child elects to work on the first issue chosen, the therapist and child might discuss it directly or choose another method, such as drawing.

The "Garbage Bag" exercise illustrates one of the general underlying themes of child therapy. An emphasis is placed upon translating abstract, psychological concepts such as affects and defenses into forms the child can more readily understand. We advise the reader to review a paper by Harter (1977) and a subsequent chapter (Harter, 1983), in which the cognitive–developmental limitations of children's understanding of emotional and psychological concepts are discussed. Harter argues that child therapists need to concretize these ideas via visualizable symbols so that the child can attach real experiences to these abstract concepts. In the "Garbage Bag" exercise, writing down the aversive or distressing episodes, incidents, or issues puts them into a concrete form to which the child can attach feelings and cognitions. Use of the paper bag to hold these feelings is another example of the concretization of a psychological concept, that is, that the child has many feelings and issues in his or her psychological world. By symbolically emptying the garbage bag of these issues, the child is provided with a concrete reminder that he or she is beginning to master these distressing feelings and is making real progress: the fewer pieces of "garbage" left in the bag are tangible proof of this progress.

There are other structured exercises that may be used to help children express feelings and thoughts about a history of maltreatment. In their manual describing a curriculum for group psychotherapy for sexually abused children, Mandell and Damon (1989) describe several "handouts" that children should complete. The content of this material is focused upon sexual abuse, but the clinician may modify it for children who have been physically abused, neglected, or psychologically maltreated. The handout "Feelings about Being Molested" (Mandell & Damon, 1989, pp. 76–77) consists of eight statements (e.g., "I would like to hide from people so I don't have to talk about it"). The intensity of these feelings must be rated by the child on a scale from "never" to "always." In the handout "I Think This Happened Because _____" children are asked to list the reasons they think they were molested and to identify the reasons the perpetrator engaged in this behavior (Mandell & Damon, 1989, p. 77). This technique helps children articulate their attributions about the maltreatment. The handout "What Will People Think of Me?" is a sentence-completion task (Mandell &

Damon, 1989, pp. 77–78). The child is asked to complete sentences such as, "I worry that I am the only one who _____." Some victimized children may respond in ways that convey their sense of stigmatization, powerlessness, or betrayal. Other handouts provide interview guides for group-therapy members in asking each other about his or her relationship with the perpetrator and details of the abuse he or she experienced. These handouts may be used profitably in individual psychotherapy or even in the assessment phase with children who may feel more comfortable approaching these issues by writing down their responses rather than verbally communicating them. A major drawback to handouts is that the child must have the requisite reading and writing skills to complete them. Asking a child who has significant difficulty with these academic tasks to complete the forms will probably engender more frustration and increase the child's resistance to participation in therapy.

There are other ways to structure these discussions of the maltreatment. Cunningham and MacFarlane (1991, pp. 136–137) used another technique, the "Tell My Story Chart," in group therapy with children who engage in sexually inappropriate behavior. The chart has relevant inquiries about the children's own history of victimization. These inquiries include the perpetrator's identity, a description of what happened, how the child felt about it, and how the abuse stopped. Again, this chart may be used in individual psychotherapy with maltreated children who have experienced other types of abuse or neglect. A tangible demonstration of the child's progress is recorded when the child marks off or places a sticker on the chart each time a question is addressed. The chart also provides concrete reminders of topics that should be discussed in therapy.

The child who constricts certain affects may be helped to express them with another technique developed by James (1989), "Feelings: Inside and Outside" (p. 93). A piece of paper folded in half so that it opens like a greeting card is given to the child. The youngster is instructed to draw a self-portrait on the outside of the card depicting the way the child thinks everyone sees him or her. Then the child is told to open the paper and draw a self-portrait of the way he or she really feels "on the inside" (James, 1989, p. 93). This concrete depiction of the child's feelings again may serve as a springboard for discussion. The therapist helps the child identify the "inside" feelings and attach verbal labels to them. This technique may be especially useful for those children who manifest the problems in the development of an autonomous and integrated self we described in Chapter 1. They may have split-off or dissociated perceptions of themselves and others, have developed a "false self," or demonstrate a pattern of "compulsive compliance." Using this instrument, they can begin to identify different and sometimes diverse aspects and characteristics of their selves, such as cognitions, feelings, attitudes, and behaviors, rather than denying them.

Specific Problems and Strategies

Sexual Concerns and Issues of Sexually Abused Children

Some sexually abused children experience pleasurable or positive physical feelings and sensations during abusive episodes. In our experience, children are often extremely reluctant to acknowledge these reactions because of embarrassment or confusion about their origins. Likewise, some therapists have difficulty understanding how children can become sexually aroused while they are being molested. Others cannot accept the fact that children have sexual feelings or show sexual responses at all. If this subject was not addressed in the evaluative phase, the therapist must ask the child, in a matter-of-fact way, whether he or she experienced pleasurable physical sensations during the episode. If, in response to more general inquiries about body sensations during the sexual assault (e.g., "How did your private parts feel when he touched you there?"), the child does not indicate he or she experienced any pleasurable feelings, the therapist should ask more pointed, albeit leading questions. The therapist might ask "Did it ever feel good when he rubbed your vagina?" Positive feelings must be acknowledged and validated as a legitimate part of the child's experience (e.g., "When he touched your vagina like that, it felt really good. Even though you were scared and didn't like what he was doing, part of you thought it felt good. Other girls who have been touched that way have told me the same thing.") Given the acute sensitivity of this matter and the child's intense anxiety about his or her response, it is often useful to provide a simple but direct explanation of sexual-response physiology and how sexual arousal occurs. For example, 11-year-old Peter, whom we first discussed in Chapter 7, eventually revealed that he experienced intense feelings of pleasure when his stepfather performed oral sex on him. Besides being extremely embarrassed, Peter thought that his physical reactions, especially his erections, were evidence of his being a "pervert" and that something was wrong with his penis. Besides empathizing with his embarrassment, the therapist provided a simple explanation of sexual response in boys. He explained how Peter's physical reactions could be understood from this perspective. Peter was relieved when he heard that the therapist had talked with other boys who had experienced the same reaction. His ability to express fears and anxiety about this issue was the first step in helping Peter reformulate this specific aspect of his maltreatment. It also provided some immediate relief from the anxiety associated with the issue.

Following some education about the normalcy of children's sexualized reactions, therapists might ask about other sexual concerns or behaviors that the child may find even more embarrassing. After receiving an explanation for what to them is sometimes confusing and perplexing behavior and learning that others have shown similar behavior, children may be increasingly willing to divulge more of their symptomatology. Typically, these sexual reactions elicit great embarrassment and shame. Let us return to the example of Peter.

> After the therapist explained the basis of Peter's physiological response to the sexual assaults by his stepfather and the reasons for his premature eroticization, Peter began to talk somewhat more openly about his sexual fantasies. He revealed that he sometimes thought of having sex with babies because they were "totally helpless." Although Peter expressed revulsion and disgust with himself, the therapist maintained his attitude of acceptance and reiterated his commitment to helping Peter with this particular difficulty. Eventually, as his anxiety abated, Peter could reexamine this issue productively in greater depth.

Peter's revelation of these fantasies provided some relief from his almost intolerable anxiety and shame associated with them. It also served as the first step in the process in which he and the therapist could examine the fantasies, reaching some understanding about their emergence (i.e., that they were a result of his premature sexualization rather than an indication that he was a deviant or perverted child). Finally, some strategies were developed to help Peter gain a sense of control over the sexual fantasies.

James (1989, pp. 96–98) describes a technique, "Guess What Other Sexually Abused Kids Worry About?," that may be used to elicit more of the child's concerns or feelings about sexual abuse. The exercise is presented as educational information about the common reactions, fears, and worries of maltreated children. The child is told to listen to what the therapist tells "other kids." The therapist also invites the child to ask questions. James uses this technique to address the concerns sexually abused children have about their body integrity. It can also be used to address any of the child's significant issues and concerns that were identified in the assessment. For example, the therapist might make the comment that many boys and girls worry about the sexual excitement they may have experienced during episodes of molestation. The therapist's comments demonstrate that these fears and worries, which the child originally believed reflected just a personal experience, are shared by many others. This new knowledge may be a catalyst that reduces the child's sense of isolation and facilitates the child's expression of his or her own anxieties and worries.

Neglected Children with Limited Verbal Skills

The techniques described above are often useful in assisting children to talk in more detail about their feelings regarding their maltreatment. However, there are some children, especially those exposed to significant neglect, who have difficulty with the verbal expression of feelings in general (see Chapter 1 for a review of this research). The therapist must help such a child learn to identify and label feelings in general before focusing upon the particular affects associated with the maltreatment. Here we review some specific techniques to teach children so they can express their feelings verbally. Again, we draw upon the work of others. Many of these techniques have a psychoeducational orientation. It is important to make these activities as much fun as possible for the child. They should be interspersed with other activities, since some children quickly become bored in sessions where the focus is exclusively upon these more educational tasks.

The clinician will usually have numerous opportunities to model the verbal expression of a wide range of feelings in therapy sessions. These statements might be made in response to the child's account of abusive or neglectful experiences or even everyday occurrences. For example, a child tells the therapist that she was picked last for a game during gym class. She recounts this in an angry tone of voice while ripping up a piece of paper but does not use the words "angry" or "mad" to label her feelings. Simple empathic statements from the therapist like, "You're really mad!" will model the verbal expression of this feeling. Playing board games affords the therapist another opportunity. Besides verbally identifying the child's feelings displayed during the game (e.g., anger or disappointment over losing, happiness about winning), the therapist might articulate his or her personal feelings about winning or losing. As discussed in Chapter 7, the therapist might become angry over some aspect of the child's behavior. Rather than acting out this anger inappropriately or suppressing it, the therapist should tell the child that he or she is angry. Similarly, the therapist should express pleasure when the child accomplishes tasks and demonstrates new skills (Urquiza & Winn, 1994).

There are other specific techniques clinicians can use to teach children to identify and label their feelings. One of the simplest is to present simple drawings of facial expressions that denote different feeling states and teach the child the verbal labels corresponding to each emotion. The therapist might start with the four basic feelings—happy, sad, scared, and angry—and then add more facial expressions as the child masters the basics. More realistic pictures may be presented, such as magazine photographs of people, so the therapist may ask the child to identify the feelings the pictures might convey. Mandell and Damon (1989, pp. 60–61) describe a technique called "Feeling Collages." Although this technique was developed for group therapy with sexually abused children, we have adapted it to individual therapy and for children subjected to other types of maltreatment. The therapist and child decide upon a feeling they want to portray in the collage, such as sadness. They then look through magazines to find photographs or pictures that depict this feeling. More fun may be generated by writing a number of feeling states on paper slips, putting them all in a bag, and then having each person draw a feeling out of the bag. Without showing each other the feeling states they are to portray, the therapist and child construct their own collages (or just one or two pictures). At the end, each attempts to identify the feeling states portrayed by the other individual's collage. Mandell and Damon (1989, p. 61) also suggest the therapist list a variety of words denoting feeling. The child must construct a collage, choosing at least one picture for each feeling listed. Again, the therapist and child try to identify the feelings depicted in one another's collages.

Mandell and Damon (1989, p. 60) describe another technique, "What Kinds of Things Make People Feel _____?," to help children identify the precipitants of common feelings like sadness or anger. Although the technique was originally developed as a work sheet, the same principle can be incorporated in a task during which the therapist and child each draw paper slips with different feelings written on them out of a bag. Then each must verbally describe a situation that would evoke this affective state. As children become more comfortable with this task, they may be asked to identify actual situations that have elicited the same feelings in them. Lists or charts of the precipitants of various feelings may be used to help identify those people, situations, or things that evoke particular feelings in the youngster, including episodes of abuse and neglect. If the child is particularly anxious about doing this, the therapist should ask the child to list the precipitants of these feelings in "other kids" before identifying idiosyncratic precipitants. Nonverbal children may be encouraged to act out the situation in a charades game format or even to draw the situation. The therapist might verbally label the child's nonverbal depiction of the precipitants and affects. Mandell and Damon (1989, pp. 61–62) developed another handout, "How I Show My Feelings," in which the child lists the ways he or she demonstrates feelings nonverbally. Again, the child with poor literary skills may portray these nonverbal expressions of feelings by using role play or pantomime. The therapist and child think of words that might convey the feelings displayed in the behavioral manifestations.

These are just samples of the creative strategies clinicians may use to help children identify and label their feelings. The therapist must remain cognizant that accomplishing this task is often a gradual and sometimes long process that runs through the entire course of therapy. The therapist who believes that this task will be accomplished after two or three sessions and working on a few handouts will be sorely disappointed. Children need repeated opportunities to practice their growing skills in this area. The therapist's efforts must be supported and complemented by parents or caregivers who model, teach, and encourage the child's verbal expression of feelings and emotions.

PLAY THERAPY TECHNIQUES
Introduction: Why Play Therapy?

In Chapter 4 we discussed how play serves as a medium through which children, with their less sophisticated verbal skills, can communicate their thoughts, feelings, and significant concerns. Besides those cognitive–developmental variables that render play a viable and meaningful communication medium, maltreated children are often too frightened to talk directly about their experiences. For these children, play provides a safer means of communication. But as we argued in Chapter 5, the therapist might have to take a more directive approach, albeit one that is gradual and sensitive, for those children who strenuously attempt to avoid exposure to the cues and stimuli associated with maltreatment.

Play therapy may be used to help children learn to articulate their feelings rather than to rely upon maladaptive affective expression. The child's impulse control is enhanced by transforming action into words. The doll play of children with anger management problems illustrates this concept and may be replete with examples of physical aggression: in the doll play, parents physically or sexually assault their children, who in turn attain vengeance or retribution by beating up or assaulting others. When confronted with these displays, the therapist should introduce more appropriate and healthy expressions of anger. This process may be initiated by the therapist verbally labeling the affect of the play character (e.g., "She's really mad!"). The therapist asks the child to have the character put those feelings into words ("What could she [the character] say when she was so angry?") and then asks the character how it feels to speak of the feelings. For children who have great difficulty in refraining from physical assaults, even in the context of pretend play, the therapist might issue a challenge in a positive and fun way. Perhaps the therapist might say, "Let's see if you can put your hands together and keep them like that while you tell him how angry you are. Let's see how long you can do that. I'm going to start timing you now." Other techniques have been developed based upon a similar premise. James (1989, pp. 165–166) describes the "Clay Bombs" exercise as a way of releasing aggressive feelings. The therapist draws a picture of the person who abused the child. The therapist and the child then take turns throwing clay "bombs" at the depiction of the individual. However, both must also verbalize the accompanying feelings as they do this.

As children grow more comfortable with the maltreatment-related material and their feelings, they become more amenable to discussing their own experiences and feelings openly. Webb (1991) notes that relief of symptoms with no transition from the play to the child's life is certainly possible, especially in work with preschool-aged children. However, the school-aged child who learns to tolerate and engage in more direct discussions of the victimization experiences seems to gain an even greater sense of mastery over these events and a greater sense of accomplishment ("I can talk directly to another person about those painful things that happened to me"). This greater sense of mastery may be particularly true for the older school-aged child who is expected to rely more heavily upon verbal communication skills than upon symbolic play in his or her natural environment (e.g., the classroom).

Although many factors influence the youngster's ability to verbalize, a principal goal of play therapy is to help the child toward better verbalization (Enzer, 1988; cited in Webb, 1991). Harter (1983) describes a four-phase model of therapy that has direct relevance for this goal. In play, the child moves from an indirect expression of his or her needs and conflicts in play to direct verbal expression. Harter's model is consistent with our description of the use of metaphorical play. Sensitive topics are first presented in an indirect and gradual way that ensures the child's defense mechanisms, such as avoidance and denial, are not reactivated. This gradual exposure decreases the child's anxiety. The youngster becomes increasingly able to tolerate more direct exposures to the material. In Harter's first phase, the characters within the play scenario talk to each other, with one character interpreting the other's behavior. For example, one character might comment that another is angry or distressed about being abused. This strategy provides sufficient psychological distance to enable the child to tolerate material that would be avoided if presented more directly. In the second phase, the therapist comments on how the child is like one of the dolls. In the third phase, the therapist tells of another child with the same name or similar appearance who is struggling with the same dilemmas or difficulties. This message is still sufficiently metaphorical and indirect for the child to accept the content of the communication. Finally, the therapist makes direct comments or interpretations without having to resort to metaphorical or disguised communications.

We now review in detail some of the more common play therapy techniques used with maltreated children.

Doll Play

Every playroom should be equipped with a set of bendable family dolls that represent mother, father, girl, boy, baby, grandparents, adolescents, and other adults. A dollhouse with furniture adds to the child's interest and encourages reenactment of family scenes. Life-size infant dolls, along with bottles and toy baby food, provide further opportunities for children to portray their experiences. Other useful play equipment for this work includes medical kits, soldiers, dinosaurs, and animals (wild and domestic).

A variant of this approach is sand play, or sand-tray therapy, a technique originally developed by Jungian analysts. An advantage of providing a sand-box or even something less elaborate, such as a large plastic rectangular container filled with sand, is that children, especially younger ones, seem to like the sand's tactile sensation. Also, they are able to hide or bury people or objects in the sand. Additionally, it is a medium with which most children are familiar, having played in sandboxes or sand trays at home, at parks, or in the kindergarten classroom.

Some maltreated children will begin to play spontaneously with this equipment and quickly reenact scenarios of their own maltreatment. For example, children may begin to portray the mother or father doll spanking or even physically abusing the child doll. These assaults may occur along with oppositional or defiant behavior by the child doll, such as refusing to eat. To encourage the child to talk about his or her affects that are related to this maltreatment, the therapist might ask the child how the doll feels when being so treated, or the therapist might speak to the doll directly. Upon hearing the child's (or doll's) reply, the therapist shows empathy with the expressed sentiment via simple statements like, "_____ [name of the doll] is really mad when her father hits her like that."

As already discussed, there are some children, especially neglected youngsters, who cannot verbalize these affects, even in the metaphor of play. They may not have the requisite verbal skills, such as internal state language, to articulate these affects. Doll play may afford another opportunity to teach the child to label these affective states. The therapist must observe the action of the play closely to detect whether the characters are giving hints or clues about how they feel. After observing the doll character lash out at others following an assault by a parent doll, the therapist might say to the child, "The doll seems really angry." Alternatively, following Harter's (1983) model, the therapist might have another doll in the play scenario make this comment. As children become more adept labeling feelings, the therapist might address the doll who is assaulting the child character, saying, "When you hit _____ [name of the child character] like that, you make _____ feel a lot of things. You make him/her feel _____." At this point, the therapist hesitates, leans over in the child's direction, and whispers, "What did he make _____ feel?" The therapist should empathize and legitimize the normalcy of the doll character's feelings just as he or she would in a more direct discussion of these experiences. Such comments convey the therapist's sensitivity to the child's internal state and place the child's feelings in a broader context (e.g., "Most kids get mad when they get hit like that"). These comments also serve to lessen the child's confusion about the origin of these feelings, and they help reduce the child's feelings of isolation and stigmatization as well. If the therapist believes the child is ready to move on to the next stage, the similarity between the doll's experiences and those of the child may now be pointed out. The therapist may ask if the child, when being abused or neglected, ever felt the way the abused doll feels (stage 2 of Harter's model). This approach may be too premature for some children, who respond to the anxiety by quickly stopping the play (play disruption) or vociferously and adamantly denying they ever felt that way. Rather than constituting evidence against the correctness of the therapist's comments, these overreactions indicate that the therapist's interpretations have generated significant anxiety and are therefore meaningful to the child (Harter, 1983). Conversely, children who show no reaction probably have not been affected in the same way, leading to the hypothesis that for them the comments may not have been that relevant. If the child's anxiety escalates significantly after these interventions, the therapist should empathize directly with that anxiety ["When we start to talk about what happened to you and how you felt, it makes you pretty nervous"]. The therapist may also explore the child's fears that are related to discussing the maltreatment. It may be necessary to revert to the more indirect comments to further allay the child's anxiety before attempting to expose him or her to more direct material in subsequent sessions.

Some children will not even use the metaphor of play to communicate thoughts or feelings about their victimization; even these indirect depictions and portrayals are too threatening, and the child will engage in repetitive or obsessional play to avoid those feelings. In Chapter 4 we described an assessment technique in which the therapist becomes more directive and presents maltreatment-related material in the guise of doll play. The therapist asks the child to "show what happens next." The clinician might use a similar technique in therapy sessions with children who attempt to avoid any form of communication about their experiences of abuse or neglect. At this time, children who have not yet played with the dolls or dollhouse might be introduced to play therapy. The therapist might draw the child's attention to the toys and suggest that child and therapist "make up a story about a family." Some children will respond but may spend most of their time arranging and rearranging the dollhouse furniture, probably to avoid significant issues. A limit should be placed on the time the child spends in this obsessional play, with the therapist making comments such as, "That looks pretty good. Let's see what happens in this family."

When a child continues to avoid any play that includes content related to maltreatment, the therapist should then seriously consider becoming more directive and begin exposing the child to some of the child's experiences of abuse. This direct approach may incorporate the doll play; the therapist might say he or she has "made up" a story about the dolls and would like the child to watch. The story should incorporate aspects of the child's own aversive experiences. However, the therapist should incorporate only those elements the child would probably be able to tolerate. Initial portrayals of actual episodes of the maltreatment, even in the metaphor of the play, may be too threatening and overwhelming and might render the youngster even less enthusiastic about this activity. For example, the therapist may want to start portraying a family whose members are of the same gender and age as the child's family. The family should be depicted in some relatively neutral activity and the child invited to "show what happens next." The child may, of course, want to stay with this neutral theme, but at least the therapist has caught the child's attention. In the next session, the therapist might present another family scenario using dolls. This time, a more emotionally sensitive element may be introduced, one that the child can tolerate. For example, the therapist might suggest that one parent is "cranky" and then ask the child to continue the action. Via the character of the child doll, the child might be asked how he or she feels when a parent becomes "cranky" and to portray what happens next. A subsequent scenario may involve the therapist portraying the child as somewhat defiant, then asking for a depiction of the parent's reactions. We have developed story stems that incorporate features of other types of maltreatment. Again, the main goal is to expose the child gradually to the disturbing material. This technique is similar to the gradual and paced approach the therapist takes when engaging the child in direct discussions about abuse-related material. Considerable time with these less threatening scenarios may have to be spent before the child can move on to more sensitive material. Rushing through this process or forcing a youngster to confront such material prematurely will lead to the reemergence of the child's maladaptive defense mechanisms and erode her or his trust in the therapist as a sensitive and benevolent figure.

Some therapists, especially those trained in a purely nondirective play therapy approach, may object to the purposeful introduction of abuse-related material into sessions. We can only counter by again stating that the external and internal pressures on maltreated children to avoid exploring and examining these issues, either directly or indirectly, are often enormous. They present a formidable obstacle to the child raising these issues. On the other hand, we strongly disapprove of forcing children to confront their pain or of continuing to expose them to material they are unable or unwilling to handle. We can only provide a relationship in an environment in which the child feels safety and accepted, then offer opportunities that, to use James's words, "gently invite the child to explore" (James, 1994, p. 85).

Puppets, Drama, and Role Playing

Like doll play, puppets, psychodrama, and role playing provide the child with a metaphorical means of communication and gradually expose the youngster to the maltreatment-related material. As in doll play, the therapist may assume a role in these activities, introducing relevant situations into the play or drama to present more material and to elicit the child's feelings and thoughts about it.

The child may spontaneously ask to play with the puppets (there should be a variety of animal and human cloth puppets, rather than complicated string marionettes) or to put on plays. Using the puppets, the child might enact scenarios of the original maltreatment. If the child does not verbally express the characters' feelings, the therapist, as the audience, may, at the performance's end, ask the puppets relevant questions about their feelings and thoughts. Another useful technique in engaging the participation of reluctant children is for the therapist to initiate a puppet show, in the same manner as was described in the doll-play section. The therapist might present an opening scene and then ask the audience (i.e., the child) for help in determining what might happen next. More emotionally salient material may be introduced in this gradual fashion. Similarly, the therapist may suggest stories for puppet plays that are relevant to the child's life and circumstances. The following case illustrates this approach.

> Seven-year-old Tara was living in a foster home after being removed from her mother, who had severely physically abused her for a number of years. For the first several months of therapy Tara was a defiant, noncompliant, and disruptive child who would not talk about her experiences. She began to show some interest in the puppets, picking them up and examining them. However, when invited to present a puppet show, she adamantly declined.
>
> The therapist decided to take the initiative and presented a puppet show to Tara. She gave Tara a "front-row seat" and told her that it was the very best seat in the house. The therapist began to enact a story about a little girl who lived with her mother but sometimes wasn't very happy. At this point the therapist stopped the action and, turning to Tara, asked her what should happen next.
>
> Tara then became a very active participant. She suggested that the mother become an "evil witch" who beat the girl. At this point, the therapist invited Tara into the show and asked her to think of a character she would like to portray. Tara assumed the role of a prince who went to elaborate lengths to ensure that the witch would not hurt anyone. He locked her in jail, threw her in a lake, and gave her "magic potions" that killed her. Despite these actions and precautions, the witch always escaped or, if dead, returned to life.
>
> In the metaphor of the puppet show, the therapist and Tara talked about the girl puppet's fear and anger, the normalcy of these affects, and the girl puppet's expectation that she was powerless and could do nothing to protect herself from the witch.
>
> Tara repeated this play regularly for several months. As her anxiety decreased, she and the therapist were able to have more direct discussions of how she had been treated in a similar manner by her own mother and of her fear that she would be returned to live with her mother.

The puppet play gave Tara the opportunity to express her fears and anxiety, initially in a disguised form and then more openly. It also provided the opportunity, in her role as the prince, to achieve a sense of mastery over a frightening situation. Although initial efforts were futile (the witch always returned to life or escaped), her puppet plays in later therapy sessions ended with the prince finally vanquishing the witch. Chapter 10 is devoted to a detailed discussion of play-therapy techniques that will allow the child to build a sense of mastery over the maltreatment.

Similarly, role plays and psychodrama provide the anxious child with some much-needed psychological distance from relevant themes. Just as hiding behind a puppet theater and speaking as puppets attenuate some anxiety, dressing up in costumes and pretending to be somebody else offer the same sense of distance and relief. Face makeup, masks, or even sunglasses may contribute to the child's sense of psychological safety. James (1989, p. 195) discusses "clowning": the therapist and child, pretending to be clowns, express emotions in verbal and nonverbal ways. In an earlier paper, Smith, Walsh, and Richardson (1985) describe a short-term therapeutic group in which the children were invited to create a pretend identity, a clown character who was a metaphorical expression of themselves. The children were encouraged to create a life story for their character. As a whole, the group constructed a story of how they came together and how they got along interpersonally. The same basic premise may be applied to individual psychotherapy. Children may be invited to participate in role plays and dramas in which they reenact relevant and sometimes painful aspects of their own histories. The therapist might suggest some relevant themes (e.g., "Let's put on a story today about a little animal who doesn't have a home"). As a character in the play, the therapist might model the verbal expression of feelings or ask how the child's character feels. Furthermore, the child should be encouraged and assisted in demonstrating ways both the child and the therapist might protect themselves or prevent further maltreatment.

Some children are enthusiastic about the idea of videotaping puppet shows or drama productions. The advantage of this technique is that the child and therapist can view the production and discuss it in detail. For example, the therapist can stop the tape at a particularly significant or interesting juncture and ask what the child's character was feeling. They might want to look at that particular portion of the tape several times to help the child identify and label the feelings accurately.

Other props may be used in these dramas and role plays to create a sense of safety for the child. We have already discussed the use of makeup and costumes. Toy telephones are useful as a means for the child to communicate with somebody she or he is not yet ready or able to address directly. The phones can easily be incorporated into the metaphor of the drama or role play.

Storytelling and Story Writing

Stories may be used in several different ways to help maltreated children uncover their experiences and express their feelings. Within the safe metaphor of the story, the child can learn to express feelings or discuss events, including those connected with a maltreatment history. Stories may also provide the child with the opportunity to master past trauma. For instance, traditional fairy tales such as *Hansel and Gretel* portray child characters as victorious over punitive and frightening figures. We discuss the use of stories to attenuate feelings of powerlessness and facilitate a sense of mastery and control over aversive events and circumstances in Chapter 10.

As a way to help the child express feelings regarding the maltreatment, the therapist might tell stories that incorporate the youngster's experiences. The therapist might also engage in a mutual story-writing task in which the clinician provides the narrative stem (see Buchsbaum et al., 1992, Chapter 4). The child is asked to answer questions to complete the narrative. In Chapter 2 we introduced 6-year-old Gary, who had been apprehended because of severe physical abuse, neglect, and psychological maltreatment. This was the young boy who misinterpreted the actions of other children on the playground. For example, he believed that their running toward him reflected a desire to hurt him. To facilitate Gary's exposure to the abuse-related material, the therapist began to write a story. *The Little Bear's Story* included some brief text and some questions for Gary to answer. Gary and the therapist completed a chapter each week. His answers were transcribed by the therapist, since Gary was only 6 years old and unable to write. The first three chapters and Gary's responses to the questions at the end of each chapter follow.

Chapter 1

Once upon a time there was a little bear who lived with his mommy bear and his uncle bear in a dark, scary cave. The little bear did not like living here because sometimes his mommy and uncle were mean to him.

QUESTION: How do you think they were mean to him?
GARY'S RESPONSE: They spanked him and said bad things to him like, "You shouldn't live here."
QUESTION: How did he feel when they were mean to him?
RESPONSE: The little bear felt sad and mad.
QUESTION: How would most little bears feel when their mommy and uncle were mean to them?
RESPONSE: They would feel worried about other worser things. Lock him in a closet, scared.

Chapter 2

Sometimes this little bear would get very angry when his mommy and uncle were mean to him. When he got angry he would have big temper tantrums – he would yell, stomp his feet, and sometimes he would pick fights with the other animals who lived in the forest.

QUESTION: How did the little bear feel when he had these temper tantrums?
RESPONSE: Mad.

Chapter 3

The little bear also got really scared when he got so mad and had these temper tantrums. He was scared that everyone would hate him and that he was the worst little bear in the whole world when he got mad and had these temper tantrums. Sometimes his mommy and uncle told him he was a horrible little bear when he had a temper tantrum and that no one loved him or wanted him when he was very mad. And they would be even meaner to the little bear when he had a tantrum.

QUESTION: Do you think the little bear was a bad bear because he got so angry?
RESPONSE: No, because he didn't do anything.

The narrative stem developed by the therapist incorporated actual episodes from Gary's life. He had been abused by this mother and her partner. Both had repeatedly told him that no one loved him when he retaliated with anger. He had also been locked in a closet. The therapist encouraged Gary to draw pictures to depict the scenes in each chapter. Drawing was another way for Gary to express profound feelings of terror and sadness about being treated so horrifically. Allowing children to use the therapist's computer to write these stories often adds another element of interest and fun. However, with young children like Gary, the therapist did the writing and transcribed his verbal responses to the questions. Gary was pleased with the "book" he had produced. Overtime, as Gary became more comfortable with this material, his anxiety abated, and later he could talk more directly about his actual experiences. Gary also had the good fortune of being placed with a foster parent who provided him with excellent care and ultimately adopted him. Now at 11 years of age, Gary is flourishing. He is a top student, has friends, and is described by his adoptive mother as a loving and caring child.

Writing letters is a technique that, like storytelling, gives the child the opportunity to express difficult feelings. The child feels more comfortable with this exercise when he or she is informed that the letters will not be mailed. Even young children who cannot read or write can participate in this exercise. The therapist functions as the "secretary" who transcribes the child's letter. The following letter was "dictated" by a 7-year-old boy whose father had physically and sexually abused his older brother and sister. Although Mike had not been abused, he was unable to see his father because contact had been prohibited by the court.

To Dad:

When will you stop abusing other kids and get some help so you can see us again? I'm mad at you because you abused Sam and Donna. Why did you feed us pizzas every time we went over there [referring to contact before the court restriction]? Thanks for the things you gave us.

Clean your house—it's a mess.

Love, Mike

The reader will readily discern that the letter is replete with ambivalence. It served as a base from which Mike and the therapist could discuss these conflicting feelings. Mike's father was murdered several months after this letter's preparation. The therapist used it again after his father's death to help Mike express his grief and conflicted feelings about his relationship with his dad.

Children may be encouraged to write letters to the nonoffending parent. Feelings of anger, betrayal, and hurt often emerge. They are often associated with the child's suspicion that the nonoffending parent had knowledge of the maltreatment while it was occurring. Their concern that the caretaker could have been more supportive can be expressed safely in these letters.

Art

Art can symbolize intrapsychic as well as interpersonal events. As Harter (1977) states, art visually and concretely portrays feelings and other abstract psychological constructs that the child may have difficulty expressing verbally. Art is a way of concretizing psychological concepts.

Many of the techniques described in Chapter 4 may be used for therapeutic purposes. Children may be encouraged to produce graphic representations of their affective states when they were being maltreated. Figure 8.1 is a poignant illustration of the feelings of sadness and powerlessness engendered in a 9-year-old boy who was physically abused by his mother. Figure 8.2 was produced by a 4-year-old child. She had been sexually abused by her mother's common-law partner, and she was now asked to draw how she felt when it happened. The third drawing (Figure 8.3) was made by a 9-year-old boy who had been sexually abused by his mother's partner. The therapist asked the boy to draw his feelings about the abuse. In the middle of the drawing is the perpetrator, with a prominent penis, and the child is on the right-hand side, throwing an egg at the perpetrator's genitals. After he produced this drawing, the child was asked to draw a picture of his face showing his feelings about the sexual abuse. He produced the angry-looking face we see in Figure 8.3, with the daggerlike teeth in the right-hand corner. These graphic representations of feelings allowed the

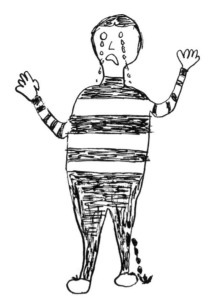

FIGURE 8.1. Nine-year-old boy's depiction of his feelings during his physical abuse.

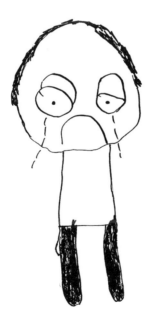

FIGURE 8.2. Four-year-old girl's depiction of her feelings during her sexual assault.

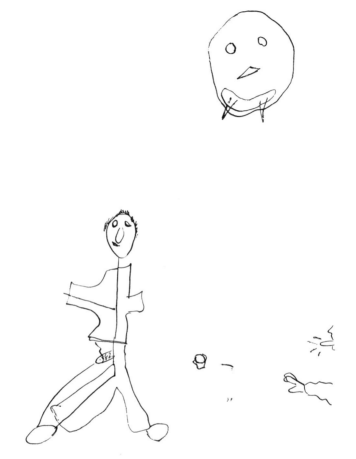

FIGURE 8.3. Nine-year-old boy's depiction of his feelings during his sexual assault.

therapist and child to label them, and the therapist was able to legitimize the normalcy of the child's rage. Asking children to draw their bodies after the maltreatment may give them the opportunity to express their concerns and worries about body integrity and health.

The other drawing techniques described in Chapter 4 may be used productively in therapy to facilitate a child's expression of his or her feelings and cognitions about the maltreatment. Children may be asked to draw their family or the perpetrator. The drawings may be quite accurate depictions of their feelings of loss, sadness, or anger, as well as of their ambivalence. The reader may wish to consult Chapter 4 for a more detailed review of these tasks.

Older school-aged children sometimes produce even more complex and sophisticated graphic representations of psychological events. In Chapter

4 we referred to 10-year-old Bob, who had been sexually abused by his mother and her common-law male partner. Bob testified in criminal court against them. Both were convicted of sexual assault and sentenced to lengthy prison terms. Several weeks after testifying, Bob was bothered by a recurrent dream. He was asked to draw the dream, which was in three parts (Figure 8.4). In the first part (Figure 8.4a) , Bob and some other boys found themselves in a prison run by a "headmistress" and a man with "skraggly hair." These people were abusive toward Bob, who was approximately 20 years old in the dream, and toward the other boys, some of whom were as young as 5 years. Bob drew a picture of himself with strap and whip marks across his chest. After Bob had produced this first picture, the therapist asked him if the man and woman in the picture reminded him of anyone. Bob immediately stated that they reminded him of his mother and her common-law partner because they had been so mean to him. In the first part of the dream, the boys and Bob escaped, and he cut off the breast of the headmistress (as exemplified by Bob's drawing of the "snippers"). The therapist asked Bob to identify on the paper how he felt when he was maltreated in this manner, and he wrote, "Mad, scared, sad, get Vengeance [*sic*]."

In the second part of the dream (Figure 8.4b), Bob broke into a gun store and stole a gun, which he fired at the headmistress. He felt "god [*sic*] [i.e., good], vengence [*sic*], mad, and powerful." In the third and final part

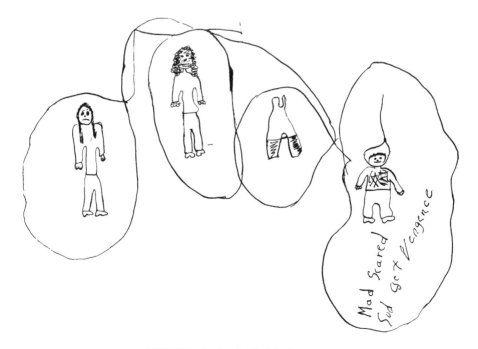

FIGURE 8.4(a–c). Bob's dream.

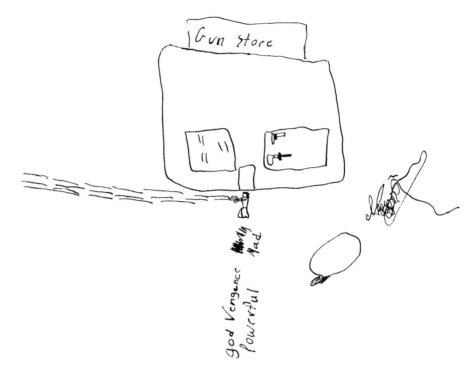

FIGURE 8.4b.

of the dream (Figure 8.4c), the headmistress came back to life. She and Bob together were involved in a car crash. The headmistress died, and he sustained a broken leg. Bob spontaneously noted after drawing this picture that he was "hurt on the inside" (analogous to the broken leg). He then began to talk directly about some of the emotional sequelae of his own abuse experiences. He also expressed confusion about why, in the dream, *he* had

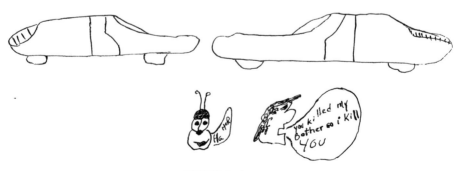

FIGURE 8.4c.

been hurt in the car crash. The therapist wondered aloud whether Bob was in the car crash because of his guilty feelings about his anger and his worries regarding the consequences of his anger for his mother (firing a gun at the headmistress and sexually mutilating her). At this point, Bob burst into tears. Bob told the therapist that he had felt "awful" about testifying against his mother, even though he knew that her abusive actions were destructive and illegal. His involvement in the car crash may well have been his symbolic attempt to punish himself for betraying his mother by testifying. Bob's dream provided some information regarding the revenge fantasies he had that included a sexual component (e.g., cutting off the breast of the headmistress). This graphic portrayal of the dream was a springboard from which Bob and the therapist could talk about his conflicted feelings regarding his testifying against his mother, Bob and the therapist were now also able to discuss more appropriate ways for Bob to express his anger.

Art provides other ways of representing complex and sophisticated psychological concepts. Nine-year-old David had been severely physically and psychologically neglected by his mother who eventually abandoned him, his older brother, and his younger sister. In her one meeting with a child welfare worker, David's mother stated she was "fed up" with the demands of her children. A consistent theme in therapy was David's confusion about the reasons for his mother's abandonment and his longing for her to return and resume caring for him. During one session, David commented that he had been thinking he would like to draw some pictures of his family. The therapist encouraged him to do so. David spontaneously said that he was going to make a "map." He proceeded to draw a picture of a house and then drew small figures of himself, his older brother Andrew, his younger sister Victoria, and his mother (Figure 8.5). On several occasions, he spontaneously referred to these figures as being "stuck" and needing to find their way back home through the "mazes." He drew an X on the map, which he claimed represented a treasure chest that contained $60,000. When asked what would be the best thing about having this kind of treasure chest, David stated that his mother would find it. She would then be able to buy "good food and good clothes" for him and his siblings. The therapist and David began to talk about his intense desire for his mother to find a job and a residence. David believed this would result in her return and resumption of parenting. He acknowledged feeling quite sad when he thought about his mother's absence. He then drew a "bridge" from his mother to the treasure chest; the "bridge" was a "shortcut" to the money and allowed her to bring the children to her home. When asked how the children would feel if their mother could find and bring them home, he said they would feel "happy," but "sad" if they were still "stuck" outside. The map was an accurate representation of David's feelings of abandonment, the difficulty he foresaw in returning to his mother's care (the "mazes"), and his feelings of

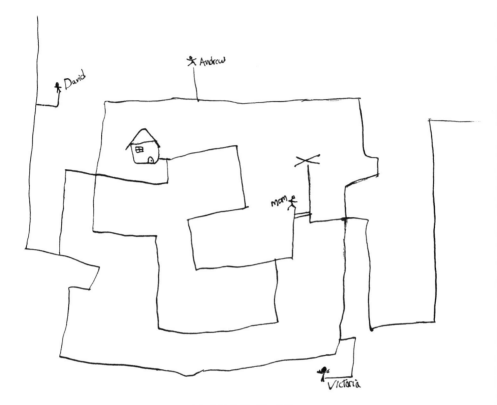

FIGURE 8.5. David's map.

sadness about separation from her. It also depicted his reliance upon a more tolerable explanation for his mother's absence. David attributed her absence to a lack of financial resources rather than acknowledging she no longer wanted to be bothered with the demands of childrearing.

FACILITATING FEELINGS ABOUT LOSSES

Maltreated children need to experience and express their feelings of loss. Failure to do so may result in their reliance upon maladaptive defense mechanisms such as projection, denial, and splitting, which create more problems in the long term. Memories of unfulfilling and unsatisfying relationships with parental figures have to be recovered and retained, rather than denied and repressed. For example, the child needs to mourn the loss of a parent that results from a legally mandated separation. The feelings of sadness and betrayal that accompany the realization that the parent was unable or unwilling to love the child in the way the youngster wanted also must be acknowledged and expressed. Obviously, examining such issues is extremely painful. The child must have alternate sources of support before he or she can acknowledge the parent's inability or unwillingness to provide the love and care the child deserves (James, 1994).

Besides defense mechanisms, there are certain cognitive–developmental factors that limit young children's ability to recognize and acknowledge their ambivalence about their parents. A hallmark of the preoperational period of thought (ages 2 to 7 years) is the child's ability to attend to only one perceptual dimension at a time, to the exclusion of all others. The classic example is the conservation experiment. Here the preoperational child insists there is more water in the taller and narrower beaker than in the shorter and squatter container. The child's judgment is dominated by the perception of the single most salient perceptual feature, in this case height (Piaget, 1952, 1967). In contrast, the concrete operational child can consider more than one attribute simultaneously and can understand the reciprocal relationship between height and volume. Harter (1977) extrapolates these principles to the development of the child's understanding of emotional concepts. Just as the preoperational child can focus on only one perceptual dimension at a time, the same child has difficulty focusing on more than one emotional dimension at a time. Harter (1983) demonstrates that 4- to 12-year-old children encounter great difficulty in understanding that they can have both positive and negative feelings toward the same person. Thus, a maltreated child may have great difficulty in comprehending that he or she can both love and hate an abusive parental figure.

How can therapists facilitate the child's acknowledgment and expression of painful and sometimes conflicted feelings? Harter (1977, 1983) describes a simple drawing technique that can help a child understand his or her ambivalent feelings. The therapist draws a circle or other shape to represent the child. A line is drawn down the middle: the two halves represent two feelings, such as love and hate. The drawing provides a concrete visualizable symbol to which the child can attach real experiences. Figure 8.6 is a reproduction of one drawing completed by a 7-year-old boy who was physically abused by his mother.

Rich was asked to draw a shape that depicted himself and to identify feelings associated with certain aspects of his relationship with his mother. Rich identified "mad" and "sad" when she hit him, and "glad" when they had fun playing games together. Identifying and acknowledging these split-off feelings can counter the child's tendency to engage in defenses like dissociation.

Readministering this may also help in gauging changes in the child's differentiation of feelings as therapy progresses. Figure 8.7 displays the feel-

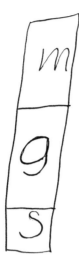

FIGURE 8.6. Graphic respresentation of a 7-year-old boy's feelings about his mother. m, mad; g, glad; s, sad.

ing circles drawn by Jonas, who was 12 years old when he was removed from his home by child welfare authorities. This action followed the disclosure of Jonas's longstanding sexual abuse by his mother and her common-law partner, Max, who was also a close relative. Max also subjected Jonas to many beatings. Jonas did the first drawings (Figure 8.7a) shortly after beginning therapy, when he wanted strongly to return to his mother and minimized his abuse. The next drawings (Figure 8.7b) were done 10 months later. They clearly demonstrate that Jonas was beginning not only to acknowledge his abuse but to recognize the many conflicted feelings he had about his mother and her common-law partner.

A therapist may use other techniques to help children uncover these memories and concretize past experiences. A child might be asked to bring photograph albums to therapy sessions. Looking at pictures of family members, especially of those who no longer have contact with the child, provides the child with concrete reminders about these relationships. By reviewing photographs, children often begin to remember specific incidents that in turn bring more significant material into consciousness. Many children in the care of child welfare authorities have been given "life books," which are a compilation of mementos, photographs, and souvenirs about the child's history. These objects are concrete reminders that allow children to acknowledge their history more openly and directly, including the negative and painful aspects they have tried to avoid and deny. Although it is often a difficult task, the therapist and child should begin to assemble a life book, if it has not already been done. The therapist may have to gather historical information from child welfare authorities and share it with the

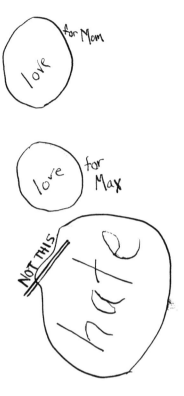

FIGURE 8.7a. Drawing by Jonas in early therapy.

child. Helping the child prepare simple genograms, or family trees, often clarifies for the youngster some of the more confusing aspects of his or her history. It sometimes elicits even more questions, some of which cannot be answered. The creation of a family tree affords another opportunity to help the child identify and express feelings of sadness, loss, and anger. These feelings may be associated with never having had, for example, a consistent father figure or even knowing his identity.

One of the most powerful exercises in uncovering these memories and feelings is to go on a "photo expedition" with the child. This procedure is particularly useful for a child with little documented history and who doesn't remember his or her previous residences or family placements. It is often useful first to gather some relevant historical information about the child from other sources, such as child welfare records. The therapist should make a list of the addresses of the child's previous residences or schools and show them to the child. To make this exercise even more concrete and real, both might visit these locales. Obviously, the therapist must exercise ex-

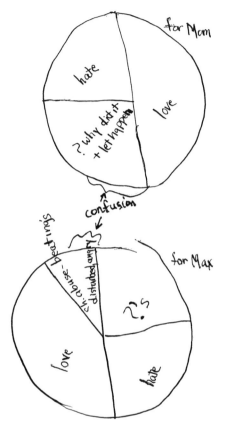

FIGURE 8.7b. Drawing by Jonas after 10 months of therapy.

treme caution and sensitivity when deciding what information the child will receive and what sites they will visit. Giving a youngster the address of his or her biological parents whose parental rights have been terminated is not in the youngster's best interests and might also contravene strict court orders prohibiting any contact between parents and child and constitute an invasion of the parents' privacy. It is usually best to limit information of, and subsequent expeditions to, former schools or residences; the therapist must be absolutely certain that these sites are no longer occupied by individuals with whom the child should have no contact. The therapist might teach the child how to use a simple camera, so the child can take pictures of each significant locale to place in a life book. Children usually love this "field trip." They frequently begin to remember past incidents or episodes when they are at a site, such as a school they once attended. Painful and powerful feelings are sometimes elicited. The therapist should help the child articulate these feelings and connect them to specific events, including maltreatment. Having a permanent record of these stimuli in the form of a photograph allows the child and therapist to reexamine these issues often.

A number of years ago one of the authors treated a 12-year-old boy who had been badly neglected. His mother had committed suicide and was buried in a distant city when James was 8 years of age. His mother's death was a significant issue, and he had never seen her grave. This fact contributed to his difficulty in putting any closure on this aspect of his life. During James's treatment, his therapist and her husband and children visited the other city for a vacation. The therapist offered to search for the boy's mother's grave and take a photograph of it. After considerable searching by all family members in the cemetery where the grave was known to be, it was found and a photograph was taken. This photograph served as a concrete reminder of his mother's death and, although painful, did much to help James express his sadness and grief about this loss.

Cunningham and MacFarlane (1991, pp. 138–139) developed a tool they call "The Loss Timeline." Children construct a graphic representation of the losses they have experienced and their ages when these losses occurred. The technique may be combined with "Color Your Life" (James, 1989, p. 196). The child is instructed to makeup legends of different feelings, each associated with a different color. The child uses the colors to identify various events on "The Loss Timeline." This is another visual depiction of the child's losses and their specific associated feelings. The child may also be helped to express feelings of loss by identifying the differences between his or her "old family" and "new family." The child lists or dictates the differences and then displays them next to each other on a piece of paper. If not particularly verbal, the child might draw scenes depicting the "old life" and the "new life," along with the different feelings and reactions evoked by each.

Kagan (1986) recommends the use of games to help children who are in alternate placements express the attendant feelings. Kagan (1986, pp. 80–92) developed "Cast Adrift," a pursuit game in which the squares graphically portray typical situations and events of being in care, such as running away from a foster home. As these examples show, a game may be created to reflect each child's particular experiences. For instance, by landing on a square that says "Removed from foster home, lose one turn," the child is encouraged to discuss the feelings he or she associates with such an event. The game may be developed by the child and therapist after they have gathered more information about the child's life through life books or photo expeditions. This material may be incorporated into an individualized game that reflects the salient facets of the child's life.

TREATMENT OF DISSOCIATION
AND MULTIPLE PERSONALITY DISORDER

The major task in the treatment of dissociative phenomena is to bring repressed feelings and experiences into the child's conscious awareness so that they may be acknowledged and explored. The child then no longer must rely upon dissociation or other defense mechanisms to guard against the overwhelming pain and anxiety associated with these experiences (Gil, 1991; James, 1989). Assisting children to express these repressed and split-off feelings has been the central theme of this chapter.

It is appropriate here to make several other comments about the specific treatment of dissociation. Other techniques can be used profitably besides those of identifying and sorting out feelings. Gil (1991) and James (1989) describe quite similar intervention plans. They recommend the therapist evaluate the child's awareness of his or her use of dissociation and help develop a label or term the youngster can use to communicate about it. Children may be helped to identify those situations in which they dissociate and to examine the functions of the dissociation. They should also be told that there are even more adaptive ways to cope with aversive experiences or feelings. James (1989) also advocates helping the child examine the advantages and disadvantages of dissociation. She suggests that the therapist explain to the youngster that he or she has used dissociation in a creative and inventive way for protection. Then the child may be asked to describe his or her idiosyncratic dissociative response or pattern and to "pretend" to dissociate in the therapist's presence (Gil, 1991). In subsequent sessions, the child may be encouraged to stop this sequence at different points while pretending to dissociate. The precipitants to this response must be identified and, as we have stressed, the painful feelings and experiences identified. James (1989) maintains that it is especially important to help children acknowledge and accept the fact that they have conflicting feelings. They must also understand that feelings and thoughts are not actions and that they should discard their expectation of being rejected or punished for having these feelings. The therapist must introduce more adaptive ways of coping with these troublesome feelings or situations rather than repressing or avoiding them. Chapter 9 is devoted to a detailed description of how to teach children healthier coping mechanisms.

The authors have not had much clinical experience in treating children with multiple personality disorder. Consequently, we would refer the reader to the work of others, which provides some specific direction besides those in our earlier comments on treating dissociative phenomenon (Braun, 1986; Gil, 1991; James, 1989; Kluft, 1984, 1996; Putnam, 1989). Among these other treatment aspects are making a contract with each personality a child may exhibit to avoid harmful actions such as suicide or homicide or to meet therapy goals, working on the problems of each personality, and mapping and understanding the structure of the personality system (Braun, 1986). Gil (1991) and Putnam (1989) recommend that the therapist encourage co-consciousness and communication among the personalities. James (1989) uses metaphors in stories "where separate parts can come together to create a wondrous whole that is appreciated by all, with no one losing. Examples might include a rainbow whose colors are all right separately, but especially beautiful, powerful, and appreciated when joined together." (p. 112). She also suggests the therapist get the child to use vivid visual imagery to accompany these metaphors. Gil (1991) has prepared a clinically rich case description of the treatment of a severely sexually abused 8-year-old girl who had developed several distinct personalities. Kluft (1996) has written a valuable article describing the outpatient treatment of dissociative disorders in children in detail but space limitiations preclude an in-depth review of this work. Kluft describes the differences between the treatment of adults and the treatment of children with dissociative symptoms, the importance of creating an atmosphere of safety in which the child feels secure, fostering cooperation among the alter personalities, and teaching the child to contain strong feelings. "Metabolism of trauma involves accessing and processing the overwhelming event held in autobiographical memory, regardless of their unascertainable historical accuracy" (Kluft, 1996, p. 481). Kluft warns therapists to refrain from exposing the child to traumatic material too prematurely; processing should proceed at a pace tolerable to the child as to avoid significant anxieties and distress.

Both Friedrich (1990) and James (1989) caution therapists against intervening in ways that inadvertently reinforce the development of more dissociative phenomena or more numerous or complex personalities. For example, by asking leading questions of maltreated children who feel compelled to acquiesce to adult demands the therapist may open the door for elaborated but misleading symptomatology. James (1989) also recommends that therapists work closely with other significant adults in the child's life so that they accept these phenomena but do not overreact in ways that make the child the center of attention. This is excellent advice from two experienced clinicians.

In this area clinicians seem to be divided between "believers" and "nonbelievers," with both sides expressing strong and sometimes vitriolic opinions. As clinicians, we must approach issues of dissociation and multiple personality disorder with an open mind. However, we must evaluate the applicability of such diagnoses to our young clients in the same rigorous, comprehensive, and individualized manner that should characterize all our clinical work. Labeling a child as dissociative or "a multiple" just because these terms are in vogue does our client and our profession a great disservice. Conversely, a failure even to entertain the possibility of the presence of these phenomena results in a failure to provide comprehensive and adequate service.

Whatever techniques are used, the therapist who helps children uncover their histories and express the attendant feelings and issues must often use exquisite timing and clinical judgment. Knowing when to expose a child to a bit more material and when to back off are skills honed by experience, training and supervision, and a critical and rigorous examination of one's work. The therapist must have the flexibility and creativity to respond to the changing and sometimes perplexing needs of these young children.

Assisting children to recount these experiences and express their feelings is only one part of the therapeutic process. Maltreated children must learn effective ways of coping with their painful memories and feelings. In the next chapter we discuss this topic in detail.

NINE

Helping the Child Develop Effective Coping Mechanisms

ABUSED AND NEGLECTED children require help in developing mechanisms to cope with feelings and cognitions regarding their maltreatment. The therapist can help a highly anxious child cope more adaptively with symptoms such as nightmares and sleep disturbance. The child who acts out anger or sexualized feelings needs assistance to bring this behavior under control. This control enhances the child's behavioral and emotional self-regulation and ensures that others are not hurt. A child who continues to act out invites rejection and condemnation, which in turn has a detrimental effect upon that child's self-esteem.

In this chapter, we describe specific techniques for targeting problems such as anxiety, nightmares and sleep disturbance, physical aggression, and intrusive sexual behavior. Given the limitations of this volume, our review must be somewhat cursory. Topics like anger management in children and, more recently, interventions for intrusive sexualized behavior have received considerable attention in the professional literature. We hope to give the reader a brief overview of the theoretical basis and a description of some commonly used techniques.

TECHNIQUES TO HELP THE CHILD COPE WITH ANXIETY-RELATED PROBLEMS

In Chapter 1 we reviewed the internalizing problems associated with a history of maltreatment. Posttraumatic stress disorders and other anxiety-related symptoms are among the most common disturbances in self-regulation manifested by maltreated children, especially those who have been sexually abused. Manifestations of increased arousal associated with a posttraumatic stress disorder include sleep disturbance, hypervigilance, difficulty in concentrating, and outbursts of anger or irritability. Dreams, flashbacks, and psychological and physiological distress associated with exposure to external or internal cues that resemble or symbolize an aspect of the traumatic event are examples of reexperiencing phenomena. Dreams and sleep disturbance often generate a great deal of distress in children and parents. A number of strategies may be employed when the clinician is confronted with these problems. Assisting the child in learning effective ways of coping with the anxiety is often a central task of treatment. Besides being exposed to the anxiety-related stimuli so that their anxiety can be extinguished, children benefit from other strategies.

In Chapter 8 we described standard techniques such as breathing and relaxation training to help children reduce the anxiety they experience during direct discussions of the maltreatment or during symbolic play. The therapist, besides incorporating and using these techniques in therapy sessions, should instruct and guide children with significant anxiety problems to use such techniques in other environments.

Relaxation Exercises

To alleviate some anxiety, the child may be instructed to use relaxation exercises while in bed. Younger children often require concrete imagery and an audiotape, whereas older children eventually learn to relax and control their response without these prompts. Sometimes older children enjoy working with the therapist to develop a relaxing scene; the therapist then records the details on tape. The material on the tape may incorporate one or several techniques the child finds useful. The child then takes the tape home and uses it to help him or her calm down. These exercises may be especially useful at bedtime, when some children are particularly bothered by intrusive memories and anxiety. Most children respond well to some parental or caregiver support when using a tape or the other techniques and are impressed when parents also use the tapes for themselves. Other techniques such as breathing and balloon imagery, described in Chapter 8, may be used in almost any situation in which the child feels anxious and overwhelmed. Other people around the child may not even realize the child is consciously working at calming himself or herself.

Visualization

Visualization is useful in assisting children to master unpleasant or frightening dreams. The therapist asks the child to recount or even draw the frightening dream to obtain more details of its content. Then the therapist instructs the child to visualize a scenario that transforms the frightening content of the dream into something more benign. For example, the child might visualize having a magic wand that changes a monster into a positive and friendly figure. Depending upon the sophistication of the child's verbal and cognitive skills, detailed scenarios may be developed that incorporate this sense of mastery. Drawing and art may be used as adjunctive strategies to visualization. The child draws the dream sequence using a cartoonlike format in which the frames of the cartoon depict the dream's progression. The youngster develops new scenes or frames that portray the child mastering the monster or other frightening figures or scenarios. This graphic depiction might then be tacked on the wall near the child's bed. Just before going to bed, the child looks at this sequence, particularly the positive outcomes, as an aid in visualizing the new outcome. To further diminish his or her anxiety, the child may employ deep breathing or other relaxation exercises while visualizing the new dream. Self-hypnotic techniques can also be taught to induce this state of relaxation.

Other frightening dreams or nightmares may be symbolically contained by having the child draw a picture of the dream and then put the drawing in a box. The youngster tapes the box shut to ensure the dream does not "escape." The child should be encouraged to "open up the box" (i.e., examine the maltreatment-related material symbolized by the dream) when he or she feels more comfortable. This process is similar to James's (1989) "Garbage Bag" technique, which was reviewed earlier. However, keeping dreams locked up forever may reinforce the child's belief that this material is so threatening it can never be examined and therefore must be suppressed. This belief may consolidate the child's use of maladaptive defense mechanisms and entrench his or her symptoms. When feeling less anxious, the child might pull a different aspect of the dream (each aspect is graphically displayed on a separate piece of paper) from the box in each therapy session and examine it. The piece of paper should be symbolically destroyed once the child has processed that particular vignette of the dream.

Rituals

There are other techniques that rely upon the concretization of abstract psychological concepts. For example, some children with increased arousal become hypervigilant. They may fear that the perpetrator will break into their homes and reassault them. Terrorized children may maintain this belief even when they know the perpetrator has been incarcerated. These children constantly monitor their environment and are acutely sensitive to any stimuli (e.g., unexplained noises) that might be interpreted as evidence they are again in danger. We have had children "freeze" their perpetrators to reinforce the belief that they—the children—are now safe. A small figure of the perpetrator is constructed by the child from plasticine or other modeling material. The child and parents or caregivers are instructed to bring this figure home and place it in a container of water so that it is totally covered. The container is frozen, and the block of ice with the figure is removed from the mold and placed back in the freezer. When feeling particularly anxious about the perpetrator escaping, the child may go to the freezer and look at the perpetrator entrapped in the block of ice. Concurrently, the child may use self-statements as a reminder that the perpetrator can no longer hurt the child. This strategy is often particularly useful for children with sleep disturbance associated with the expectation that the perpetrator will return at night and reassault them. They might spend several minutes just before going to bed looking at the block of ice while using relaxation exercises or self-hypnotic techniques.

Other children make up their own rituals to instill a sense of safety. They may have to tour the house to ensure that the doors and windows are locked, or they may check under beds and in closets. Some children may insist upon sleeping with their parents. We try to discourage the last as much as possible since it inadvertently conveys the notion that the child is unable to master the anxiety. Also, sharing their sleeping arrangements sometimes engenders frustration in parents, who are thus deprived of their privacy. However, children who are absolutely insistent may be accommodated by sleeping on the parents' bedroom floor in a sleeping bag or on a small cot, but not in the parental bed. Each night the parent should encourage the child to move the makeshift bed a little further from the parents'; out of the bedroom, into the hallway, and eventually into the child's room. Giving the child a night light, particularly one that he or she has chosen, may reduce some of this anxiety at bedtime, as can relaxing and soothing experiences such as having a hot bath or listening to music.

Cognitive–Behavioral Techniques: Self-Statements

The therapist may use cognitive–behavioral techniques profitably to help children master other anxiety-related symptoms such as intrusive memories and thoughts. Any reader unfamiliar with this approach should review standard texts in the field (e.g., Kendall & Braswell, 1993) for its theoretical underpinnings and for detailed descriptions of specific techniques. Some of the basic elements of cognitive–behavioral therapy are incorporated into the techniques we describe in this chapter.

At the risk of overly simplifying cognitive–behavioral therapy, it is possible to describe its principal goal as teaching children how to "stop and think." A major class of interventions within the cognitive–behavior therapy area is self-instructional training. According to Kendall and Braswell (1993), "Self-instructions are self-directed statements that provide a thinking strategy for children with deficits in this area and serve as a guide for the child to follow through the process of problem solving" (p. 124). A central theoretical notion inherent in self-instructional training is the relationship between behavior and language. We argued in Chapter 2 that the development of internal-state language aids in the child's regulation of behavior and emotion. Vygotsky (as cited in Kendall & Braswell, 1993, p. 10) postulates that a crucial step in a child's ability to control his or her behavior voluntarily occurs when the child internalizes verbal commands. The influence of self-talk or self-statements is clear when we think about learning to perform some new task or skill. We may even talk to ourselves aloud (overt self-statements) to provide ourselves with guidance and direction (e.g., "Now I have to press this key in order to call up the information on the computer"). Then we move on to covert self-talk or self-statements where we "quit talking out loud and begin to think the instructions to ourselves" (Kendall & Braswell, 1993, p. 184).

Let us return to the problem of intrusive thoughts and memories in maltreated children. Self-statements may be an especially useful technique. Intrusive memories and thoughts about the maltreatment (i.e., "flashbacks") are often particularly frightening and distressing; children feel they have little, if any, control over their affective states. One of the first things a therapist can do is to provide a simple yet direct explanation of this phenomenon and make it clear that many other children have experienced similar reactions. The child should be taught to use self-talk or self-statements to reduce anxiety, such as, "What happened to me is over and this is just a flashback," or, "This has happened to other kids too–I'm not crazy!"

Children then may be encouraged to develop self-statements that in turn can be combined with other techniques to counter anxiety. In Chapter 7 we briefly introduced 11-year-old Derek, who was sexually assaulted once by an adolescent male babysitter. He was referred to therapy because of anxiety-related symptoms, including nightmares and intrusive memories of this one-time assault. Derek was bothered by intrusive memories of the sexual assault, particularly of the scene in the bathroom, where he had been forced to perform oral sex on the adolescent babysitter. The bathroom served as an external cue that quickly elicited his anxiety, which was reflected in these intrusive memories and a sense of reliving the experience. In Derek's words, sometimes just being in the bathroom made him feel as if "it was happening all over again." His anxiety-related symptoms were an example of the localized effects described by Finkelhor (1995).

To assist Derek, the therapist suggested that he say "Stop!" to himself as soon as he became aware of the intrusive memory of the assault. The therapist and Derek developed a self-statement Derek could use after telling himself to "stop": "This is just my memory–I'm not really being abused again!" The self-statement was combined with simple muscle and deep-breathing relaxation exercises. Other self-statements incorporated the fact that Derek had prevented further occurrences of the abuse by quickly disclosing the incident to his parents the day after it had happened ("I took action, and it didn't happen again!"). Derek was directed to visualize himself as the major-league baseball player he especially admired to reinforce and consolidate his growing sense of mastery over the situation. This visualization served as a concrete reminder to Derek of his own excellent athletic abilities and that the sexual assault had not diminished in any way his outstanding performance in baseball and other sports. The salience of the visualization and self-statements about his mastery and numerous other strengths was increased after Derek was instructed to place a baseball card of his hero in the bathroom. This card served as a concrete prompt for Derek to begin the "stop and think" process. It also served as a cue for visualizing his own substantial strengths and as a reminder that they had not been deleteriously affected by the assault. Given his excellent adjustment prior to the assault and the support afforded by his family, therapy with Derek was short-term (6 weeks).

Some children have been so severely abused and terrorized that they experience overwhelming and debilitating anxiety that deleteriously affects many areas of their functioning. Anxiety that has been generalized to many different stimuli in their environments is now pervasive. These children begin to avoid such stimuli to reduce their discomfort. An intervention that must target a number of different symptoms in different environments frequently requires the collaboration of other significant people in the child's life and is usually of much longer duration than Derek's. This approach was used in the following case.

> Steve was a 13-year-old boy who, from 9 to 12 years of age, had been sexually abused by his father. The abuse was horrific and included the father anally raping Steve on numerous occasions. The father also used physical violence to gain his son's compliance and ensure his silence, and threatened to kill him and his mother if he ever disclosed. Steve disclosed the abuse several months after his parents separated and the father left the home. The police subsequently charged his father with a number of counts of sexual assault, and a court order was issued prohibiting any contact between Steve and his dad.
>
> Steve showed symptoms of a posttraumatic stress disorder when he was seen in the initial assessment. He was having frequent dreams of the abuse and many flashbacks of the incidents. He also showed symptoms of increased arousal, including disrupted sleep and difficulty in concentrating in the classroom. Steve was especially hypervigilant, constantly monitoring his environment to ensure his father was not following him or lurking around the home. His anxiety had escalated to the point where he was terrified of leaving his home. He would not go outside and refused to attend school. Steve claimed

that he saw his father near the school grounds after he had been charged and believed his father would attack him because he had disclosed. His father's threats to kill him and the physical violence to which Steve had been subjected gave these fears a solid basis in reality. Steve was terrified of leaving his mother at home because his father had also threatened to kill her. Steve's anxiety about this issue had been compounded by his witnessing several episodes of marital violence before his parents separated.

Intervention incorporated many of the elements we have described in this chapter. Relaxation exercises resulted in an improvement in Steve's sleep. A major emphasis was placed upon helping him leave his home and return to school. To initiate the process of gradual exposure and desensitization, Steve was instructed to spend 3 minutes on his front steps several times each day while engaging in deep breathing and muscle relaxation exercises. Steve insisted on keeping the front door fully open so that he could get into the house immediately if his father appeared. The amount of time spent outside and the distance from his front door (which he finally allowed to be closed) increased and continued to be paired with relaxation. With the help of his therapist, Steve began to develop self-statements emphasizing his progress and mastery of the anxiety (e.g., "I'm now halfway down the block–I'm doing really well!"). Other self-statements, which focused on concrete strategies he could use to protect himself if his dad ever appeared, began to counter his feelings of powerlessness (e.g., "I'll run right into the house, lock all the doors, and tell Mom"). After several weeks, Steve could walk around the block and approach his school, a short distance from his home.

Steve required further practice with these techniques before he could resume classes. In particular, he identified those situations at school that quickly evoked strong feelings of anxiety (e.g., being outside on the school grounds). Not only was he instructed to use the relaxation techniques in these situations; he and his therapist devised "a plan of action" that Steve would use if his father ever came to school. According to this plan, Steve would go immediately to the school office and tell the staff of his father's presence in the school. Steve and the therapist had previously rehearsed what he would say if this sitaution arose. Self-statements such as "I know what to do now if he ever shows up" helped decrease his anxiety. Fortunately, the school vice principal agreed to be part of the treatment team. Not only was she willing to talk with Steve when he became especially anxious but together they developed a specific plan that she or her designate would implement if his father ever came to the school (e.g., calling the police to report that the father had broken the no-contact order). These plans attenuated some of Steve's anxiety and increased his feelings of mastery and control over a terrifying environment.

This case example highlights the need to involve significant people in the child's life during the treatment program. Besides the vice principal,

Steve's mother played a critical role in assuring him that she could protect herself. There were times when she had to be firm, such as insisting he attend school even when he was anxious. To have allowed him to remain at home would have done nothing to help Steve surmount his anxiety. Moreover, these strategies were only one component of treatment. Much emphasis was placed on helping Steve articulate his rage, sadness, and feelings of betrayal, as well as reformulate the meaning of these experiences.

Some abused and neglected children experience symptoms of depression. In Chapter 8 we described strategies to help children recover and express memories related to their histories of maltreatment, abandonment, and family dysfunction. Another component in treating depression is to encourage the child to reexamine and reformulate the meaning of the abusive or neglectful episodes. This topic is discussed in the next chapter.

EXTERNALIZING BEHAVIORS: PHYSICAL AGGRESSION AND INTRUSIVE SEXUAL BEHAVIOR

Our review of the effects of maltreatment indicate that physical aggression is not an uncommon symptom in abused or neglected children. These children require intensive assistance to prevent them from victimizing others and ensure they learn healthier ways to express their angry feelings, which in turn makes it easier for them to form more rewarding interpersonal relationships. This is a broad topic and we can only highlight some of the more important approaches and techniques; we rely primarily upon a cognitive–behavioral approach. Besides the work by Kendall and Braswell (1993), the reader may want to refer to the descriptions of anger management programs prepared by Lochman, White, and Wayland (1991), as well as a review of anger management control techniques for children completed by Stern and Fodor (1989).

We have also pointed out that sexualized behavior is another common sequelae of childhood sexual abuse. Children who engage others in this behavior need the same kind of intensive help as physically aggressive youngsters. Although this area has not received enough professional attention, there are some valuable resources the reader may wish to consult for detailed descriptions of treatment approaches (Cunningham & MacFarlane, 1991; Friedrich, 1990; Gil & Johnson, 1993; MacFarlane & Cunningham, 1988). Here we review the application of cognitive–behavioral principles to treat physical aggression and sexually intrusive behavior exhibited by some maltreated children. In Chapter 6 we described the critical role parents play in this process, especially in supervising and limiting their children's inappropriate behaviors.

Clinicians sometimes struggle with the problem of how to treat child victims who exhibit "victimizing" behavior (physical aggression or sexually intrusive behavior toward other children). Their reluctance to address this behavior actively may be due to their greater experience and familiarity with treating victims rather than perpetrators. Clinicians may also not understand that a child's victimizing behavior may well reflect unresolved issues engendered by his or her victimization. Unfortunately, the traditional division of clinicians into those who treat victims and those who treat perpetrators has done little to encourage the development of a service-delivery approach that integrates features of both domains. Intervening with both victimization issues and physical aggression and sexually intrusive behavior is consistent with our philosophy of providing comprehensive treatment services. A clinician's failure to intervene when a child shows victimizing behavior may represent the clinician's inadvertent collusion with the child's reliance upon this behavior. It places other children at risk and does little to help the youngster develop more appropriate coping mechanisms (Cunningham & MacFarlane, 1991). Conversely, the failure to address these victimization issues precludes an opportunity for the child to uncover, express, and reformulate the meaning of the the victimization and its relationship to the child's maladaptive coping mechanisms. For example, victimized children need to express their feelings of powerlessness and inadequacy as a first step in finding more adaptive ways to cope with these effects. To provide truly comprehensive services that address the different facets of the maltreated child's functioning and adaptation, the therapist must be prepared and able to address both sets of issues.

Self-Monitoring

Before they are taught to control their anger, children may benefit from learning some self-monitoring skills. First, they may be taught to identify their angry feelings. Some children are not able to recognize accurately the point at which they begin to get angry and may only realize they are angry after they have hit someone. Control of these feelings may improve if they can identify their anger at an earlier point and implement techniques before their anger escalates to the point where an aggressive outburst becomes likely. Children may be helped to identify the somatic cues to their anger (e.g., flushed face, increased muscle tension) by having them graphically depict such somatic cues on an outline of their bodies. Some children may be able to identify the cognitions or self-statements that occur as they become angry (e.g., "I'm so angry I'd like to knock his head off!").

Similarly, children should be taught to identify and recognize their sexual feelings. This is even a more difficult task than having children identify their anger. Typically, we do not talk with our children about the fact they have these feelings. Children have an even smaller common vocabulary to describe their sexual feelings than that describing their anger, so they have fewer terms they can share with adults. Furthermore, there is considerable debate about the role of sexual arousal in generating sexually intrusive behavior in preadolescent children (Hall, 1993). There is no consensus regarding whether every child who is sexually intrusive has been influenced by strong feelings of sexual arousal. Even if some are aroused, they usually do not have the terminology and words to communicate these internal feelings and experiences.

The therapist should help the child understand the difference between anger (a feeling) and aggression (the overt behavioral expression of this anger via physical attacks or other means). Children should be told that anger is a normal feeling experienced by all of us. However, children should learn we do not have the right to express angry feelings in whatever form we desire, as in beating up someone. They should know that the same notion applies to sexual feelings: such feelings are normal, but their presence does not give us the prerogative to act them out in any way we want. There are various ways to help the child differentiate between anger and aggression. Besides verbal discussions, the child might cut out magazine pictures of people showing angry feelings and contrast them with pictures of individuals behaving aggressively (Cunningham & MacFarlane, 1991). Cunningham and Mac-Farlane (1991) also suggest that the child and therapist use puppets or role plays to illusrate concretely the difference between these two concepts. For example, the youngster is asked to enact one scene showing the puppet displaying angry feelings in healthy ways (e.g., talking about his or her anger) and then another scene in which the characters express anger aggressively. Obviously, the therapist cannot ask young children to find pictures of people acting out sexual feelings in inappropriate ways. Instead, therapist and child might discuss what would constitute healthy and age-appropriate sexual expression for the child.

Drawing the distinction between having a feeling and expressing it in destructive or unhealthy ways highlights a broader issue confronting therapists who work with children with externalizing behavior. What are the therapist's values and beliefs regarding physical and sexual aggression? It is important to address this issue, since these values invariably affect one's clinical work. For example, one of our basic values in working with children who present significant problems with physical aggression is the importance of introducing nonaggressive and noncoercive means of conflict resolution. Therapists who do not introduce the child to alternate means of expressing anger may convey a tacit approval of the child's continued reliance upon physical aggression. Such a misconception may lead to serious consequences for the child and others. For those children with poor ego controls and barely functional defenses, a therapy process that encourages catharsis only does not serve recovery well. We strongly encourage the reader to review an article by Ryan (1989) for a more detailed exposition of this argument. She maintains that therapists must introduce accountability into therapy by limiting the child's demonstrations of power and control that victimize others. According to Ryan (1989), therapists must confront a child's irrational thinking (e.g., "I'm going to kill the person who abused me") and offer rational alternatives to aggressive displays. Given our adherence to the value of nonaggressive ways of resolving conflict, we work actively and intentionally in therapy to promote the same approach in the children we treat. Therapists should describe the underlying beliefs that guide their treatment plans when discussing recommendations and the proposed therapy plan with parents or caregivers. Parents need this information so they can give informed consent to treatment.

The issue of values becomes even more contentious when the therapist talks with children about the difference between "healthy" sexuality and "inappropriate" expression of sexual feelings. Although therapists must examine and identify their own values, they must also consult closely with parents or caregivers about their values and what they want conveyed to the child. Are parents even aware of their sexual values, particularly as they relate to their children? If it is a two-parent family, have they discussed this issue with each other and reached a consensus? What do they believe constitutes acceptable sexual behavior for their children: may the child masturbate, or is this totally unacceptable? As we noted in Chapter 6, these are central issues that must be addressed before any direct work with the child is initiated concerning distinguishing between "appropriate" and "inappropriate" sexual practices. If the therapist promotes one set of values and the child is exposed to a different or even contrary set at home, the child is placed in an untenable position. Moreover, this situation undermines the parent's authority. Therapists must be especially sensitive to religious or cultural variables that may play a significant role in the development and maintenance of sexual mores in the family. They must attempt to seek an agreement with the parents about what is acceptable sexual expression for their child. However, we should note that sensitivity and respect for parental values concerning sexuality does not always translate into the therapist's wholehearted endorsement or acceptance of such values. We have had a few occasions when we reached a fundamental disagreement with a family. One set of parents believed that any sexual behavior, thought, or feelings constituted incontrovertible proof of sin. They thought that even raising the issue of sexuality would further eroticize their child, and they would not permit, during sessions, any discussion of the child's sexuality. These parents maintained this stance despite long and protracted discussions with the therapist and clear evidence that the boy was increasingly making sexually aggressive advances toward younger children. Eventually the therapist had no choice but to withdraw from the case because of this fundamental difference with the parents. He had to notify child welfare authorities of the real risk the boy posed to other children and the parent's refusal to permit the therapist to address it directly.

Another important self-monitoring task for many children is to learn to identify the precipitants (i.e., the situations, events, feelings, somatic cues, and cognitions) that preceded the emergence of aggression or sexually intrusive behavior in them. This task is a major component of the relapse-prevention approach. The basis of relapse-prevention is understanding the chain of events that precedes a particular pattern of behavior one wants to change. By identifying these precipitants, the child can take alternate action to interrupt such preceding events and initiate strategies to prevent their progression to physical or sexual aggression.

The therapist should attempt to determine if the child can identify any precipitants but must remain aware of possible limitations of this approach. First, treatment approaches based upon a relapse-prevention approach were developed with adolescent and adult offenders. Can we apply this model to young children, particularly considering their cognitive and developmental differences? Are young children aware of precipitants, especially more abstract kinds such as their cognitions and feelings? Harter (1977) notes that young children, even those in the stage of concrete operational functioning (7- to 11-year-old range), have difficulty in identifying and understanding their feelings, because affects are less directly observable. Other factors compound children's difficulty in examining internal psychological factors that influence behavior. Less sophisticated verbal skills, a shorter attention span, and embarrassment about the content of physically aggressive or sexually intrusive fantasies, as well as a corresponding reluctance to disclose these fantasies render the identification of precipitants a difficult enterprise for young children. Moreover, although in the adolescent/adult model sexual fantasies are considered to be significant precursors to sexualized behavior, at this point we have little empirical knowledge about the conscious, identifiable sexual fantasies of preadolescent children and what role they play in sexualized behavior (Cunningham & MacFarlane, 1991).

How can the therapist help identify precipitants? Asking children to "brainstorm" about all the situations that evoke anger is often useful. The list may be divided into different categories, such as "people who make me angry" and "things [events/situations] that make me angry." Children who cannot read or write may provide the therapist with a verbal report and then draw the particular precipitant. Having children identify and describe in detail a specific situation in which they became physically aggressive may assist in identifying precipitants. Precipitants to aggressive or other maladaptive behavior also include cognitions, which may have special relevance for maltreated children. In Chapter 2 we reviewed how maltreated children, many with insecure attachments and a consequent lack of basic trust in the

world and other people, often misperceive and misinterpret social information and behavior as evidence of hostile threat or intent. They may fail to
attend to relevant cues in social situations and then will react in an aggressive, externalizing manner to guard against the perceived threat and also
to compensate for these feelings of powerlessness and inadequacy.

Gil and Johnson (1993, pp. 244–245) have developed a technique called
"Cartoons" to teach sexually intrusive children self-observation skills. The
technique is used to identify behavior sequences, including the precipitants
and consequences of sexual behavior. Children are asked to draw pictures
("cartoons") of themselves in a series of frames or squares that depict the
progression of a particular behavior. Children should draw what they felt
and thought, and what was going on before they engaged another child
in sexual behavior. Then they should draw the actual event. Subsequent
frames illustrate the consequences of their behavior. We have found this
to be a valuable technique in helping children with physical-aggression
problems as well as intrusive sexualized behavior. Like many others, the
technique relies upon the notion that school-aged children need assistance
in making abstract concepts, such as cognitive, emotional, and behavioral
precipitants, recognizable and tangible. The therapist can provide this assistance by giving these concepts visualizable and concrete form.

Self-Instructional Training and Problem Solving

After assisting the child in recognizing his or her anger or sexual feelings
and identifing some precipitants of these patterns, the therapist should introduce other cognitive–behavioral techniques. Among such techniques are
those that incorporate self-instructional training (Kendall & Braswell, 1993)
and interpersonal cognitive problem solving (Spivack, Platt, & Shure, 1976).
The child is taught to use self-instructions and self-talk to guide himself
or herself through the various steps of problem solving. In this way, the
child's responses are preceded by deliberate thought, and self-regulation of
emotions and behavior is enhanced. The therapist should guide the child
through the steps in problem solving outlined below to prevent an episode
of physical aggression. The same strategy may be used to help children refrain
from engaging in sexually intrusive behavior.

Initial Inhibition of Impulsive Responses

The youngster is taught to "stop and think" when he or she becomes conscious of the emergence of angry or sexual feelings and cognitions that pre-
cede inappropriate behavior. Other precipitants might include particular
situations (e.g., teasing by other children, being alone with younger children). A common practice is to label these precipitants as "red flags" that

signal situations that represent potential problems. The child is encouraged to say "Stop!" and to follow this statement with another self-statement such as "I'm getting angry now. I'd better think about what I'm going to do next." A visual depiction of this instruction in the form of a small stop sign may serve as a useful reminder to the child. Other prompts for inhibiting the aggressive or sexual response, such as having the child count to 10 or "freezing" like a statue, may be suggested (Kendall & Braswell, 1993).

Problem Definition

Using self-talk, the child formulates a definition of the problem (e.g., "I'm getting real mad now, and I don't want to end up hitting him").

Choice of a Goal

Typical goals for aggressive children might include self-statements like "I'm really mad when he's teasing me. What can I do to make sure I don't hit him?" Self-statements for sexually intrusive children might include "I'm feeling like I'd like to touch someone's private parts. What can I do to make sure I don't get in trouble?"

Alternative Thinking

Alternative thinking refers to the child's ability to generate multiple alternate solutions to a problem situation. These alternatives typically include physical aggression ("I could hit him") and others that are probably more adaptive ("I could walk away and find someone else to play with when he teases me"). Children with sexually intrusive behavior have devised alternate solutions such as playing a computer game or drawing (to be described below). In this stage, the emphasis is upon generating alternatives rather than evaluating their utility.

Consequential Thinking

In this phase, the child is taught to evaluate the immediate and long-term consequences of the alternatives already generated. Kendall and Braswell (1993) recommend that the child evaluate the possibilities in terms of their emotional and behavioral consequences for the child and for the other person. The child might ask himself or herself, "What would happen if I did this?" (referring to the behavioral consequences). Then the child may evaluate the emotional consequences by asking himself or herself how the other person would feel. Based upon this evaluation, the child may next decide upon a solution and implement it. The child can also be encouraged to devise a backup plan.

Self-Reward

The child is encouraged to use a self-reinforcing statement to reward himself or herself for appropriate problem solving (e.g., "I did a great job–I didn't end up hitting him!" [or touching his private parts]). Self-statements may also be used to counter the frustration that may emerge when the child encounters difficulties. For example, rather than immediately giving up, the child might engage in self-talk that counters the frustration and encourages persistence. The child might use alternate self-statements such as, "Well, I made a mistake. It's not the end of the world, and I should try another way of doing this," rather than saying, "Boy, I made a mistake. I'm really stupid."

Practice and Rehearsal

An important component of practice and rehearsal approach is to provide the child with numerous opportunities to practice these general problem-solving skills. After the therapist has walked the child through the above steps, role playing with the child can start. The therapist may want to choose scenarios that are not particularly difficult to solve to ensure the child achieves some initial success. As the child becomes more comfortable with the approach and attains even more success, the therapist may begin to present situations and scenarios that present greater problems. Among these situations are those that the youngster has identified as precipitants to aggressive displays. The therapist may then present actual scenarios that have been particularly troublesome for the child in the past. The therapist might play the role of another child who frequently teases the child, which in turn prompts the youngster to hit the other child to stop the teasing. The therapist should be extremely cautious about presenting role play scenarios that include sexualized interactions between the child and another person. Children find such scenarios too arousing, and their anxiety rapidly escalates. It is better to talk about these situations rather than to role play them.

Besides teaching the general process of problem solving, the therapist should assist the child in developing specific plans to cope with especially difficult situations. The child may be having physical altercations with a certain child or group of children. The therapist and child should develop alternate ways of coping with this situation, engage in thinking of ways to evaluate the consequences of each alternative, and then rehearse and practice the child's specific response. The same approach may be taken with sexually intrusive children. They require specific plans to cope with those situations in which they are more likely to act in a sexually inappropriate manner. Gil and Johnson (1993) recommend that children develop substitute behaviors to distract them from sexual thoughts and feelings. These activities should be ones that the child likes and finds pleasurable (e.g., video games, puzzles). They should help expend energy but should not involve body contact or physical aggression. Participating in these substitute activities with parents may motivate the child to refrain from engaging in sexual behavior (Gil & Johnson, 1993). Children should try the problem-solving approach and different alternatives in their real environments between sessions and then report the results during their next session. "Homework" might consist of recounting observations of the other person's reactions to their nonaggressive stance, the success of the alternative solution, and personal feelings and reactions (e.g., pride at not hurting somebody).

A fun element and the provision of more opportunities to practice and rehearse the problem-solving approach and specific plans may be introduced by writing different scenarios on index cards. The child and the therapist take turns choosing a card and rehearsing the steps. These same scenarios may be incorporated into a simple pursuit board game. When either lands on specially designated squares, he or she must respond to the provocative situation described on the card using the steps described above. Either misses a turn if he or she is unable to generate alternate solutions or a specific plan. The therapist's involvement in these tasks makes them much more a shared activity and enables the therapist to model the problem-solving approach.

A similar approach may be applied to actual interactions with the child. For example, the child may behave in a way that angers the therapist. The therapist may verbalize aloud, using the problem-solving steps to develop an appropriate response to the child's provocation. Similarly, the therapist may encourage the child to use the problem-solving approach when he or she is angry with the therapist. As reviewed in Chapter 2, some chronically abused and neglected children are not lucky enough to have had a relationship with a primary caregiver that fostered these self-regulatory skills. The therapeutic relationship can provide such a child with the opportunity to engage in a process wherein the therapist helps the child develop the capacity for self-regulation. For example, in Chapter 7 we discussed the tendency of children with ambivalent–resistant attachment organizations to become angry when they believe their needs are not being met. Besides helping the child inhibit impulsive responses by the imposition of external limits or through self-statements, the therapist assists the child to define the problem in the relationship verbally with the therapist and to identify the associated affects (e.g., "I'm mad at you because you won't let me stay longer in the session"). Children with poor internal-state language may need considerable help in identifing and expressing these feelings. The therapist then helps the child choose a goal and generate alternate solutions to the problem.

The therapist should be aware that many maltreated children, especially those whose internal-state language was compromised at a very young age, require a great deal of practice to develop these internalized controls.

We stressed in Chapter 6 that the therapist must incorporate parents or caregivers in the treatment program. Their participation is especially important because it is often in the home environment or community that the child exhibits externalizing behavior. Kendall and Braswell (1993) recommend that therapists encourage parents to express social recognition and praise when they observe the child using the problem-solving approach. Parents must be particularly attuned to those situations in which the child is likely to become aggressive or is at risk for engaging in sexually intrusive behavior. The parent may then have to prompt the use self-instructional skills via simple statements like "This looks like a good time to stop and think" (Kendall & Braswell, 1993, p. 189). A nonverbal prompt such as a hand signal also may be useful. Its added benefit is that although the child recognizes the cue, others are unaware of the significance of the communication. Parents who model the problem-solving approach in their daily lives exert a potent and positive influence upon their children. Children who have lost control should be given in a time-out until they have themselves under control again. The parent should present the time-out as an opportunity for the child to calm down and gain control (Kendall & Braswell, 1993). The time-out interrupts the behavior, thus permitting the child to exercise control rather than being used punitively.

The various elements of self-monitoring, self-instructional training, and problem solving discussed above may appear complex and confusing to some child clients and their caregivers. Over years of working with children who have difficulties with expressing anger in particular, we have evolved a concrete model that can help clients understand the basic elements of these interventions. We call this model the "Anger Mountain" and find that children readily identify with it, particularly when they exhibit massive tantrums and rages. An Anger Mountain, as illustrated in Figure 9.1, is drawn and colored in by the therapist and the child and then explained to the child's parents or caregivers.

Line *A* on the drawing of the Anger Mountain represents the current status of the child's anger and tantrums. A child may seem calm, but an apparently minor stimulus may well generate instant, soaring anger. Because of the immediacy of the child's anger, there is no time to divert the impending tantrum and manage it more thoughtfully. Furthermore, the child takes a long time to calm down. By the time the child is calm again, both child and caregivers are exhausted and feel inept and overwhelmed. To begin the intervention, the child and caregivers are instructed to focus first on helping the child calm down sooner. This task may involve introducing reinforcments for the child to calm down, such as not permitting the youngster to come out of the room until he or she is calmer. This approach is a better alternative than having the child wait for a set period or trying to talk the child out of his or her anger. These last two interventions some-

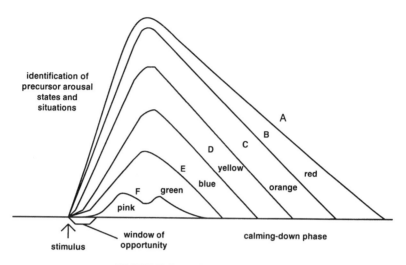

FIGURE 9.1. Anger Mountain.

times inflame a child's tantrum further. As the child and the caregivers discover that the child is able to become calm sooner, the tantrums are likely to lessen in severity, as illustrated by lines *B* through *F*. The goal is not to eliminate the anger but to moderate it so that it is manageable, as illustrated by line *F* or possibly even line *E*.

Once the child begins to learn to calm down, both the child and caregivers begin to feel less overwhelmed. A small window of opportunity to avert a tantrum then appears in the anger outburst. The child begins to be aware that he or she is angry and can then begin problem solving and planning constructive ways of expressing the anger. The precursors of the outbursts may also be identified. These precursors may include the child's recognition that some situations will produce heightened anger in him or her or that various physiological states such tiredness, hunger, illness, and excitement will increase his or her reactivity. In our experience, many children can easily rate the level of their anger by using different colors on the Anger Mountain and see their progress as the colors change. Children the feel more successful and more in control of regulating the expression of this affect.

Developing Empathy and Perspective Taking

Another important component of the cognitive–behavioral approach to anger management is the individual's ability to take the perspective of the other person (empathy). Although there are many determinants of aggressive behavior, empathy deficits have been cited as one variable associated with its emergence (Feshbach, Feshbach, Fauvre, & Ballard-Campbell, 1983). Children may be inhibited from hurting others by becoming aware of the potentially harmful consequences of their actions. Inhibition occurs when they have a cognitive and emotional appreciation of the psychological and physical pain evoked by their aggression. Similarly, Cunningham and MacFarlane (1991) propose that sexually intrusive children must develop an appreciation of the effects of their behavior upon others. This empathic understanding contributes to their ability to stop and later refrain from the sexualized behavior.

Unfortunately, maltreated children, especially those who have suffered prolonged and serious abuse or neglect, may encounter significant difficulty in empathizing with the needs and feelings of others. In Chapter 2, we reviewed how some maltreated children's difficulty in establishing a "goal-corrected partnership" with a primary caretaker impairs their subsequent social relationships. These relationships become characterized by an absence of reciprocity, sharing, and sensitivity to others' feelings and needs. Furthermore, a maltreated child's exposure to the psychological distress of others may be threatening, since these reactions begin to remind the child of his or her own pain. By successfully excluding these affective states from consciousness through avoiding, ignoring, and dismissing the feelings of others, the child avoids personal distress. Children must confront their own pain before they can acknowledge that of others.

Helping children develop empathy for others is often a slow process. Although the therapist may introduce some activities to initiate this process, children require considerable practice in honing these skills. Again, the involvement of parents or caregivers is critical. These adults should prompt such children to consider the consequences of their actions for other people. Cunningham and MacFarlane (1991) present many techniques designed to encourage a sense of empathy. The reader is well advised to review this valuable resource for creative ideas and suggestions: we briefly describe several techniques below.

The therapist may begin by helping the child identify his or her needs in different situations before attempting to identify the needs of other people. Cunningham and MacFarlane (1991, pp. 184, 186) describe an activity they call "What Would You Need If?" It invites children to respond to questions like, "What would you need if you were lost?" or, "What would you need if you were caught in an elevator?" Subsequent questions deal with the needs of children who have been maltreated: "What would you need if you were physically abused?" "Sexually abused?" (Cunningham & MacFarlane, 1991, p. 184). In a subsequent exercise, "What Do They Need?," children are asked to identify the needs of people in various situations as portrayed by magazine pictures (Cunningham & MacFarlane, 1991,

p. 186). Another exercise, "Identifying the Feelings of Others" (Cunningham & MacFarlane, 1991, p. 186), involves children in looking at pictures of people in various situations and then identifying the people's feelings. The children are invited to speculate about the possible situations and events that might have led to these affective states. This exercise is another opportunity to teach children to identify and label feelings accurately as well as to sensitize them to the feelings of others.

There are many other opportunities to help the child develop a greater appreciation of the feelings and needs of others. In play scenarios in which the child assumes the role of a hurt or threatened character, the therapist might request the character to verbalize his or her feelings or reactions. Empathic statements from the therapist model this skill and reinforce the notion that one's actions do have consequences for other people.

After the therapist and child gave engaged in these preliminary exercises for the development of empathy, a focus should be placed upon identifying the common reactions of people subjected to physical aggression or intrusive sexual behavior. This may be a relatively straightforward task for children who have already uncovered their own feelings about their victimization. By drawing upon their own experiences, they can now answer questions regarding the feelings of persons who have been physically or sexually assaulted. Other children may need more concrete stimuli to become more familiar with common maltreatment effects. A particularly useful video, *Good Things Can Still Happen,* has been produced by the National Film Board of Canada (Scully, 1992). This 22-minute video depicts common reactions of boys and girls (cartoon characters in the video) who have been sexually abused. There is a pause in the video between the segments that portray these different reactions. The therapist and child should watch the video together, with the therapist asking the child to identify each character's feelings and reactions. For those child victims who have not yet clearly articulated their feelings, viewing the video can reduce their sense of isolation and serve as a catalyst for more discussions about the child's reactions (e.g., "Have you ever felt like that kid in the video?"). The video also helps develop or consolidate children's appreciation for the effects of abusive behavior, including their own, upon others.

Older school-aged children may benefit from reading newspaper accounts of real children who have been physically or sexually abused. Again, they should be asked to identify the possible reactions and feelings of these other child victims. Puppet plays may be used to depict a character being hurt or somehow maltreated. As the audience, the child, using the puppets, indicates how the victimized character might feel and is encouraged to show and verbalize these feelings.

Once the youngster becomes more comfortable with talking about physical aggression or inappropriate sexualized behavior, the therapist should

begin to focus on the reactions and feelings of the person the child assaulted or involved in sexual behavior. The therapist should request a verbal
account of what the child did to the other, with a particular focus upon
the youngster's perception of the other child's feelings and reactions. Children with limited verbal skills or who are reluctant or embarrassed to talk
more directly about these issues may be asked to draw a picture of the incidents and of the other child's facial expressions that depict that individual's
feelings. Again, the therapist must assist the child to identify and articulate
these affects. Here the trick is to avoid evoking an overwhelming sense of
shame or guilt about the behavior. The therapist should focus upon the
child's behavior rather than personally attacking the child and conveying
a sense that he or she is a replica of the perpetrator who hurt the youngster.
Statements like "When you hit other kids, you're doing just what [name
of perpetrator] did to you. You're turning out just like him!" erode a child's
self-esteem. They transmit the notion that the child is condemned to repeat
the past, only this time as the aggressor. Furthermore, these comments
reduce the child's trust in the therapist and might render the youngster even
more unwilling to disclose this problem behavior because of his or her fear
of more insults or personal condemnation. Therapists need to take physical aggression or intrusive sexual behavior seriously, but they must confront
the child about these patterns and their effects upon others in a respectful
way.

Exploring the actual feelings and reactions of maltreatment victims raises
a central question: "What is wrong with physical aggression [or intrusive
sexual behavior]?" This issue may be addressed directly by identifying as many
negative consequences as possible for both the victim and the perpetrator.
The negative consequences for the victim should be listed on one side of
a piece of paper and those for the perpetrator (e.g., loss of self-esteem, external consequences) on the other.

The therapist should attempt to convey the notion of coercion to children. Children should be encouraged to think of times when they felt forced
to do something, including episodes from their own victimization. They
should be prompted to articulate the associated feelings, either verbally or
through other means such as drawing their facial expressions. The child
should be informed that children cannot give consent, since they are not
aware of many consequences of sexual behavior with others. Role plays may
be developed depicting different types of coercion; in them, the child is
asked to portray his or her reaction. We mentioned earlier that the therapist must avoid pretending to physically or sexually abuse the child in role
plays. Such activity usually elicits intense anxiety from the child; it is better
to role play this abuse more indirectly, using puppets or small dolls. A list
may be developed of numerous ways to coerce people, such as resorting
to physical threats and psychological coercion. The use of developmental

status as a means of forcing others into inappropriate activities may be illustrated with examples of older children using their greater knowledge to trick younger ones into sexual activities. Also, it should be explained that differences in physical size may be sufficient to obtain younger children's compliance. To accentuate the potency of physical size as a way to gain compliance, we have marked a child's height on a blackboard. Then we have invited the child to estimate the height of the child he or she victimized. While the clinician assumes the child client's height, the child is instructed to crouch down to the level of the other child's height. Then the child is asked to look up at the therapist and state how it feels to be in such a position, especially if one is being threatened. The therapist must be especially sensitive to the child's anxiety in this exercise, since it puts the child in a submissive position, thereby replicating elements of the original victimization. Before beginning the exercise, the therapist should explain its purpose and instruct the youngster to signal if he or she becomes especially anxious and needs to stop at any point. A distinction should be drawn between the current situation and those that led to past victimization by pointing out that the therapist will do nothing to hurt the youngster. As an alternative, dolls may be used to represent the individuals, since doll play usually does not pose as great a threat to anxious children.

We reviewed earlier the importance of consequential thinking in problem solving. The child's understanding of the consequences of harmful or coercive behavior for others may be incorporated into self-statements (e.g., "She would probably feel really scared if I touched her private parts"). These self-statements may then be used by the child to prevent further episodes of inappropriate behavior.

Children should be encouraged to put empathic feelings into action once they develop an appreciation of the effects of their behavior on others. In our earlier discussion of problem solving and self-instructional training we reviewed strategies that enable children to engage in more fulfilling and healthier interpersonal relationships. The therapist might introduce some other techniques to consolidate these skills and abilities. "What Would You Do If?" presents a number of scenarios to which the child is invited to respond (Cunningham & MacFarlane, 1991, pp. 201, 203); for example, "If you lost a game at school, what could someone say to make you feel better? What could you say to someone who lost a game at school?" (Cunningham & MacFarlane, 1991, p. 201). Subsequent questions focus upon the child's own sexual molestation history and how others might respond to make the child feel better; also, what the child might say to someone else with this history. Appropriate questions may be developed for children with a histiry of physical abuse and neglect; the children themselves may be invited to develop the questions. Using the format originally developed for group therapy, each child picks and responds to a card on which one of the "What Would You Do If?" scenarios is written. A similar format may be used in individual therapy, or the therapist might create a simple pursuit board game: when either therapist or child lands on specially designated squares, he or she must pick one of the cards on which these scenarios are written. The child may take another turn as a reward for an appropriate response that displays an empathic appreciation of the needs of others.

After completion of these exercises, which focus upon more general responses to others' distress, the therapist may assist the child in identifying ways of making amends to the person the child hurt or victimized. One useful technique is to have the child to compose a letter of apology. These letters may be mailed, but only with the explicit permission of the parents or legal guardians of both children. The client child should state how he or she feels about hurting the other individual and describe what happened to validate the other person's experience. The child should be encouraged to assume responsibility for his or her actions, absolve the other person of any blame, and express some concern for that person. The therapist should act as a "secretary," transcribing the dictation of those children unable to write. The benefits that will accrue to the other individual, such as feeling validated and believed, should be discussed with the child. Children should be asked to put themselves in the other person's place and describe how they would have felt if their own perpetrator had apologized as they are now doing. It is also important to identify the benefits to the child who has apologized. These benefits include feeling better about oneself because one's guilt feelings are alleviated, as well as the realization that one can take responsibility for one's behavior.

The letters and discussions may serve as rehearsals for actual sessions in which the child apologizes to the other child (again, of course, with the permission of the legal guardians of both children). This session should be held after the child has developed some genuine appreciation of the effects of his or her actions. Having a child flippantly or smugly "apologize" does nothing to validate or legitimize the other child's concerns or issues. We have treated children who have devised other creative ways of making amends to younger siblings whom they have physically assaulted or sexually abused. One 11-year-old boy decided to allow his 7-year-old brother unrestricted use of his prized baseball glove for an entire week to make amends for his physical assaults toward the younger boy. Actions like these may be the first step toward a healthier and more fulfilling relationship between the child and the other individual.

"Recording Friendly Deeds" (Cunningham & MacFarlane, 1991, pp. 198, 200) is an excellent exercise to develop positive social skills and counter negative self-esteem, especially when it is based upon negative and harmful interactional patterns with others. Children may be told that although their physical aggression or intrusive sexual behavior indicates they made a mistake in the past, they are still able to relate in caring ways to others. This exercise is designed to provide children with proof of this statement. As a homework assignment, the child is given the task of performing a "friendly deed" a certain number of times in the intervening week. The child is given a simple chart on which to record the identity of the person who is the object of the caring act, the deed itself, and the other person's response. Children who cannot write may depict this information in simple drawings. Having the child observe and record the other individual's reactions enhances the child's concept that his or her actions have effects on others and that these effects can be positive and beneficial. We have asked parents or caregivers to initial each friendly deed the child completes that week, just as the parent might do for regular school homework assignments. Doing so ensures that parents become aware that their children can succeed and are not condemned to repeat physical or sexual aggression. The therapist should provide a great deal of praise and reinforcement for the friendly deeds completed in the intervening week. The child then completes another cartoon sequence (described above) that describes the deed and the consequences, as well as the child's feelings, cognitions, and situational variables that preceded the initiation of these friendly actions. This exercise provides the child with more practice in understanding that behavior has precipitants. However, as we noted elsewhere, younger children who have little insight into their behavior may encounter some difficulty in identifying these precipitants. The therapist may instruct those with poor peer relationships, in how to complete a friendly deed for another child.

Helping Children Acknowledge and Discuss Their Externalizing Behavior

Children are sometimes reluctant to acknowledge behavior problems, especially sexualized behavior. Because discussing such difficulties may pose a significant threat to children's fragile self-esteem, they attempt to avoid these issues by an outright refusal to discuss them or by disruptive behavior designed to deflect the therapist's attention. One strategy we have used with some success is to help these children identify some of their strengths. The therapist might point out that although the child has engaged in some inappropriate behavior, the he or she has many positive characteristics and can do some things well. This approach is eventually helpful in assisting highly anxious children to confront their problems with physical aggression or sexually intrusive behavior directly. Cunningham and MacFarlane (1991) devised a number of activities designed to bolster the self-esteem of children who molest other children. The "Me Badge" (Cunningham & MacFarlane, 1991, pp. 59, 60) is a nonthreatening exercise that most children can do. A circular piece of cardboard is divided into four sections. The child is to identify (or draw pictures of) positive characteristics. These characteristics might include something the child likes to do, something he or she is good at doing, something the child does to help the family, and something that is very special to the child. This concrete and visual depiction may be kept handy and shown to the child as a reminder of these strengths when the child feels threatened by discussions of his or her problema behavior.

To help children acknowledge problems, "Five Things I Do Well" (Cunningham & MacFarlane, 1991, p. 73) instructs them to list five things they do well (or draw if they are unable to write) on one side of a folded piece of paper. They then list five things they would like to do better on the other half of the paper. The therapist points out that everyone has strengths as well as areas that need improvement. This exercise gradually exposes children to the process of acknowledging their difficulties (by having them identify things they would "like to do better"). If the child does not acknowledge having problems with physical aggression or sexual behavior, the therapist might point out this lapse matter-of-factly and wonder aloud why the child did not do so. Children might be asked to think of the "worst thing that could happen" if they were to acknowledge the problem. This approach helps them identify the source of their anxiety. By empathizing with their fears and then correcting particular distortions (e.g., the therapist will think negatively of a child if he or she becomes aware of the child's behavior) the therapist may help overcome a child's reluctance to explore these issues.

Cognitive–behavioral techniques may be employed to counteract these negative self-statements, which inhibit children from engaging in an open and direct account of their difficulties. Cunningham and MacFarlane (1991, p. 55) describe a strategy, "My Inner Critic," in which children are asked to identify their negative self-statements, including those related to their sexual behavior. Children with other behavioral difficulties such as physical aggression may be encouraged to identify the negative self-statements associated with these problems (e.g., "I'm a bad kid, and everyone hates me because I beat up other kids"). When they become aware of making these covert self-statements, they are instructed to visualize a stop sign. They are then to say "Stop!" to themselves and replace the negative self-statement with a more positive one (e.g., "I made a mistake, but I'm learning how to control my temper"). The therapist may have to prompt the child to use this strategy or provide tangible reminders of the child's strengths (using the "Me badge") when the youngster becomes especially anxious. These strengths should be incorporated into self-statements; the child should use them when he or she feels especially threatened by explorations and discussions of his or her problem behavior (e.g., "Even though I sometimes beat up other kids, there are some things I do well – I'm good at math and there are times when I can be nice to people!").

Children need repeated practice to learn to implement this technique. The therapist can help children practice changing their negative thoughts into positive ones by presenting a variety of self-statements, including those associated with problem behavior. The children are then asked to replace these negative thoughts with positive ones. For children who remain reluctant to acknowledge their behavior directly, the therapist may present a more detailed scenario that involves a child who also does not want to talk about embarrassing or shameful behavior. This scenario introduces sensitive material somewhat indirectly via recounting a hypothetical child's behavior (similar to the third stage of Harter's model of therapy described in the previous chapter). The child is asked to identify some negative thoughts of this other child, as well as the positive self-statements that might replace them.

Treating the Victim and Victimizing Behavior

The question that sometimes arises concerns the timing of different sets of interventions directed at victim and victimizing behaviors. In what order should they be addressed? Should each issue be addressed in a discrete phase of treatment, or can the issues be examined simultaneously? There is probably no hard-and-fast rule. The therapist must use clinical judgment about the timing of interventions pertinent to each broad class of issues. For example, a victimized child who engages in serious physical or sexual aggression toward others will probably require immediate and intensive intervention to stop this behavior so as to ensure the safety of others and contain the child's own anxiety about behaving so inappropriately. Gil and Johnson (1993) and James (1989) comment that in many cases these issues may be addressed simultaneously, rather than separately in different phases of therapy. Gil and Johnson (1993) note that children may be asked to articulate, in role plays, the feelings associated with being both a victimizer and a victim. Eventually, the therapist will be able to show the child the connection between his or her feelings of inadequacy and helplessness, which were engendered by the victimization, and the subsequent development of aggressive strategies by the child. Even within one session, therapist and child may be able to address the victimization issues and still have time to spend on the victim issues.

TEN

Reformulating
the Meaning
of the Maltreatment

Ep ISODES OF ABUSE and neglect often affect a child's appraisal of the world and the youngster's place in it. In Chapter 2 we reviewed the meanings the child imputes to the maltreatment and the important role these meanings play in the child's subsequent adaptation to trauma. Child maltreatment victims need the opportunity to understand what has happened to them and to critically examine and reformulate some of their assumptions about and interpretations of the experience. They usually must establish a relationship with the therapist before divulging their interpretations of the maltreatment. Youngsters must feel some degree of safety and trust in the relationship, since considerable shame and embarrassment are often associated with these underlying assumptions and perceptions. Issues pertaining to the meaning of the maltreatment continue to emerge as children uncover more memories and become more cognizant of their feelings.

In this chapter, we discuss three major issues concerning the reformulation of the meaning of maltreatment. First, children must attain a sense of mastery over the past maltreatment and begin believing they can reduce the likelihood of future assaults. Second, therapists must assist child victims in reconceptualizing the meaning of the maltreatment, especially as it pertains to their child's own sense of responsibility. Third, efforts have to be directed at helping youngsters develop a more positive sense of self-esteem.

BUILDING MASTERY

Maltreatment frequently engenders feelings of helplessness, powerlessness, and inadequacy. Besides acknowledging these feelings and finding more adaptive ways of expressing them, children need to move from a position of powerlessness to one of effectiveness. This change diminishes children's feelings of inadequacy regarding their past victimizations and increases their confidence in protecting themselves from future assaults. The therapist has many ways of helping to develop this sense of mastery. These methods range from indirect, metaphorical play techniques to strategies that engage the child in more direct discussions and explorations of these issues.

Posttraumatic Play and Reparative Metaphors

There has been a long tradition within the fields of psychoanalytic and psychodynamic therapy regarding children's play as an attempt to allay anxiety by mastering situations. Sigmund Freud used the term "repetition compulsion" to "describe the unconscious need to reenact early traumas in the attempt to overcome or master them" (Goldenson, 1984, p. 632). Traumatized children play frequently reflects the repetition of these themes. For example, children who have been involved in motor vehicle accidents often reenact repeated car crashes in which the occupants are seriously injured and ultimately rescued by police. Children who have undergone painful and invasive surgeries pretend they are doctors and perform countless operations on dolls or stuffed animals, thereby converting a passively experienced event into one over which they have control and are able to reduce anxiety. Besides providing the child with a metaphorical or symbolic way of becoming the victorious survivor who is no longer the passive victim of uncontrollable forces, play is an opportunity for the therapist to introduce more adaptive ways of mastering fears and anxieties rather than allowing the child to rely upon strategies such as physical aggression.

Some children spontaneously begin to enact scenarios of abuse or neglect using play. They may depict it in an even more disguised form by using animal rather than human characters. The content of the victimization may be portrayed metaphorically: the animals or humans are attacked by monsters rather than physically or sexually assaulted. After enacting the play scenario, the child may use the play to depict a solution. For example, Peter, portraying himself as Superman, was a powerful figure who rescued animals from threatening figures (Chapter 7). He used this play to transform himself from the passive victim of severe and longstanding abuse into a figure who was now invincible and invulnerable to the assaults of others.

There are other children who enact the traumatic or victimizing experience in their play but cannot resolve or master the situation. Terr (1990) cautions that reenactment without resolution reinforces the child's sense of helplessness and of being at the mercy of forces beyond his or her control. These feelings of terror and helplessness may be accompanied by further behavioral regression. Terr argues that therapists need to intervene actively after a repeated number of these play scenarios have been acted out (8 to 10 sessions). Intervention is necessary to help the child assume a more active role in the play and generate alternate resolutions, thereby promoting in himself or herself a sense of symbolic mastery and control over the frightening or painful event. Terr (1990) describes many useful strategies to modify such posttraumatic play. These strategies include disruptions in the actual play sequence, such as asking the child to make physical movements like standing up or taking deep breaths. Verbal statements from the therapist about the play and comments upon the action may interrupt the child's self-absorption and rigid reenactment. Terr (1990) also recommends more active interventions. Play sequences may be modified by asking the child to take a specific role and to describe the character's perceptions and feelings. The therapist may manipulate the characters by moving them around. Even more directive and specific prompts may be provided by asking the youngster to respond to questions like, "What would happen if the little girl asked somebody for help?" The therapist might prompt the child by saying, "Let's make this little girl really powerful. Let's think of some ways she could get away from that monster. She could _____," with the therapist turning to the child and inviting a response. Terr (1990) suggests that encouraging the child to differentiate between the traumatic event and current reality may allow the child to modify the play. Videotaping the play and then watching it together is another opportunity to stop the play at important junctures and encourage the child to think of ways to solve the dilemma that appears at each juncture.

The therapist may suggest play scenarios that are not as disguised as those discussed above, so as to expose the child to more direct representations of the victimization experiences. For example, the therapist might say, "Let's make up a story about a little girl whose dad hits her alot." Some children will enact extremely aggressive solutions to being hurt. Some clinicians argue that these actions are permissible, since they are fantasy enactments. We have some trouble with allowing children to continue using these harmful and destructive solutions, even in the metaphor of the play. Although aggressive play scenarios may increase a child's sense of mastery and power, they may also promote reliance upon hurting and exploiting others that may be manifested in other environments. The therapist might suggest alternate strategies in the context of the play to increase the child's sense of safety and personal effectiveness and to restore his or her self-esteem. The therapist might say, "Rather than hitting that monster, what could the little girl say to the monster?" or, "Is there anyone else here that the boy could ask for help?" Alternate strategies may be generated and presented in a game-like format. The child might be told, "Let's think of as many ways as we can that the girl can use to protect herself from that guy who is trying to hurt her." Following the problem-solving approach outlined in Chapter 9, the therapist then encourages the child to think of the various solutions' consequences for both the perpetrator ("How do you think he'd feel if he got stabbed by a knife when he tried to hurt the girl?") and the child/hero ("How do you think she'd feel if she tried to kill him? What do you think would happen to her if she killed him?").

Storytelling also may impart messages about constructive and healthy ways of gaining mastery over traumatizing events. Mills and Crowley (1986) discuss the use of therapeutic metaphors in general with children, and Davis (1990) has written a book of metaphorical stories for abused children. Useful material may be found in both works. Individually tailored metaphorical stories may be used to help youngsters develop adaptive responses to abusive situations. The same general technique we just described with doll play may be used in storytelling. The therapist begins by recounting a metaphorical description of an abusive situation and then asks the child "to make up the ending." Gardner's "Mutual Storytelling Technique" may be used if the therapist wishes to introduce a healthier response to the abuse (Gardner, 1971). With this technique, the child tells a story and the therapist repeats it with the same theme and characters. However, the therapist introduces a healthier resolution than the one initially proposed by the child. Applying this technique to metaphorical stories about maltreatment, the therapist tells the story again but modifies the child's ending to propose a more constructive solution that does not rely upon aggression.

Developing Realistic and Viable Self-Protection Strategies

Children may be better able to tolerate more direct discussions of these issues after participating in these play activities. Through these activities, they will have become desensitized to anxiety-provoking issues and will have started to build up confidence and feelings of mastery by resorting to fantasy. Although the therapist must allow these initial fantasy attempts to emerge, the failure to introduce other means will reinforce the notion that the child must rely upon these fantasy measures in real-life situations. Children should have realistic expectations about their ability to care for and protect themselves, such as understanding that adults have ultimate responsibility for ensuring their safety. Moreover, the therapist needs to promote more realistic and viable strategies for the child to reduce the probability of future victimization. This knowledge may further attenuate a child's anxiety and feelings of powerlessness; now the child has a better idea of what he or she could actually do. In Chapter 9 we described how Steve's anxiety began to decrease after he developed a specific and viable plan he could implement if his father tried to reassault him.

To initiate this process, therapists should comment upon the previous methods or strategies youngsters used to protect themselves during the abuse. These strategies are often valiant attempts by young and inexperienced children to alert others to the terrifying things that are happening to them. One 5-year-old girl would knock on her bedroom wall, which adjoined her parents' bedroom, whenever her stepfather sexually abused her. She explained to her therapist that she was trying to give her mother a "signal" about what was happening. The mother recalled that she had sometimes heard the knocking but usually was so tired she fell asleep. Children should be told that they had done the best they could have done, given the situation and their lack of knowledge and experience about how to deal with traumatizing events.

The need for directly educating children about maltreatment was demonstrated in a study of the characteristics of sexually abused and nonabused children's conceptions about personal body safety (Miller-Perrin, Wurtele, & Kondrick, 1990). A vignette describing the violation of personal body safety was presented to 25 boys and girls aged 5 to 12 years who were entering a treatment program for sexual-abuse victims. They were matched with a group of 25 nonabused children. The sexually abused children were more likely to describe the vignette situation as involving abuse or rape and were more likely to provide a correct definition of sexual abuse. However, 25% of the sexually abused children were still unable to label the situation accurately as abusive, even though they had entered treatment for sexual assault. Only half of the sexually abused group and 28% of the nonabused group could provide a correct definition of sexual abuse. Although children need to be able to recognize and identify different situations as abusive or even neglectful, it is often a difficult for them to do so. Some situations are quite clear, as such flagrant acts of physical or sexual abuse. Others may be somewhat more ambiguous, especially for younger children. For example, some sexually abused children have learned to equate sexualized interactions with manifestations of love and nurturance. They may not see these situations as exploitative.

Cognitive–developmental variables also influence children's understanding of concepts that are typically presented in abuse-prevention programs. Tutty (1994) has prepared an excellent review of the developmental issues related to child sexual-abuse prevention. She notes that developmental factors, such as a child's difficulty in understanding abstract and subtle concepts, affect how readily the child appreciates ideas like "good touch" versus "bad touch." Teaching children to oppose the wishes of an adult, especially familiar adults in a caretaking position, is another common task in sexual-abuse prevention programs. Here again, developmental factors affect children's understanding of the issue. Damon (1980; cited in Tutty, 1994, p.

181) found that children aged 5 to 6 believe authority figures have an inherent right to be obeyed because they are larger, more powerful, stronger, and have higher status.

Daro (1991) reports that the empirical findings regarding the effectiveness of child sexual-abuse prevention programs are mixed. Tailoring material to a child's cognitive characteristics and learning abilities, presenting material in a stimulating and varied manner, and providing lots of opportunities to rehearse prevention strategies through staged interactions were all especially useful in helping children learn the concepts and skills of self-protection. Therapists should incorporate these characteristics of successful prevention programs in interventions to be used in individual therapy. The information should be presented in different and stimulating ways; for example, the therapist might write descriptions of different scenarios on cards. The therapist and child then take turns discussing each scenario and deciding whether it might constitute an act of abuse or neglect. Rather than trying to provide children, especially younger ones, with an exhaustive list of all the potentially abusive or exploitative situations they might encounter, a more useful and viable strategy is to teach children to tell an adult when a situation confuses them (Daro, 1991). The effectiveness of this simple strategy is indirectly supported by the reports of adult sexual offenders. They have stated that they are deterred by a youngster who indicates an intention to tell a specific adult about an assault (Budin & Johnson, 1989; Conte, Wolf, & Smith, 1989).

Our clinical experience has convinced us of the importance of providing children with many opportunities to rehearse what they would actually do or say in these situations. The therapist should present various situations, some of which may replicate selected aspects of the child's past episodes of victimization. Then the child is asked the respond to these situations. Scenarios may be presented in a more tolerable form, such as puppet plays, to children who remain particularly anxious about dealing directly with this material. The therapist may begin the play by enacting a situation in which the characters might be victimized. Then the child is requested to step in as the puppeteer and demonstrate an adaptive solution. An emphasis should be placed upon how the child might disclose the situation to a trusted adult, including the actual words the child would use. Children should identify those adults to whom they feel they could disclose this information. We have constructed simple pursuit games in which children must answer hypothetical questions regarding personal safety when they land on specially designated squares. The scenarios might include some that deal with other aspects of personal safety (e.g., "If you got lost in a department store, what would you do?") and others that focus upon victimization episodes. The therapist should develop scenarios that parallel the child's own past experiences. Participants get an extra turn if they can provide an adaptive solution to these dilemmas. Allowing each participant to take two extra turns if he or she can also act out the response introduces even more fun and provides additional practice. Again, the therapist must pay careful attention to the nature of these responses and intervene to correct any unrealistic or inappropriate solutions.

Another way of helping children gain a sense of mastery over their past victimization is to have them help others who are struggling with similar issues. This approach is particularly applicable to older school-aged children who have the cognitive and verbal skills to engage in these projects. The knowledge that one can now help others has a positive effect upon a child's self-esteem. This project is usually best introduced near the latter phase of therapy, when children feel better about their experiences and have learned some adaptive ways of handling their reactions. We have invited maltreated children to "help other kids who are beginning therapy" by preparing brief pamphlets that describe the common reactions and feelings associated with a maltreatment history. These pamphlets help children consolidate their understanding of their own reactions and raise their self-esteem. We have been impressed with the enthusiasm and eagerness of children to assist others. Some have even volunteered to meet with the other child. The sharing of similar experiences is one of the great strengths of other treatment approaches, such as group psychotherapy. On several occasions, we have invited children to prepare a video in which they talk about their own experiences and the coping mechanisms they used. We also give the child a copy of the videotape. With explicit permission from the child and his or her legal guardians, we have shown these videos and pamphlets to other children, who then experienced a reduced sense of stigmatization and isolation. Of course, the therapist must ensure that the child who receives the video has no knowledge of the child who prepared the pamphlet or, even more important, who appears on the video.

CHANGING THE MEANING OF THE MALTREATMENT

Therapists must correct some of the cognitive distortions children have about their victimization experiences for them to be able to reformulate the meaning of the abuse. One of the most predominant issues is the child's feeling of responsibility for the perpetrator's actions. The adult would not have beaten, neglected, or psychologically abused the child if he or she had been more worthy or better behaved. If the child had not asked questions about sexuality or where babies come from, he or she would not have been sexually assaulted. These internal attributions reinforce a child's feelings of stigmatization, shame, and guilt and add to the his or her overall level of psychological distress and depression.

Modifying Attributions of Responsibility

Any therapist who treats maltreated children should read Lamb's (1986) article on the issues of blame and responsibility. She points out that many therapists reassure sexually abused children they are blameless so that they, the therapists may present themselves as trustworthy, helpful individuals. Lamb contends that although this view seems just and proper, it may have detrimental effects. The gist of her argument is that these statements confer victim status on children and diminish their sense of power and control. According to Lamb, sexually abused children may feel they made some choices that led to a continuation of the abuse. By saying it is not their fault, the therapist removes any sense of efficacy they may have experienced. Lamb recommends that therapists help abused children understand that the abusive situation is one containing many choices. Children should be assisted in understanding that they made the best choice they were able to in the abusive situation and that they now can make different choices. Lamb also maintains that simple statements such as "It's not your fault" run counter to the sense of responsibility children may have felt in these interactions. Offering premature reassurances of blamelessness may well invalidate the child's phenomenological experience and erode the child's growing perception that the therapist is sensitive to feelings and issues (Friedrich, 1990).

How then do we help children change their belief that they were responsible for the maltreatment? For example, some children may have engaged in behavior that contributed to a continuation of the sexual abuse; such as going back to the perpetrator's home or seeking extra rewards or privileges for complying with sexual activities. The therapist should point out that they are not "bad children" but that they had not learned enough about the world to make the proper decisions. The therapist should explain that although the child had returned to the perpetrator's home, the adult still had ultimate responsibility for his or her actions; the adult was older, more knowledgeable, and more able to exert power and control over the child. Acknowledging that the child made a mistake by returning to the perpetrator's home may seem somewhat heartless and cruel. However, by doing so the therapist is suggesting that the youngster can make different decisions in the future that could reduce the risk of further exploitation.

Characterological or internal attributions of blame (e.g., "I was abused because I was a bad kid") can be ameliorated by the therapist stating that no matter what the child did, he or she did not deserve this kind of treatment. The therapist should coach the child to use appropriate self-statements when he or she is bothered by these internal attributions (e.g., "He was a grown-up, and he shouldn't have done those things to me"). Another effective way of concretizing this concept is to use role playing. Court scenarios are especially useful. A scenario may be introduced in which the child is asked to defend the perpetrator and the therapist assumes the judge's role. As the judge, the therapist might ask the child for an explanation of the perpetrator's behavior—will the child attribute responsibility to the child victim or to the offender? If the child blames the victim, the judge proposes an alternate explanation. For example, the child may say that his or her acting-out behavior was the cause of the physical abuse. The judge might then say that even if the child had been behaving inappropriately and needed discipline or limits, nothing would have justified that kind of treatment. Similarly, the child may refer to the physical pleasure he or she derived from the perpetrator's sexual assaults or attribute the adult's actions to the child's questions about sexuality. Again, the judge (i.e., the therapist) might remark that even though the child was curious or even aroused, these feelings did not justify the adult's behavior. This kind of scenario may lead to a discussion of the normalcy of children's physiological/sexual arousal and that it can never be used as a rationale by adults for involving children in sexual behavior. As the judge, the therapist should explain the concept of consent and that the child did not have the requisite knowledge to agree to the perpetrator's advances. Roles may be reversed, so that the therapist plays the offender or the offender's legal counsel, who presents several rationalizations for the perpetrator's behavior. The therapist gently prompts the child (as the judge) to think about what the offender is saying and whether it truly justifies the offender's actions toward the child. The child may well derive some sense of power and mastery by successfully countering the therapist's (i.e., the perpetrator's) arguments and rationalizations and then handing out an appropriate sentence.

There are other strategies that can be used to reinforce the notion that the child was not responsible for the victimization. By reviewing salient aspects of a parent's historical difficulty in caring for him or her, a child's attributions of personal responsibility are counteracted. We have requested that child welfare workers who had been involved with the child at a very young age meet with the child. The welfare workers recount the reasons for their agency's involvement and describe the difficulties parents had in caring for the youngster. Although painful, these realistic portrayals also facilitate the child's acknowledgment of profound feelings of loss associated with the parental inability or unwillingness to care for him or her. Usually, children must begin the process of acknowledging parental difficulties and their own feelings of loss before they can accept such sensitive historical information. Presenting the information when a child still adamantly denies the parent's problems and tenaciously clings to hope that the parent will reform often strengthens the child's defenses of denial and avoidance.

Some children persist in maintaining that they should have physically fought the perpetrator or defended themselves from the assaults. A failure to modify these unrealistic expectations leaves the child with no alternate strategies that have a better chance of ensuring his or her future safety. Although he or she identifies and empathizes with the child's wish to have been strong and powerful, which typically underlies such fantasies, the therapist should point out sensitively that the child probably would not have been successful in defending himself or herself by this means. The therapist should assist the child to develop alternate ways of dealing with this kind of situation. Children should articulate what they might have said to the perpetrator or might have done to ensure their safety, rather than relying upon unrealistic strategies.

Children deserve a simple, yet straightforward, explanation of the perpetrator's behavior to help attenuate their feelings of responsibility and make sense of the perpetrator's behavior. Often the explanation is frightening, confusing, and at times bizarre to the child. This task seems simple but is often difficult. As is true of every other aspect of human behavior, multiple factors contribute to abusive or neglectful behavior; it is difficult to provide a simple, yet honest, explanation. It is probably wise to provide children with a simple and direct explanation for their parent's behavior without attempting to incorporate all the causative factors or subtle influences. Learning of these aspects would overwhelm the child with excessive information. For example, it may be helpful to say "Your dad has a big problem using drugs, and it's real hard for him to stop. When he uses those drugs, he has trouble making meals or making sure you get to school on time" may be helpful. Saying that the perpetrator is "sick," although an easy solution, often creates even more difficulties. The idea of sickness diminishes the notion that the perpetrator was responsible for his or her actions. The child may feel sorry for the perpetrator and guilty for having disclosed the assault and getting a "sick" individual into trouble. The youngster may also feel guilty about having strong feelings such as anger toward someone who is ill. Other explanations such as "She really loves you but she has all these angry feelings too" may be incomprehensible to young children. They have difficulty understanding that people can experience opposing feelings simultaneously (i.e., love versus anger) (Harter, 1977).

Modifying Attributions That the Maltreatment Is Inevitable and Pervasive

The therapist should encourage the child to identify relationships that are not abusive or exploitative to counteract the child's belief that maltreatment is inevitable (i.e., stable attributions) or pervasive (i.e., global attributions). Using information from life books or other historical information as cues, the child can develop a list of positive interactions/relationships. The child and therapist should focus upon specific and concrete evidence of the child having been well treated, such as a birthday party organized by an otherwise neglectful parent. Some children with horrendous histories may have had few, if any, positive past experiences they can identify. The therapist may have to focus more on the here and now and have the child identify ways in which he or she is being well cared for. In Chapter 8 we described how children may be encouraged to identify the differences between their "old family" and the "new family." Besides describing the actual changes, children can be helped to do the same regarding the feelings and cognitions and/or assumptions evoked by these different experiences. For example, some severely neglected children now in foster care will identify very concrete changes, such as being adequately fed. The therapist might ask the child how it feels when she or he is fed and then direct a series of questions designed to help the child reformulate basic assumptions about the world: "When your foster parents give you food, how do you think they feel about you? Do you think other people will feed you, or is everyone going to be like your parents, who didn't give you enough to eat?"

The therapist may draw upon his or her personal interactions with the child to initiate a similar process: "When I kept the promise I made to you that we would paint this week, how did you feel? Do you think other people will keep their promises in the future?" Children might maintain a written log or record of the "friendly deeds" that others have done for them. Illiterate youngsters might draw pictures that depict these positive interpersonal experiences and bring them to therapy sessions. These pictures supply more data for the therapist to use to introduce an element of discontinuity into the child's internal working model of others. This disconinuity begins to counter their tendency to misattribute hostile intent to others, as described in Chapter 2. This process is long and gradual for many children who have such entrenched beliefs and perceptions; and, as mentioned before, the therapist will have greater success in modifying them if the help of others is enlisted.

Countering Victimization as the Defining Characteristic of Self-Image

Children may regard their experience of victimization or maltreatment as a core component of their self and personality. Rather than looking at other aspects of their functioning or personality, they tend to regard themselves solely as "victims" of abuse or neglect. Unfortunately, such a self-view exacerbates their feelings of powerlessness and inadequacy and leads to even lower self-esteem. The therapist's task here is to help the child understand that he or she is not alone. Others have been victimized, survived, and even done well. This history of victimization should not be the defining characteristic of the child's personality or life (James, 1989; Urquiza & Winn, 1994).

James (1989) describes some creative techniques to address this issue. Using "The List of Bad, Mean, Rotten Things That Can Happen to Kids" (James, 1989, pp. 170–172), the therapist conveys the notion to the child that "bad things happen to other kids, that what happened to them is just one of several terrible things that could have happened, and that things could be worse" (James, 1989, p. 170). In this technique the child or therapist writes on strips of paper all the negative experiences that might happen to children. The child is invited to place the strips in order so the very worst experiences are on the top, with the others below in descending order of how awful the child perceives them to be. James (1989) reports that this is a particularly useful tool for group therapy, in which children can compare their lists. They begin to understand that their own experience of victimization may be viewed in the context of a range of experiences with which children must cope. In fact, there might be other, "worse things" that could happen. James also notes that repeating the exercise at later points in treatment is a good way for the therapist and child to see how the youngster's perspective has changed. Another technique developed by James (1989, pp. 173–175), "The Elderly Child Remembers," helps the child acknowledge the maltreatment and place it in its proper perspective. The child is invited to imagine himself or herself in the future as an elderly individual who is talking about his or her life to other elderly friends. The therapist instructs the child to describe the feelings about having been abused or traumatized years ago and how the child "got stronger, and then how you went on in your life to be successful" (James, 1989, p. 174). This exercise allows children to imagine themselves as survivors of maltreatment. It introduces the possibility that they can be successful, thereby challenging their expectation that they are condemned to suffer forever because of the maltreatment.

In Chapter 8 the use of life books and historical information was described. The therapist might point out that the child has had some happy times and has achieved some successes, although no attempt should be made to deny or minimize the trauma and associated feelings the child has experienced. Photographs of the child winning an award or even just having fun with other children may be used to support this view. The therapist might use statements like "Even though your mom didn't pay you any attention and you had to come to a foster home, these pictures show me that you've been able to do some pretty neat things." Such statements underscore the point that the child should not look at the victimization as the sole defining characteristic of his or her life. Similar to James's (1989) technique of "The Elderly Child Remembers," the child may be asked to describe some of the major accomplishments and positive events the child foresees for himself or herself in the future. This exercise may be done verbally or through other means such as drawing or role playing. It instills a sense of hope and counteracts the child's feelings of despair, hopelessness, and depression.

Physically Abused Children's Concerns about Body Integrity

Children will require assistance in exploring and reexamining other aspects of the maltreatment. Children who have been physically assaulted may harbor fears about their health and body integrity. Some children have been scarred or disfigured (e.g., burns, scars from facial injuries). These marks serve as continual reminders of the maltreatment (Urquiza & Winn, 1994). The feelings elicited by these stimuli should be discussed directly, and the therapist should openly empathize with the child's anger, sadness, and loss connected to the assaults. Compounding children's distress is anxiety about what to say to people who ask about their obvious injuries or scars. The therapist and child should rehearse what the youngster will say; the child's responses should be designed so as not to elicit fear, rejection, pity, or even more intensive questioning. Some children may be particularly anxious about others seeing their scars, since they expect people to reject them automatically. Children might complete a homework assignment in which they observe the reactions of others to their scars or disfigurement and then recount their observations in the next session. The therapist might pose questions such as "Did everyone laugh at you?" "Did they still let you play with them?" "When kids asked you what happened and you told them what your dad did, did they laugh at you or blame you?" The therapist should encourage the child to engage in self-talk and use self-statements such as "If they don't want anything to do with me because I have a scar, then it's their problem, not mine!" The therapist should also acknowledge the child's specific accomplishments despite a disfigurement, scar, or handicap. This approach may help the child develop an identity that is more balanced and not based solely on body image (Urquiza & Winn, 1994).

Sexually Abused Children's Concerns about Sexuality and Sexual Functioning

Sexually assaulted children are sometimes fearful of sexually transmitted diseases such as HIV/AIDS or are concerned about their genitalia and sexual functioning. These children need prompt medical attention, including being tested for HIV and other diseases. Although stressful, a medical examination of the child's genitalia may reassure the child that he or she has sustained no permanent damage. Positive test results will exacerbate the child's distress, especially if HIV is diagnosed in the child. At this point, the therapist and child are dealing not only with the direct sequelae of the assault but with the complex issues arising from a diagnosis of a terminal illness.

We discussed in Chapter 8 how children who have been sexually assaulted worry about their sexual adequacy and functioning. The therapist should provide direct information about sexuality, including the anatomy, purpose, and functions of the genitalia and an explanation of normal sexual response to help them reformulate their experiences. Boys should be educated about the physiological basis of reactions like erections. The difference in the size of the genitalia between the adult male perpetrator and the boy may also be a source of worry, with the child feeling that he is in some way inadequate. Again, the therapist should provide information about sexual development and puberty to allay these concerns. This concern may also be true of boys who have been sexually abused by adult females.

In Chapter 4, we briefly discussed the Rorschach responses of 10-year-old Bob, whose mother had sexual intercourse with him. He divulged to his therapist that he was worried something must have been wrong with his penis when he had intercourse with his mother 2 years earlier. He thought it was "too small" for his mother's vagina. He had felt that his penis was being "swallowed up" and had been damaged in some way when she inserted it into her. Bob feared he would never be able to satisfy a female partner sexually when he was older. His anxiety decreased when the therapist explained to him that his genitalia had not been harmed or injured in any way (this had been confirmed by an earlier medical examination). The therapist and Bob talked about puberty and its concomitant physical changes, including those of the genitalia. This, discussion, combined with information about normal sexual response, alleviated some of Bob's anxiety about not being physically able to satisfy a sexual partner when he was older.

Bob also revealed to his therapist that he was worried he might reexperience some of the flashbacks about the sexual abuse when he was older and involved in a sexual relationship. Rather than discounting this fear as unrealistic, the therapist empathized with Bob's anxiety. He suggested to Bob that working hard in therapy now was the best thing he could do to minimize the likelihood of future problems. The therapist avoided giving Bob any outright guarantee that he would never have any problems in later life.

Therapy terminated approximately 2½ years later. Bob contacted the therapist again when he was nearly 15 years old because he was having some problems with his father. Bob and the therapist began a short course of sessions to address this particular difficulty. The therapist took the opportunity to inquire about Bob's sexual adjustment. Bob reported that while he was not yet sexually active, he was no longer bothered by the intrusive memories of having sexual intercourse with his mother that characterized the initial phase of therapy several years earlier. Bob was hopeful that his positive adjustment would continue. However, given the horrendous abuse he had suffered at the hands of his mother and her common-law partner, there is no guarantee that Bob will remain asymptomatic, especially as he moves into the next developmental stage of forming romantic and sexual relationships.

Children may worry about their sexual orientation if they were abused by someone of the same gender. Telling a child with this concern that it is nonsense may do a real disservice if the youngster is indeed developing a homosexual orientation. Again, glib and easy reassurances should be avoided as much as possible. The therapist should explain the development of sexual orientation to children, emphasizing that no one, including doctors and therapists, knows all the factors that lead to a particular sexual preference. Children may refer to their own sexual excitement and arousal as "proof" that they are gay. A discussion about the basis of sexual arousal may attenuate some of this anxiety and provide a more balanced perspective on this issue. Urquiza and Winn (1994) note that children who are confused about their sexuality may feel compelled to engage in sexual relationships with members of the opposite sex to prove they are "straight." The authors recommend offering the child support and encouraging the child to refrain from initiating sexual relationships until he or she is emotionally and physically ready for the experience.

REPAIRING AND RESTORING SELF-ESTEEM

Helping children feel better about themselves is necessary to counteract their feelings of stigmatization, inadequacy, and depression. Like most of these tasks, it is one that runs throughout the course of therapy. The clinician must be alert to any opportunity to bolster the child's self-esteem. In Chapter 9 we described some specific strategies (e.g., "Me Badge," "Five Things I Do Well") to use to challenge the child's model of the self as unworthy and inadequate. We reviewed the use of positive self-statements to counter negative ones. These strategies are particularly useful in situations where the therapist wants to help the child explore and examine some of the more troublesome aspects of behavior and functioning. In Chapter 9 we also examined strategies children might use to gain better self-control and regulation of their behavior and emotions. Such improvements have a positive effect upon children's self-esteem, especially if the behavioral changes are accompanied by the child's greater acceptance by and involvement with other people, including peers. In this chapter, we have examined how to instill in the child a sense of mastery and self-efficacy concerning past and possible future maltreatment episodes, which may also have a positive effect upon the child's self-esteem; the child no longer regards himself or herself merely as a passive victim. Changing their assumptions about the maltreatment, such as taking personal responsibility for the actions of the perpetrator, enables children to see themselves in a different and more positive perspective.

What are some other activities that will consolidate this healthier sense of self-esteem? We again refer to the child-development literature to sensitize we clinicians to the developmental variables that may have significant implications for our interventions.

Providing Children with Behavioral Evidence of Their Strengths

Harter (1983) describes a four-stage sequence of the development of children's concept of the self. The first stage corresponds to Piaget's preoperational stage of thought (in children 2 to 7 years of age). In this stage, the self is defined by behavior and observable attributes. In the second stage, corresponding to the Piagetian concrete operational stage of thought (ages 7 to early adolescence), the child begins to integrate these behavioral descriptions as trait labels (e.g., smart, popular). However, Harter (1983) notes that children at this age engage in all-or-none thinking. Thus, a child may conclude that he or she is not a good athlete because of difficulties in one or two athletic activities, despite other indicators of skill. In adolescence, abstractions emerge (third stage), and then single abstractions become further integrated into higher-order abstractions (fourth stage).

One implication of this developmental sequence is that therapists must provide the behavior evidence upon which trait labels are constructed. Relying upon trait labels (e.g., "You're a smart kid") may not have as great an impact as citing the specific behaviors that form the basis of such statements. When Peter began to play Chinese checkers with the therapist (see Chapter 7 for a more detailed description of this vignette), he immediately said he would never learn to play the game. The therapist empathized with his fears and provided Peter with gentle encouragement at least to try. This approach was in contrast to simply telling Peter that the clinician thought he was "smart" and could do it. Peter lost the first game, but the therapist identified several of Peter's moves that showed good judgment and forethought as concrete evidence of Peter's intellectual ability. Peter began to request the game as a routine part of subsequent therapy sessions. The therapist often had to identify other behavior that showed evidence of good abilities to help Peter improve his profoundly low self-esteem. He was taught to use self-statements that identified his specific strengths and abilities whenever he began to feel badly about himself.

The therapist should acknowledge specific aspects of the child's participation in the therapeutic process to raise the child's self-esteem. Statements like "You really worked hard in therapy today. Even when you became so upset and started to cry about how your mom was never around for you, you kept on talking about it" are much more meaningful than vague and diffuse statements such as "You did well." The therapist should use examples of the child's interaction with the therapist as further evidence of progress: "When you got really mad at me today because I wouldn't let you do the finger painting, you used words to tell me how mad you were rather than trying to hit me." This content may be incorporated into the child's positive self-statements, which he or she might employ at particularly difficult moments in therapy.

Encouraging the Child to Try New Activities

The therapist should encourage the child to try new activities during therapy sessions to provide even further opportunities for success. Sitting passively and allowing the child to engage in the same activity month after month just reinforces the notion that the child is incapable of doing anything else. Although Peter was somewhat resistant, the therapist gently encouraged him to try playing Chinese checkers. The trick is to suggest an activity that the therapist believes the child can handle with some success. Difficult material that the child cannot master will prove to be another frustrating and demeaning experience. With younger children or those whose self-esteem is profoundly low, shorter activities may be a better choice than those that take a long time to complete. While waiting to see if they will be successful, their anxiety will escalate so significantly they may refuse to continue. Young children with little play experience should be taught how to play using plastic building blocks, or, they may be taught how to paint. We have successfully taught older school-aged children to use the personal computer in our offices to write and compose stories or letters to their perpetrators. The process of learning to use a computer or mastering other skills (e.g., learning to operate a video camera when taping a session) enhances a child's feelings of adequacy and self-esteem.

The therapist should encourage the child to develop new interests outside therapy as well as during therapy sessions.

After being placed in a foster home, Bob expressed a strong interest in playing organized hockey, an opportunity he had never previously had. However, he was anxious about joining a league because he barely knew how to skate and believed he could never match the skills of the other boys. Fortunately, his foster parents sought out a team that accepted him, and the coach gave Bob extra instruction in the fundamentals of the game, such as skating and stick handling. The therapist encouraged and supported Bob in this new activity, and they explored some of his distorted cognitions about joining a hockey team. He expected that spectators would laugh at him if he fell on the ice and that he would never get a goal. Bob was encouraged to develop alternate self-statements to use when he was bothered by these thoughts. This strategy, as well as the generous support and encouragement of his foster parents and the one-on-one instruction from his coach, contributed to Bob's persistence with hockey. His self-esteem received a real boost when he won the trophy for the most improved player at the end of the season.

This concrete demonstration of Bob's ability helped challenge his model of himself as a passive, powerless child who could do nothing to change his life. This example also illustrates the importance of working closely with the significant people in the child's life to ensure his or her exposure to multiple and positive experiences.

Some maltreated children, especially those who have been neglected, begin to fail dismally at school; in these cases the therapist might advocate individual tutoring for such a child. Academic tutoring may increase children's academic skills and decrease their frustration and disruptiveness in the classroom. These improvements, in turn, promote a child's social adjustment and counter the development of negative self-concepts (the FAST Track Program of the Conduct Problems Prevention Research Group, 1992). The therapist should consult closely with the tutor about the child's presentation or progress in tutoring sessions.

The child might start a scrapbook that includes drawings or even photographs of his or her new abilities and strengths so as to concretize these accomplishments. Again, the emphasis should be on the specific and observable evidence of these gains. The therapist should instruct the child to be alert for evidence of new strengths between therapy sessions and to depict them in the scrapbook for the next session. This exercise may become a routine part of therapy, with the child identifying at least one strength per week. Therapists eventually should encourage children to look for new strengths in the social-skills area, such as concrete examples of their helping other people (see Chapter 9 for a description of the "Recording Friendly Deeds" exercise). The first example of an interpersonal strength from a 9-year-old boy in foster care occurred when he got a drink of water for a younger child who was also in care. A running account of the child's progress in therapy may be kept by identifying one positive thing the child does in each session or in the intervening week. This "positive" may then be written down on a large piece of paper. As these "positives" are added to over the course of weeks and months, they give the child a visual record of all the things he or she has accomplished. At termination of therapy, we have given children these often large sheets of paper as a souvenir of the progress and gains they have made.

Board games are useful to help children who have problems with self-esteem. They can be encouraged, like Peter, to learn games with which they are unfamiliar, so as to boost their sense of mastery and adequacy. Their reactions to losing and winning are often good reflections of their self-esteem, as is other behavior, like cheating. We have a few comments about the choice of games before we discuss these patterns and the therapist's responses in greater depth. Games should not be so complicated and involved that they take hours to complete. There should be a good chance of finishing the game within the therapy hour and, ideally, to have time left over for other activities. There must be a selection that range from simple games that even young children can master to the more complex to challenge older school-aged youngsters. Children who are particularly anxious about their abilities may choose to play games in which success is solely dependent upon luck. They should be allowed to do so but then encouraged to attempt games that have elements of skill.

Maltreated children share a number of common reactions to games, with which the therapist must be prepared to intervene. Some children with low self-esteem interpret losing a game as further evidence of their inadequacy or stupidity. If they do agree to play a game, they quickly begin to verbalize fears about losing. The therapist should articulate and empathize with the feelings of anxiety. The therapist might ask a child to identify the "worst thing that would happen if you lost this game." Common fears include fear of the therapist's reaction (e.g., "You'll think I'm dumb," "You'll laugh at me") or feeling even worse about themselves if they lose. The child should be instructed to observe the therapist's behavior keenly at the game's end to see if any of these expectations are fulfilled. This course is preferable to providing a blanket reassurance that the therapist will not denigrate the youngster. The therapist might suggest a few practice games before they play "for real." This approach may be especially important for children who are trying new games or who are especially anxious. It can be explained that some games, just like many other activities, require practice to become proficient. After playing several of these practice games, the therapist may remain concerned that the child has not had enough practice and will lose badly. Proposing that the child accept a handicap (which may not be the right choice of words for some children) is one way to avoid crushing defeats that exacerbate a child's low self-esteem. As an example of such a "handicap" the child may have fewer board pieces to move. To ensure that the child is not insulted by this suggestion, the therapist might use the game of golf as an example, explaining how handicaps are regularly assigned to different players. Additionally, the therapist might say that he or she does not want to take advantage of the child's lack of experience or practice, since that would not be fair.

Some children will beg the therapist to let them win the game. The therapist should comment empathically about the child's anxiety, conveying an understanding that losing poses a real threat to the child's self-esteem. However, the therapist should also tell the child that he or she is not going to throw the game. Allowing children to cheat reinforces their expectation that they will never attain success through their own efforts. Consistent with the findings of developmental research reviewed above, children need concrete and authentic experiences to raise their self-esteem, not experiences they know are based upon dishonesty. The rest of the world, particularly other children, may not be as benevolent as the therapist and will quickly re-scind invitations to the child to participate in games after the youngster tries to cheat. Intervening with cheating in this manner may prevent such unfortunate occurrences in the future, thereby improving the child's social skills.

Children may begin to cheat during the game to preserve their fragile and tenuous self-esteem in the face of losing. Again, the therapist must intervene as soon as the transgression is noticed and bring it to the child's attention. Asking if the child cheated (especially when the therapist knows it occurred) is often misguided, since the child will usually deny it. Then the therapist is left in the situation of trying to decide what to do next. Cheating should be presented as a statement of fact rather than an inquiry, if the therapist is certain the child has cheated. The child should be helped to reflect on why he or she might have cheated. Questions regarding how the child might feel if he or she loses are often useful in identifying a child's need to win at any cost to preserve a shaky sense of self-esteem. The therapist should tell the child firmly that cheating is not allowed: that it is not fair, and that if the child cheats while playing with other children, he or she will probably be thrown out of the game. Moreover, the therapist should tell the child that by allowing cheating, the therapist would be colluding with the child's negative self-image: "If I let you cheat, what I'm really telling you is that I don't think you're able to win by yourself. I think you can win without cheating, so that's why I'm not going to allow you to do it." There may be no choice but to end the game and refuse to play if the child persists in cheating despite these explanations and discussions. This decision should be explained in terms of concern for the child: "We have to end the game now since you're continuing to cheat. I don't want you to think that this is the only way you're able to win. That wouldn't be good for you, so we're going to stop the game." The therapist might offer to play the game in the next session to provide the child with another opportunity to handle this anxiety more adaptively. Other children may attempt to change the rules in the middle of the game to ensure they will win. This play should be prohibited, with the therapist providing the same rationale as that used to limit cheating. Modifications of the rules should occur before a game begins and only after both have discussed and reached an agreement about the proposed changes.

These interactions with the therapist are often a novel experience for children who have never heard an adult tell them he or she thinks they are capable of success. These new expectations, and the therapist's firm yet non-punitive stance toward behavior like cheating, constitute experiences that help a child modify the internal working models of others and the self in a more favorable and positive direction. Therapy can be a powerful tool when it integrates skillful attention to relevant content with sensitive use of the relationship as a medium of change.

ELEVEN

Termination of Therapy

THE TERMINATION of therapy is a process that all children and therapists confront, but it often receives insufficient thought or attention. Many maltreated children come to regard their therapists as significant figures. Ending therapy provokes strong reactions in both clients and therapists. Attending closely and carefully to feelings and cognitions evoked in the child by termination of therapy can transform this therapy phase into one that further promotes growth. Termination offers another opportunity to help the child reexamine historical issues, especially those related to loss. It is also an opportunity for the child to develop healthy and adaptive coping mechanisms to deal with this inevitable component of human relationships.

CRITERIA FOR TERMINATION OF THERAPY

Therapy should be terminated when the treatment goals have been met. This aim highlights the importance of conducting a comprehensive assessment from which realistic goals are derived. Goals guide our ongoing clinical work and serve as markers against which we evaluate the success of our interventions and whether we can begin the termination process. Of course, original treatment goals may undergo some modification during therapy as the child reveals more about the maltreatment and responds idiosyncratically to interventions. We stated in Chapter 4 that goals should be reevaluated regularly to determine their ongoing appropriateness and the child's success in meeting them. This is especially important in long-term psychotherapy, in which there may be a greater tendency for the case to drift without clear objectives or direction. Regular reviews also contribute to the child's own sense of progress and enhance self-esteem.

Some therapists believe that although treatment goals have been met, psychotherapy must continue to prevent the emergence of future psychological or behavioral symptoms. The rationale seems to be that more of a good thing will protect the child from future problems. This notion that psychotherapy can effectively address issues emerging much later is misguided. Therapy can increase the probability of more adaptive future functioning via the development of healthy coping mechanisms and a reformulation of victimization experiences. Participation in successful therapy also establishes the expectation in children and families that subsequent difficulties can be faced rather than ignored or denied. These positive therapy experiences increase the chances that clients will not interpret a subsequent return to therapy as a personal failure to be avoided. However, issues related to the maltreatment may emerge later, albeit in somewhat different forms; as a result of life experiences (e.g., revictimization) or the individual's progression through different developmental phases. Developmental transformations of these original issues could not have been successfully treated earlier since they had not yet emerged. Individuals may need another course of therapy at this later time. In Chapter 2, we reviewed the case of Chris, who reentered therapy when he began adolescence. Adolescence was a catalyst for the evocation of issues pertaining to sexual identity and homosexuality, themes related to Chris's history of sexual abuse by his father. The therapist was unable to treat these specific issues when Chris began therapy at 9 years of age, since they had not attained any prominence or significance during that earlier stage of development. Again, we cannot treat what has not yet emerged. Attempting to do so results, at best, in therapy with vague and diffuse goals. At worst, it results in a process that wastes both the therapist's and the child's time. A sense of accomplishment derived from attaining the original therapy goals is significantly diminished or obviated when the child is informed that more therapy is necessary. A more reasonable course is to terminate but give the child and family an open invitation to recontact the therapist if future problems emerge. Through this "family practice" model (described more fully in Chapter 5), the accomplishments of the child in a course of therapy are recognized. Concurrently, it acknowledges the real limits of psychotherapy in providing absolute immunity to the effects of the maltreatment throughout the remainder of the life span.

Although the major criterion for termination is the achievement of treatment objectives, changes in the youngster's therapy presentation may provide clues that the child is less dependent upon therapy; ending can then be considered. Dodds (1985) describes some of these changes. The child's interest in attending therapy sessions begins to wane. The child starts to come late, misses appointments, or asks to leave early. The child may comment that there is nothing more to talk about or nothing interesting to play. These actions may be accompanied by a greater focus than usual on matters outside therapy, such as school activities and friends. The child begins to recount what he or she would be doing if not at the therapy session. Discussions about these other matters may reflect a greater interest in nontherapeutic issues, particularly if the youngster is not encountering any problems in these areas. Salient themes that characterized the earlier play are often no longer present. There is a greater emphasis upon playing for the sake of playing than upon using it to communicate about maltreatment-related issues. Older school-aged children begin to make direct statements about the therapeutic relationship. They may acknowledge the therapist's role in their recovery or comment on their sense of being heard. The child may spontaneously start to reminisce about past therapy events or ask directly when therapy will end. Changes in the therapist's interactions with the child may also be apparent. The therapist may make more statements that review and encapsulate past therapy events, and he or she may encourage the child to take greater risks outside therapy. If the therapist notices these changes, it may be appropriate to reevaluate the child's progress in meeting treatment goals as the first step of the termination process.

PREPARING CHILDREN FOR TERMINATION OF THERAPY

The child should receive adequate preparation for the termination of therapy whenever possible; the therapist should broach the subject with the child well ahead of the expected final session. How much time will be needed for termination depends on factors such as the nature, intensity, and duration of the therapeutic relationship and the child's typical pace and rhythm in processing issues (Carek, 1979). Children traumatized by previous losses will also need sufficient time to cope adequately with the end of therapy. Carek (1979) suggests that termination over two to three weeks may be adequate if the therapy has been more short-term. One or 2 months or more are usually required for children in long-term therapy (1 year or more). Flexibility is necessary, however. Although a child may have been involved in intensive, long-term psychotherapy, the youngster may have been disengaging for some time before termination is raised as an issue. As a rule, 4 to 6 weeks is adequate.

One way to approach termination is to remind the youngster of the original reason for therapy and to inquire whether the child thinks that reason still exists. The therapist might remark that treatment cannot continue forever and that it is time to think about when the child might stop coming, since he or she has made many improvements. The therapist must discuss the reasons for termination in some depth, even if the child professes a firm understanding that termination is needed because goals have been met. Given our strong orientation toward cognitive–developmental variables, we believe the therapist must provide specific and concrete examples of the youngster's gains. These gains must be contrasted with the condition of the child that led to the initial therapy referral. While we must acknowledge that the relationship is ending, we can also point out that termination is a "commencement": the child is leaving the old, but his or her gains are great enough for the youngster to begin something new (Allen, 1942). We sometimes use the term "graduation" with older school-aged children. We explain that ending therapy is somewhat similar to leaving a valued and trusted teacher at the school year's end because of the child's successful completion of the term. Although this event is characterized by feelings of sadness, it is also a time to feel proud of one's accomplishments.

Ross (1964) recommends that therapists do not allow children to make the final decision about the actual termination date. To do so might place an unfair responsibility on the child, leading to an impasse if the child sets a distant date. The therapist should suggest a date and then seek the child's approval. Many clinicians choose termination dates that coincide with other transitions in the child's life, such as the end of the school year. The child may regard termination as a change similar to others in which relationships end before new ones commence. This approach seems to help children through the process. However, Sandler, Kennedy, and Tyson (1980) argue that termination of therapy at the start of school vacation may lead the child to rationalize that the separation is not final and is due solely to the vacation. This rationalization plays into the child's attempt to deny and avoid painful feelings of sadness and loss. The therapist must remember that there are no rigid rules regarding timing. Clinical judgment must be used to decide what best meets the child's needs.

The frequency of sessions may be tapered off during the termination phase. This tapering process may help the child become comfortable with the idea of functioning more independently without the therapist's regular assistance. For example, sessions may at first be biweekly and then less frequent as the final date approaches. If the child has had no opportunity to deal more independently with the challenges and problems of daily life before therapy ends, the child's self-confidence may be eroded and accompanied by significant anxiety. In the termination phase, the therapist should continue to encourage the child to use skills that foster more independence and provide positive feedback and reinforcement for these efforts. These measures are particularly important if independence was a central therapeutic issue in the preceding treatment phases.

HELPING THE CHILD EXPRESS FEELINGS ABOUT TERMINATION OF THERAPY

Children usually have ambivalent feelings about the termination of therapy. They feel pleased with their accomplishments up to this point and look forward to devoting the time now occupied by therapy to other activities. They feel sad at the prospect of no longer seeing the therapist, especially if the therapeutic relationship was a principal means of change. Termination may reelicit many feelings about relationships that were evident in earlier therapy stages. For the child with an ambivalent/resistant attachment history, dependency needs may reemerge. The child may demand more frequent sessions, ask for the therapist's home phone number, and request assistance for tasks previously handled with ease. These demands may be accompanied by displays of anger, with the child vehemently protesting the therapist's decision to end therapy. A youngster with an avoidant attachment history may rely upon defenses that characterized his or her earlier functioning. Rather than openly and directly acknowledging the sadness and loss evoked by termination, the child may employ defenses such as denial or avoidance. The child may even refuse to acknowledge that the relationship will end. Many maltreated children have experienced numerous losses, with people leaving their lives without explanation. They had no opportunity to express feelings of loss, abandonment, and anger, which increases the probability that these issues and feelings will emerge during the termination phase. Other children may resort to the same internal attributions that were apparent at the initiation of therapy; the child has done something to anger or alienate the therapist, or the child is unworthy of the therapist's commitment.

The termination of the therapeutic relationship provides an excellent opportunity to help children consolidate their ability to cope adaptively with these feelings. Reminding the child of the number of remaining sessions at each session's start may counter the child's tendency to deny the reality of the impending termination. The child should be encouraged to verbalize the feelings evoked by termination, with the therapist empathizing with and validating their normalcy. Modeling affect expression may occur as the therapist articulates his or her personal feelings about ending the relationship, although not to the extent that the child feels burdened. Dodds (1985) reminds us that we do not want our child clients to feel responsible for either causing our feelings or for helping us deal with them. Some children feel especially hesitant to verbalize their anger because they do not want to alienate the therapist further. Telling the child that anger is a normal and expected reaction to separation and loss may enable the child to acknowledge similar feelings.

Other techniques besides encouraging the child to verbalize his or her feelings associated with termination may be used. The child may draw facial expressions that depict the feelings, present puppet plays that focus on issues such as separation, or use some of the other techniques described in Chapter 8. Common reactions of "other kids" in the same situation may be discussed to expose children to this painful material. A book or pamphlet describing his or her experiences in therapy, including the ending phase, may be prepared by the child. We must be cautious about maintaining an exclusive focus upon the negative feelings connected with terminating therapy. Assisting the youngster to identify the positive feelings associated with termination is necessary to promote a more balanced perspective on ending the relationship.

Although the therapist involved the child in a discussion of the reasons for ending therapy when termination was first addressed, the reasons will probably have to be clarified often during this phase. The child may need repeated explanations that therapy is ending because of the child's progress and not because of any personal animosity towards the child. Again, it is helpful if the therapist and child review the specific changes the youngster has made. Vague statements like "You're doing a lot better!" may be virtually meaningless to a young child who needs observable evidence of improvement. The cumulative record of weekly accomplishments kept throughout the course of therapy (Chapter 10) might be reviewed. Reminiscing about therapy provides another opportunity for the child to express feelings about specific therapeutic experiences and interactions with the therapist. Reminiscing also allows some closure in the relationship and consolidates the youngster's perception that he or she has made gains. Confirming that the child can return to therapy if needed also attenuates some of the child's sense of loss and pain. A small ceremony is a concrete reminder of the relationship's importance and is a way of acknowledging and celebrating the child's growth. Children usually enjoy planning a small party for the last session. We have had children invite family members to these celebrations, which have included cake and other favorite foods. By giving the child a small gift such as a book or a certificate to proclaim the child's participation and progress in therapy, the therapist also concretely affirms the relationship's importance to both child and therapist.

During termination, the child may begin to regress or show symptoms that had originally led to therapy. This behavior reflects the child's distress about leaving therapy. The therapist should focus on helping the youngster express the underlying feelings rather than interpreting the behavior as a need for further treatment and then quickly postponing termination. The problems usually disappear as the child resolves his or her feelings about termination.

Parents or caregivers also require help during the termination phase, and they should be encouraged to express any worries or concerns. Many fear that they or their child will not be able to cope without regular assistance from the therapist. They may be particularly distressed if the child temporarily regresses during termination. Parents see this regression as evidence that the child needs more therapy. While empathizing with this anxiety, the therapist should review the progress they and their child have demonstrated over the course of therapy. Possible steps to be taken should

future problems arise may be reviewed. Parents also experience some allevi-
ation of their anxiety when informed that they are welcome to recontact
the therapist if necessary.

PREMATURE TERMINATIONS

Unfortunately, not every termination occurs in this planned fashion. Therapy may end unexpectedly because of a family move to a new location. The
therapist should attempt to have at least one final session with the child
to explain the real reason for the termination and to emphasize the therapist's regard for the youngster. This session also may allow the child to
express some feelings about the impending separation. If even one session
is impossible, the therapist might send a short letter to the child to clarify
the reasons for termination and convey best wishes for the future.

Just as in the other phases of therapy, termination evokes feelings in
the therapist as well as in the child. We conclude this book by a consideration of this important topic.

TWELVE

Personal Implications for the Therapist

W E WOULD LIKE to discuss the personal implications for the therapist of this intense work with often very damaged, maltreated children. No matter whether the child demonstrates localized or developmental effects, the therapist needs to hear and respond to painful descriptions of abusive events. For some therapists, this can be a difficult and provocative task. Lyon (1993) recently described the marked reactions of hospital staff to adult patients' accounts of violence and abuse. She relates that some reported nightmares, intrusive and repetitive images, and somatic symptoms such as headaches, nausea, and sleeplessness. The staff workers' reactions to patients' accounts of victimization were intensified by their own personal history of victimization or psychological difficulties. Lyon (1993) speculates that these reactions might be a type of secondary posttraumatic stress disorder and suggests several ways to alleviate them.

Many children with a history of an insecure attachment organization attempt to provoke the therapist into rejecting or abusing them. Such a therapist response would confirm their expectations about how others will respond to them. In several chapters of this book we described how these children exhibit provocative behavior that can be hostile and outrageous and may continue unabated for lengthy periods. Others may treat the therapist as a nonentity for long periods, much as Peter did, as described in Chapter 7. Work with such children can be physically and emotionally exhausting and usually engenders in the therapist a range of strong reactions. According to Schowalter (1985), every therapist has reactions to the children he or she sees in therapy. However, the topic of therapists' personal reactions to their child clients has received little attention in the child-therapy literature.

COUNTERTRANSFERENCE

Countertransference is a concept that focuses on therapists' reactions to their clients. Schowalter (1985) defines countertransference as "the unconscious influence that a therapist's past needs and conflicts have on his or her understanding, actions or reactions within the treatment situation" (p. 40). Friedrich (1990) defines countertransference more simply as "reactions to our clients that are based, in part, on who we are and what we bring to the therapy process" (p. 269). Schowalter (1985) suggests that such reactions are more likely to occur in child therapy than in adult therapy. They are also more likely when the child client is the same age as the therapist's own children or when the client's problems are similar to those of the therapist or his or her children. Friedrich (1990) asserts that a substantial percentage of therapists have their own histories of victimization. A history of victimization does not necessarily make a therapist a more aware and effective clinician. Moreover, the client's therapy cannot vicariously resolve the therapist's own problems or issues with maltreatment. Friedrich (1990) stresses that it is crucial to be aware of our own personal issues and how these might interfere with a child's therapy; the therapist's effectiveness is based in part on personal maturity and integrity. During the client's therapy, the therapist must always be aware of his or her personal reactions to the client, since these reactions can help or hinder the therapy progress. A therapist's reactions and issues may arise not only from early childhood roles or from early victimization but from current relationships and possible victimization within those relationships.

Reactions may be intense and varied. James (1994) describes feelings that are common to foster and adoptive parents and therapists in their work with damaged and maltreated children. These feelings include resentment, anger, betrayal, and hurt. They arise from the daily interactions with a child who cannot trust others. Additionally, Pearce and Pezzot-Pearce (1994) describe other feelings that are perhaps more specific to working with the child in therapy. These feelings include frustration, helplessness, and hopelessness, all arising when the therapist faces a damaged child whose problems seem almost insurmountable. A therapist must be attuned to these feelings and reactions to avoid being overwhelmed and giving up on a youngster. Alternatively, the feelings might result in an array of defensive strategies by the therapist such as denying that the child has significant problems. In either situation, therapy will not be helpful to the child.

The therapist's awareness of his or her feelings and reactions and of the active strategies to cope with them are necessary to avoid inappropriate responses to the child. A therapist might terminate therapy prematurely with a hostile and provocative child who fights the procress of engaging in a working relationship. In such a situation, the therapist would probably come to anticipate therapy sessions with dread and show little enthusiasm. This reaction would be particularly likely if the therapist had no understanding of the reasons for the child's provocation. This reaction by the therapist would confirm for the child that he or she is bad, uninteresting, and unlovable and would intensify the child's attempts to distance himself or herself from the therapist. Similarly, a therapist might anticipate sessions with a lack of interest if the child repeatedly excludes the therapist from an active role in the therapy. Again, children might interpret the therapist's lack of enthusiasm as proof that they are unlovable and unworthy of attention. At other times, a therapist might prematurely discontinue therapy if the situation seems simply unworkable and so overwhelming that chances of improvement are slim. Alternatively, a therapist might have difficulty ending therapy if the child seems so dependent that the youngster cannot function without the therapist. Therapy might then be prolonged well past the time when the child is making active use of the sessions and can function without them. Therapists might also extend sessions because they enjoy and very much like a child or feel sad about losing an enjoyable client or one with whom they identify strongly.

When faced with a child who is hurting, particularly because of parental maltreatment, a therapist may experience "strong rescue fantasies." Some therapists are so overwhelmed by such fantasies that they consider becoming a foster or adoptive parent to a maltreated child. In our experience, this reaction is often typical of therapists early in their child-therapy careers. Such a step requires extremely careful consideration of the impact for the child, the therapist, and the therapist's family. A therapist who takes a child home in a foster care or adoptive capacity clearly cannot function as that child's therapist. Children who display developmental effects are generally very hard on family life. They often require 24-hour care and sometimes extraordinary structures in the home to keep them and others safe. If a therapist decides to foster or adopt, he or she, like any other parent or caregiver, must also adopt realistic goals and be prepared for the stress, exhaustion, and turmoil that may well follow. We do not want to present an overly negative picture of parenting maltreated children; many foster and adoptive parents have derived great satisfaction and rewards from raising youngsters with these histories. Our point is that despite their training, knowledge, and expertise, therapists will not be immune to the challenges, demands, and attendant reactions that others experience with these children. Therapists must be attuned to the reactions described above to guard against making decisions about the child and therapy that are based more on the therapist's feelings and needs than on those of the child.

Friedrich (1990) outlines reasons for therapists' troublesome reactions to their child clients' histories of sexual abuse. Some of these reasons probably apply to therapists' reactions to physically and emotionally abused and neglected children. Therapists might think of such children as second-class citizens who should have known better and are culpable for their own victimization. Other reactions of therapists include their confusion about dominance and sexuality, the blurred lines between the therapist's various roles (e.g., advocate, therapist, case manager, agent of the court or of child welfare services), therapists' personal issues with sexuality or physical violence, their difficulty in accepting failure, and their tendency to view a situation in unequivocal and rigid terms. This tendency includes the need to see different people (i.e., perpetrators) in rigid good-and-bad terms, rather than to empathize with the child's ambivalence toward his or her relationship with the perpetrator.

Although therapists may experience many reactions and feelings that stem from their own professional and personal issues, other feelings may be evoked by the child's presentation. Therapists' reactions to the child often provide crucial information about the motives and personality dynamics of the child. The therapist has a greater likelihood of noticing these feelings after extensive experience with many other youngsters and a wide range of responses to child clients. For example, a therapist's intense negative reactions to a specific child may suggest that the child strongly needs to distance and provoke or ignore others. The therapist can use such reactions to generate working hypotheses about the child that need validation through careful and more objective assessment and observation. The therapist must be ready to evaluate these responses critically and use them to further enhance the progress of the child's therapy.

COPING STRATEGIES

Given the challenging issues that maltreated children present in therapy, there are several strategies therapists might use to cope more effectively with their own reactions. Using these strategies not only helps the therapist but maximizes the benefits of psychotherapy for the child. Below we outline some of these strategies.

Be Aware of Personal Issues

As was evident in the preceding discussion, it is crucial that the therapist be aware of individual issues, concerning the child client that might impact on the therapist role. Not only must the therapist be aware of these reactions but he or she must recognize their source, which might be the therapist, the client, or a combination of both. The therapist must be aware of any personal biases and attitude he or she may have. A therapist who is very uncomfortable with children might be strongly advised to work in a different area, perhaps with adult survivors, especially if the therapist is aware he or she has difficulty in dealing with children who are aggressive and provocative, highly dependent and clingy, or markedly regressed and self-abusive. A therapist who has a strong aversion to perpetrators might be cautioned against working directly with children who display physical or sexual aggression. The strong feelings evoked by the behavior of such children might contribute to the therapist's condemnation of the child in unhelpful or even destructive ways. The therapist also must be aware of any bias he or she may have toward a child who repeatedly overidealizes a perpetrator. A therapist who cannot acknowledge a child's positive feelings for a perpetrator excludes an important issue from therapy.

Therapists working with maltreated children must work closely with child welfare services and the justice system at many points in their careers. Although a therapist may agree to see a child only after child welfare workers have investigated the case, the child may make further disclosures during therapy that the therapist is compelled to report to the appropriate authorities. The therapist may have to be a source of support for children and families who are going through the process of police interviews and criminal hearings; the therapist may also have to testify personally in criminal proceedings. Family court involvement may also be required. Despite the efforts of all concerned, temporary or permanent guardianship orders may be necessary, and the therapist is often called on to provide evidence about their advisability. Any therapist working with maltreated children must have a knowledge of these systems and the salient legal statutes. Therapist's must feel comfortable working with personnel in these areas, attending court and providing testimony, and participating in an adversarial system. If not, the therapist should again select another area of practice or gain the necessary knowledge and experience under the supervision of a skilled practitioner to prepare for these roles, which are usually neglected in our formal training.

Therapists who have significant personal issues with maltreatment or sexuality should carefully evaluate whether it is appropriate for them to work with maltreated children. A therapist who is personaly involved in an abusive relationship might overidentify with the child client and have trouble maintaining an objective and accurate perception of the case. The same applies to a therapist who is abusive toward his or her own children, who has a personal childhood history of maltreatment, or who has personal issues relating to sexual identification or sexual functioning. For example, a therapist who detests homosexuals might have extreme difficulty in responding to a young boy's concerns that he is gay because he was sexually abused by a male perpetrator. This therapist might downplay the boy's concerns and glibly reassure the child that he is not gay without empathizing with the boy's anxiety. The youngster might be criticized by the therapist for even voicing such concerns. Such an attitude in a therapist would deter the active exploration of the boy's feelings and worries. A therapist who has sexual difficulties might have a real problem in listening to a child's account of his or her sexual arousal. Again, the therapist's verbal and nonverbal responses might inhibit their open discussion about such issues.

The above are just a few examples of how a therapist's own issues might influence the conduct and course of therapy. They highlight the potential damage and disservice therapists might do to child clients if the therapists are unaware or unwilling to examine themselves closely. This personal examination should not, of course, be shared with the child. There are several avenues the therapist can use to address his or her issues and biases. Apart from regular self-examination, the therapist should consult with other professionals about case issues and his or her personal reactions and issues. These steps may be taken informally, or they might be a component of a formal supervisory relationship. Supervision is available in most agencies, but independent practitioners should ensure that consultation and/or supervision opportunities are built into their practices. Finally, the therapist should consider a self-referral to therapy if the issues and biases arising from his or her personal background and/or current functioning have a negative impact upon clinical work. A break from clinical practice with maltreated children may also be necessary.

Obtain Appropriate Training and Experience

Any therapist who wants to treat maltreated children effectively needs extensive knowledge and experience in many areas, such as general child development and a thorough understanding of psychopathology and family functioning. As we advocated earlier, the field of developmental psychopathology provides an excellent conceptual framework for understanding children, the developmental tasks and challenges they face, and the myriad variables that influence their developmental outcome. The practitioner must have a broad knowledge of maltreatment sequelae and the dynamics responsible for these effects, including the transactional model. Additionally, the therapist must have an extensive repertoire of clinical skills. Given the complexity and demands of this work, therapists with limited and narrow training or those who are just beginning to explore this area of work should seriously evaluate whether they have the requisite skills, experience, and knowledge to function independently. One or two workshops will not provide the depth and extent of experience and knowledge required to treat these children. Novice or inexperienced therapists should seriously consider working in an agency where rigorous training and close supervision are available. They might also have the opportunity to work as cotherapists in family or group therapy. Alternatively, novice therapists may contract with a skilled practitioner for training and supervision. Either approach will ultimately serve both therapists and clients well.

The extensive knowledge base and array of clinical skills discussed above are necessary to ensure that therapists can meet the complex and diverse needs of maltreated children. Without a thorough understanding of the reasons for the child's reactions, the therapist may become discouraged and frustrated and may begin to personalize the child's negative reactions in therapy. These reactions may lead to inappropriate and possibly harmful behavior by the therapist that will reinforce the maltreated child's internal working models. Seeing maltreated children in therapy can be a long and arduous task and can negatively affect the therapist's view of his or her own competency. A theoretical paradigm is crucial to understanding the child's presentation and the process of therapy so that the therapist's sense of self-worth does not depend solely on client success, or "cures."

Set Realistic Treatment Goals

By developing a clear conceptual framework that will help in understanding the child, a therapist will be more realistic in setting treatment goals. Therapists must realize that for many children, change will be extremely slow and sometimes imperceptible. For some children, a truly positive outcome is unrealistic. The latter is the situation in the following example.

> Trudy was a 12-year-old girl referred for assessment and therapy after apprehension because of severe sexual abuse by her mother, uncle, and brother. Trudy was living in a receiving group home with three siblings at the time of referral. She was highly indiscriminate, kissing strangers who came to the door and climbing into strangers' laps in shopping malls. During assessment, Trudy appeared emotionally needy and somewhat intellectually limited. Given these limitations, the goals in the residential treatment facility where she was later placed were focused mainly on life skills. The treatment staff hoped Trudy could learn to protect herself and become less indiscriminate. They were especially worried about early pregnancy.
>
> Trudy engaged in therapy and benefitted from it. With individual, residential, and family therapy and the ongoing involvement of child protection personnel, Trudy had her only baby after she was 18 years of age, and she avoided being abused again by family members. These were significant achievements. Once she became a mother, however, Trudy was overwhelmed by the dependency needs of her child. She chose partners who abused both her and her child, but she also sought help for both of them. The child eventually was placed under the permanent guardianship of child welfare authorities. Despite its very negative outcome after approximately 12 years from first referral, the case may still in some ways be considered successful. Given her indiscriminate style of relating, which placed her at

risk for further victimization, without intervention Trudy would probably have been seriously hurt or killed by someone before adulthood.

Although Trudy's case may seem extreme, it is not unusual. Children whose early years are replete with maltreatment may never come to truly trust other people. Intense and long-term relationships may be difficult. The therapist's awareness that some children may always struggle with issues of intimacy and trust is a prerequisite to establishing realistic goals. This awareness is particularly necessary in determining placements for children who cannot remain in their biological homes. It is a common attitude among some foster and adoptive agencies that "love" alone will heal broken children. This attitude is particularly apparent when the children are very young. Many people cannot imagine that a 2- or 3-year-old child might already have a markedly impaired capacity to trust and respond to warm caregiving. This attitude can be detrimental with children who are so damaged it is unlikely they will ever tolerate dependent and close relationships (James, 1994). Repeated and futile attempts at having them adopted further damage these children and engender considerable distress and conflict in the families in which they are placed. It may be more productive to place such children in long-term treatment foster care with no eventual plan for adoption. Furthermore, such placements should be undertaken with the expectation that some of these very damaged children may completely exhaust the resources of the caregivers in their specialized placements every 3 to 4 years. The decision to place a child in long-term treatment foster care is not an abrogation of responsibility. It may instead, be a realistic decision based on a thorough understanding of the child's needs. The child may do better in the foster-care situation, where there is less expectation to "bond". Over time, some degree of trust in the foster parents may develop and may eventually result in an adoption if such a step can be tolerated by the child. Other children may be unable to respond to interpersonal overtures even in foster care. Such children may require a staffed residential setting where there is less pressure to form emotionally intimate relationships. Again, this type of placement does not imply failure; it may be a very realistic response to the child's needs.

Realize That Multiple Experiences Are Necessary to Produce Change

The therapist must recognize that many maltreated children require multiple experiences of exposure to the sensitivity and caring they have rarely, if ever, had (Graziano & Wells, 1992; Pearce & Pezzot-Pearce, 1994). Several experiences of this kind maximize a child's chances of recovering from victimization and is consistent with the basic tenets of developmental psychopathology. As argued in Chapter 5, the direct psychological treatment of maltreated children is just one component of a total strategy to reestablish the child's progress along an adaptive developmental trajectory. The therapist is not the sole "fixer" who makes children better, and a positive or negative outcome is not the therapist's sole responsibility. A positive outcome results from the combined efforts of many people who provide the child with sensitive caring in daily interactions. These people include the therapist, natural parents and extended family, foster parents, adoptive parents, and teachers, among others. All must work together to offer the child repeated experiences that will begin to alter his or her internal working models. Any therapist working with maltreated children must keep this in mind to avoid feeling discouraged, a sense of failure, and an overwhelming sense of responsibility for every aspect of those children's lives. The therapist can also advocate for and facilitate this cooperation among the individuals involved, provided they adhere to the notion of the importance of multiple experiences for recovery.

Many children require other professionally based interventions besides psychotherapy. Youngsters may display impairments across broad domains of functioning. These impairments may be sequelae associated with the maltreatment or they may have origins that are independent of the maltreatment but serve to moderate its impact. As therapists, we must realize we do not possess all the skills and knowledge required to intervene effectively with this diverse set of problems. One of the best steps we can often take is to refer our clients to other professionals who have the expertise to intervene successfully in those areas beyond our limits of knowledge, training, or competence.

A therapist must also remember that a particular course of psychotherapy with severely maltreated children is unlikely to resolve all issues totally because the child's perception of the maltreatment may change as a function of different developmental stages and the diverse experiences and situations encountered subsequent to the maltreatment. A child's return to therapy several years after its termination is consistent with the family-practice orientation described in Chapter 5 and should not necessarily be considered a treatment failure. In fact, the child's return may attest to the strength and importance of the relationship, and it is not uncommon to have maltreated children return intermittently for further work. In Chapter 2 we described Chris, who requested further contact with his previous therapist to address his sexuality issues. Although these issues were related to his early abuse, they became salient with the onset of puberty. Cameron, the subject of the case history below, has maintained an ongoing, although at times sporadic, relationship with his therapist for a number of years.

Cameron was a 5-year-old child referred for counseling by his mother and child welfare worker. He had been badly physically abused by a stepfather. His mother had fled the home to protect Cameron, leaving behind his younger half-sister. Cameron was highly anxious and eventually required long-term therapeutic foster-care placement and permanent guardianship. The latter occurred even though his mother continued to have contact with him. For 13 years Cameron attended counseling with his therapist at various times. Initially, weekly therapy lasted approximately 1 year, followed by decreasing contact. There were several subsequent periods of no contact for 1 to 2 years. However, he requested contact at the onset of each major developmental stage. Child welfare authorities and his therapist accommodated him, since he always used sessions to articulate and work through issues related to his early history. Currently, Cameron sees his therapist approximately eight times a year. He has successfully completed high school, lives independently, and plans a university education.

Although Cameron's requests for more therapy were appropriate and proved to be of real benefit, some therapists might interpret them as failure. This is clearly not so. With this ongoing input, Cameron did better than was expected in the initial course of therapy. The case might be exceptional, since both the child and therapist continued living in the same city and all parties were agreeable to an ongoing relationship. Even if the child and a particular therapist do not resume their relationship, a course of therapy may make a child more open to later work with other therapists.

Other children may call intermittently to "touch base." These attempts to reach their therapists demonstrate the strength and importance of the initial therapy work. We have received calls from adolescents and young adults who had been seen in therapy many years previously. They are quite good at remembering the therapist's name and phone number. One of us received a call from a 22-year-old man who had been seen in therapy 12 years before. He had continued to carry the therapist's card he was given just before he moved to an adoptive home in a distant city.

Establish Positive Relationships with Coworkers

As work with maltreated children can be exhausting and trying, it is important to establish supportive relationships with coworkers. These relationships provide therapists with emotional support and the opportunity for case discussion and consultation. These contacts are especially important if the child and family trigger personal issues in the therapist. Support is often readily available if the therapist works as part of a team, particularly in a program that focuses on the evaluation and treatment of maltreated children. In such a situation, all team members face similar issues with their clients. They can provide a ready recognition of the difficulties associated with this field of practice, thereby reducing fellow therapists' feelings of isolation and helplessness. Team members need to offer and accept support from others. A team in which members vie to be the most effective or competent therapist may exacerbate rather than reduce these feelings.

Obtaining emotional support, supervision, and consultation may be a greater problem for independent practitioners. They find the same issues provocative but may not always have colleagues readily available for support or discussion. It is crucial that these therapists make provision for regular opportunities for consultation or supervision. This contact may be achieved by contracting with a skilled therapist or by meeting regularly with several therapists for group supervision. Either avenue will provide much-needed support.

Have a Sense of Humor

Work with damaged, maltreated children requires knowledge, skills, energy, and dedication. Even with these assets, therapists may be very sobered by the issues their young clients present. It is important to retain a perspective about this work, combining it with a sense of humor. This attitude may prevent intense feelings of hopelessness and early burnout.

Humor may be used in several ways. It might be used with clients directly, although care is needed in the timing and type of humor. Humor should not be used to minimize childrens' pain or to demean them sarcastically. Early in therapy, a child may be unable to respond to humor. Progress may be evident when a child starts to regard the therapist's comments as benign rather than negative. Further progress is evident when the child begins to use humor, even teasing the therapist in a playful and trusting manner.

Humor has a valuable role in a therapist's relationships with colleagues. At times, humor may ease tense and critical situations and provide sufficient release so therapists can again address difficult issues. Although they should recognize their own personal strengths and weaknesses, therapists should not be so serious that they can never laugh at themselves. Of course, the reverse is not always ideal. A therapist who jokes constantly may become quite wearisome to clients and colleagues. The constant use of humor may trivialize the intense and significant difficulties that clients and therapists face.

Limit the Number of Cases and Diversify Your Caseload

Given the intense emotional demands of this type of work, therapists may find it useful to limit the number of maltreated children they see, particularly when some of the children display significant attachment difficulties and developmental effects. Because of the intensity and complexity of maltreatment cases, some therapists focus exclusively on this area. The books and journal articles they read, workshops they attend, and cases they take on are those involving abuse. Therapists who do so may easily become overwhelmed, emotionally fatigued, and exhausted. Other clinical interests furnish diversity and enrichment that are critical in countering eventual burnout. Therapists should take care to balance their caseloads with clients who have different problems or demands. Having some variety in his or her roles, such as a cotherapist will ease the demands placed on the therapist. These strategies are particularly important if clients provoke personal issues for the therapist. Prioritizing time and workload demands can be effective strategies to prevent burnout. Setting these priorities allows the therapist to remain interested and energetic, which ultimately benefits more clients. Moreover, therapists who have a breadth of different experiences and clinical knowledge, as well as specialized training in assessing and treating victims of maltreatment, may bring a more sophisticated understanding to these cases.

Run a Safe Practice

Some therapists so identify with the helping role that they assume all clients want help and will usually appreciate and reciprocate the kindness displayed toward them. This is a naive view, particularly if therapists do not consider their own safety. Child clients are usually accompanied to sessions by adults, some of whom are extremely hostile. Although therapists often recognize that adult clients may present a risk, many do not regard their child clients similarly. Care is needed in dealing with the adults, but it is also necessary with child clients, especially those who are older. In our experience the risk is negligible, although therapists should be cognizant of several simple precautions.

Risk can have several sources, but relatively simple techniques can reduce the risk to physical safety. These techniques may include an office design with access control, glass panels or windows near the office door (with blinds for privacy), and a buzzer or phone alarm system that can be activated easily. Within the office, a therapist may place furniture so as to permit easy exit if required. Office equipment such as scissors and letter openers should be placed out of easy reach if volatile clients are expected. It may be worthwhile to alert other personnel if a therapist is worried about safety with a particular client. The door may be opened a bit, but the therapist must be careful not to compromise the client's confidentiality or privacy. Although this strategy was discussed in Chapter 7 as a way to ease a child's safety concerns, it may occasionally do the same for the therapist. Another risk is the allegation of misconduct with the child. In Chapter 7 we explained that a therapist should use caution in touching a child who might misinterpret intent because of his or her abusive history. Allegations of misconduct decrease with competent practice, although all therapists who work in this area are at some risk because of the nature of the problems clients present. Good case notes and documentation are not only useful in formulating a case, they also provide an element of safety in that a clear and comprehensive record of treatment issues and therapist's responses exists. Although some strategies such as a having buzzer alarm may never need to be used, they are worth the consideration and effort.

Make Use of Ongoing Educational Opportunities

Although in a number of professions in many jurisdictions there are formal requirements for ongoing education to maintain certification or licensing, it is not always the case. Regardless of existing policy, therapists would do well to use ongoing educational opportunities such as workshops, courses, and training and supervisory relationships. Therapists should carefully choose experiences that will meet their needs, as identified through a careful self-examination of their own practice. Educational opportunities provide new ideas arising from recent research and from the clinical experience of others. These new concepts augment and broaden the therapist's clinical-skills base and stimulate fresh and creative ways of conceptualizing issues and problems; they validate as well as some of what the therapist already does. Educational experiences can reduce the isolation that is part of the constant daily work with abused and neglected children. Contact and interchange with colleagues in various educational settings also attenuate this sense of isolation. Conferences and workshops give therapists the opportunity for self-reflection away from the intense demands of clinical practice. If the educational opportunities are carefully chosen, they are well worth the time and financial investment.

Keep Your Personal World Healthy and Separate

Working as a therapist can become all consuming for some people. It is crucial for therapists to maintain a personal world that is healthy and separate from their clinical work. Although this may apply to any therapist, it is particularly important for those who work in the highly demanding field of child maltreatment.

We believe it is essential for therapists to maintain personal lives in which they have other interests that replenish the interest and energy needed to deal with difficult and challenging cases. Therapists must set priorities concerning their time and workload so that their work does not significantly restrict or entirely consume the time for other pursuits and nonwork relationships. These outside interests include not only taking holidays but leaving some weekends, evenings, or other times free. Therapists must take particular care to nurture their relationships with friends, partners, spouses, children, and families. Besides providing emotional satisfaction and support, these relationships increase the therapist's feelings of self-worth and impact positively on a therapist's professional life. These relationships provide multiple experiences for the therapist that directly parallel those the therapist and others provide for the maltreated child. They help therapists maintain a balanced perspective about their work and provide recognition of other supports and satisfactions in their lives.

Why do we and hundreds of other therapists work with abused and neglected children? There seem to be numerous reasons that would encourage clinicians to look elsewhere for professional and personal satisfaction. The stories of many children are horrifying, and some children have been so damaged that the gains from psychotherapy and other interventions are minimal at best. The intellectual challenges inherent in this work have always attracted our attention. Treating these children and their families often defies easy and pat solutions. The clinician must attempt to conceptualize these cases in a comprehensive and rigorous manner and then develop and apply creative interventions.

Moreover, there are emotional rewards. Most of us are in the business because we truly want to help others. We can help many maltreated children, even when the results are not spectacular and when treatment requires intensive and long-term commitment. The rewards do not lie in helping children lead problem-free lives; that goal eludes all of us. The reward comes from assisting children to become open to the whole range of human feelings and experiences, gain some mastery over their emotions and thoughts, and put their histories of abuse and neglect in the proper perspective. We would like to end this book with a final case example.

An 11-year-old boy who had been severely physically abused was referred for psychotherapy. Shaun had been beaten so badly by his father that he was hospitalized for 2 weeks with multiple and serious injuries. He had been beaten on many previous occasions. Over the 2-year course of therapy Shaun struggled with acknowledging his ambivalent feelings toward his father. Like many such children, he presented an overidealized depiction of his dad and minimized his own rage and sadness. Eventually he was able to acknowledge anger and profound grief about never having had a loving father. By the end of 2 years, Shaun had made considerable progress. Although he still had some problems with interpersonal relationships, he and the therapist agreed to terminate therapy. In the final session, Shaun thanked his therapist, remarking that the therapist had helped him "become human again." When asked what he meant, Shaun stated, "You helped me feel again."

It was a compliment the therapist will never forget.

References

Aber, J. L., & Allen, J. P. (1987). The effects of maltreatment on young children's socioemotional development: An attachment theory perspective. *Developmental Psychology, 23,* 406–414.

Aber, J. L., Allen, J. P., Carlson, V., & Cicchetti, D. (1989). The effects of maltreatment on development during early childhood: Recent studies and their theoretical, clinical, and policy implications. In D. Cicchetti & V. Carlson (Eds.), *Child maltreatment: Theory and research on the causes and consequences of child abuse and neglect* (pp. 579–619). New York: Cambridge University Press.

Abidin, R. R. (1995). *Parenting Stress Index – Professional Manual* (3rd ed.). Odessa, FL: Psychological Assessment Resources.

Achenbach, T. M., & Edelbrock, C. (1983). *Manual for the Child Behavior Checklist.* Burlington: University of Vermont Press

Ainsworth, M. D. S. (1989). Attachments beyond infancy. *American Psychologist, 44,* 709–716.

Ainsworth, M. D. S., Blehar, M. C., Waters, E., & Wall, S. (1978). *Patterns of attachment: A psychological study of the strange situation.* Hillsdale, NJ: Erlbaum.

Ainsworth, M. D. S., & Bowlby, J. (1991). An ethological approach to personality development. *American Psychologist, 46,* 333–341.

Alessandri, S. M. (1991). Play and social behaviors in maltreated preschoolers. *Development and Psychopathology, 3,* 191–206.

Alessandri, S. M. (1992). Mother–child interactional correlates of maltreated and nonmaltreated children's play behavior. *Development and Psychopathology, 4,* 257–270.

Alexander, F., & French, R. M. (1946). *Psychoanalytic therapy.* New York: Ronald.

Alexander, J., & Parsons, B. V. (1982). *Functional family therapy.* Monterey, CA: Brooks/Cole.

Alexander, P. C. (1992). Application of attachment theory to the study of sexual abuse. *Journal of Consulting and Clinical Psychology, 60,* 185–195.

Allen, F. H., (1942). *Psychotherapy with children.* Lincoln: University of Nebraska Press.

Allen, J. (1988). *Inscapes of the child's world.* Dallas: Spring.

American Humane Association. (1984). *National study on child neglect and reporting.* Denver: Author.

American Psychiatric Association. (1987). *Diagnositc and statistical manual of mental disorders* (3rd ed., rev.). Washington, DC: Author.

American Psychiatric Association. (1994). *Diagnostic and statistical manual of mental disorders* (4th ed.). Washington DC: Author.

Ammerman, R. T., Cassisi, J. E., Hersen, M., & Van Hasselt, V. B. (1986). Consequences of physical abuse and neglect in children. *Clinical Psychology Review, 6*, 291–310.

Arce, A. (1982). Discussion: Cultural aspects of mental health care for Hispanic Americans. In A. Gaw (Ed.), *Cross cultural psychiatry* (pp. 137–148). Bristol, UK: John Wright.

Asher, S. R., & Coie, J. D. (Eds.). (1990). *Peer rejection.* New York: Cambridge University Press.

Axline, V. (1964). *Dibs: In search of self.* New York: Ballantine Books.

Axline, V. (1969). *Play therapy* (Rev. ed.). New York: Ballantine Books.

Barahal, R., Waterman, J., & Martin, H. (1981). The social–cognitive development of abused children. *Journal of Consulting and Clinical Psychology, 49*, 508–516.

Barnett, D., Manly, J. T., & Cicchetti, D. (1991). Continuing toward an operational definition of psychological maltreatment. *Development and Psychopathology, 3*, 19–29.

Baron, R. M., & Kenny, D. A. (1986). The moderator–mediator variable distinction in social psychological research: Conceptual, strategic, and statistical considerations. *Journal of Personality and Social Psychology, 51*, 1173–1182.

Beeghly, M., & Cicchetti, D. (1994). Child maltreatment, attachment and the self system: Emergence of an internal state lexicon in toddlers at high social risk. *Development and Psychopathology, 6*, 5–30.

Bellak, L. (1993). *The Thematic Apperception Test, the Children's Apperception Test, and the Senior Apperception Technique in clinical use* (5th ed.). Boston: Allyn and Bacon.

Belsky, J. (1980). Child maltreatment: An ecological integration. *American Psychologist, 35*, 320–335.

Belsky, J. (1993). Etiology of child maltreatment: A developmental–ecological analysis. *Psychological Bulletin, 114*, 413–434.

Belsky, J., Rovine, M., & Taylor, D. G. (1984). The Pennsylvania Infant and Family Development Project: III. The origins of individual differences in infant–mother attachment: Maternal and infant contributions. *Child Development, 55*, 718–728.

Bentovim, A., van Elberg, A., & Boston, P. (1988). The results of treatment. In A. Bentovim, A. Elton, J. Hildebrand, M. Tranter, & E. Vizard (Eds.), *Child sexual abuse within the family: Assessment and treatment* (pp. 252–268). London: Wright.

Berliner, L. (1989, November). *Evaluation and treatment of children with sexual behavior problems.* Paper presented at the Adolescent Offenders Conference: Prevention, Treatment and Management, Vancouver, British Columbia, Canada.

Berliner, L., & Wright, R. J. (1987). Treating the effects of sexual abuse on children. *Journal of Interpersonal Violence, 2*, 415–434.

Black, M., Dubowitz, H., & Harrington, D. (1994). Sexual abuse: Developmental differences in children's behavior and self-perception. *Child Abuse and Neglect, 18*, 85–95.

Bowlby, J. (1969). *Attachment and loss: Vol. 1. Attachment.* New York: Basic Books.

Bowlby, J. (1973). *Attachment and loss: Vol. 2. Separation: Anxiety and anger.* New York: Basic Books.

Bowlby, J. (1980). *Attachment and loss: Vol. 3. Loss.* New York: Basic Books.

Bowlby, J. (1982). *Attachment and loss: Vol. 1. Attachment* (2nd ed.). New York: Basic Books.

Bowlby, J. (1988a). *A secure base: Parent–child attachment and healthy human development.* New York: Basic Books.

Bowlby, J. (1988b). Developmental psychiatry comes of age. *American Journal of Psychiatry, 145,* 1–10.

Bowman, B. (1989). Culturally sensitive inquiry. In J. Garbarino, F. M. Stott, & Faculty of the Erikson Institute, *What children can tell us* (pp. 92–107). San Francisco: Jossey-Bass.

Brady, C. A., & Friedrich, W. N. (1982). Levels of intervention: A model for training in play therapy. *Journal of Clinical Child Psychology, 11,* 39–43.

Braun, B. G. (1986). *Treatment of multiple personality disorder.* Washington, DC: American Psychiatric Press.

Bretherton, I. (1985). Attachment theory: Retrospect and prospect. In I. Bretherton & E. Waters (Eds.), Growing points in attachment theory and research. *Monographs of the Society for Research in Child Development, 50*(1–2, Serial No. 209), 3–36.

Bretherton, I. (1987). New perspectives on attachment relations. In J. Osofsky (Ed.), *Handbook of infant development* (2nd ed., pp. 1061–1100). New York: Wiley.

Bretherton, I. (1990). Open communication and internal working models: Their role in the development of attachment relationships. In R. A. Thompson (Ed.), *Socioemotional development: Nebraska Symposium on Motivation, 1988* (pp. 57–113). Lincoln: University of Nebraska Press.

Bretherton, I., & Beeghly, M. (1982). Talking about internal states: The acquisition of an explicit theory of mind. *Developmental Psychology, 18,* 906–921.

Bretherton, I., Ridgeway, D., & Cassidy, J. (1990). Assessing internal working models of the attachment relationship. In M. Greenberg, D. Cicchetti, & E. M. Cummings (Eds.), *Attachment in the preschool years* (pp. 273–308). Chicago: University of Chicago Press.

Briere, J. N. (1989). *Therapy for adults molested as children: Beyond survival.* New York: Springer.

Briere, J. N. (1992). *Child abuse trauma.* Newbury Park, CA: Sage.

Briere, J. N. (1996). *Professional Manual for the Trauma Symptom Checklist for Children (TSCC).* Odessa, FL: Psychological Assessment Resources.

Briere, J. N., & Runtz, M. (1988). Multivariate correlates of childhood psychological and physical maltreatment among university women. *Child Abuse and Neglect, 12,* 331–341.

Broder, E. A., & Hood, E. (1983). A guide to the assessment of child and family. In P. D. Steinhauer & Q. Rae-Grant (Eds.), *Psychological problems of the child in the family.* New York: Basic Books.

Buchsbaum, H. K., Toth, S. L., Clyman, R. B., Cicchetti, D., & Emde, R. B. (1992). The use of a narrative story stem technique with maltreated children: Implications for theory and practice. *Development and Psychopathology, 4,* 603–625.

Budin, L., & Johnson, D. (1989). Sex abuse prevention programs: Offenders' attitudes about their efficacy. *Child Abuse and Neglect, 13,* 77–87.

Bullard, J. B., Glaser, H. H., Hagarty, M. C., & Pivchik, E. C. (1967). Failure to thrive in the "neglected" child. *American Journal of Orthopsychiatry, 37,* 680–690.

Burgess, R. L., & Conger, R. D. (1977). Family interaction patterns related to child abuse and neglect: Some preliminary findings. *Child Abuse and Neglect, 1,* 269–277.

Burgess, R. L., & Conger, R. D. (1978). Family interaction in abusive, neglectful, and normal families. *Child Development, 19,* 1163–1173.

Burke, A. E., Crenshaw, D. A., Greene, J., Schlosser, M. A., & Strocchia-Rivera, L. (1989). Influence of verbal ability on the expression of aggression in physically abused children. *Journal of the American Academy of Child and Adolescent Psychiatry, 28,* 215–218.

Caffaro-Rouget, A., Lang, R. A., & van Santen, V. (1989). The impact of child sexual abuse. *Annals of Sex Research, 2,* 29–47.

Calverley, R. M., Fischer, K. W., & Ayoub, C. (1994). Complex splitting of self-representations in sexually abused adolescent girls. *Development and Psychopathology, 6,* 195–213.

Canino, I. (1988). The transcultural child. In C. J. Kestenbaum & D. T. Williams (Eds.), *Handbook of clinical assessment of children and adolescents* (Vol. II, pp. 1024–1042). New York and London: New York University Press.

Carek, D. J. (1979). Individual psychodynamically oriented therapy. In J. D. Nospitz (Ed.), *Handbook of child psychiatry* (Vol. 3, pp. 35–57). New York: Basic Books.

Carlson, V., Barnett, D., Braunwald, K. G., & Cicchetti, D. (1989). Finding order in disorganizations. In D. Cicchetti & V. Carlson (Eds.), *Child maltreatment: Theory and research on the causes and consequences of child abuse and neglect* (pp. 494–528). New York: Cambridge University Press.

Carson, M. L., & Goodfield, R. K. (1988). The Children's Garden attachment model. In R. W. Small & F. J. Alwon (Eds.), *Challenging the limits of care* (pp. 115–125). Needham, MA: Albert E. Trieschman Center.

Caruso, K. (1987). *Projective storytelling cards.* Redding, CA: Northwest Psychological.

Cassidy, J. (1988). Child–mother attachment and the self in six-year-olds. *Child Development, 59,* 121–134.

Cassidy, J., & Berlin, L. J. (1994). The insecure/ambivalent pattern of attachment: Theory and research. *Child Development, 65,* 971–991.

Cassidy, J., & Kobak, R. (1988). Avoidance and its relation to other defensive processes. In J. Belsky & T. Nezworski (Eds), *Clinical implications of attachment* (pp. 300–326). Hillsdale, NJ: Erlbaum.

Chu, J. A., & Dill, D. L. (1990). Dissociative symptoms in relation to childhood physical and sexual abuse. *American Journal of Psychiatry, 147,* 887–892.

Cicchetti, D. (1989). How research on child maltreatment has informed the study of child development: Perspectives from developmental psychopathology. In D. Cicchetti & V. Carlson (Eds.), *Child maltreatment: Theory and research on the causes and consequences of child abuse and neglect* (pp. 377–431). New York: Cambridge University Press.

Cicchetti, D., & Barnett, D. (1991). Attachment organization in maltreated preschoolers. *Development and Psychopathology, 3,* 397–411.

Cicchetti, D., & Beeghly, M. (1987). Symbolic development in maltreated youngsters: An organizational perspective. In D. Cicchetti & M. Beeghly (Eds.), *Atypical symbolic development* (pp. 47–68). San Francisco: Jossey-Bass.

Cicchetti, D., Cummings, E. M., Greenberg, M. T., & Marvin, R. S. (1990). An organizational perspective on attachment beyond infancy. In M. Greenberg, D. Cicchetti, & E. M. Cummings (Eds.), *Attachment in the preschool years* (pp. 3–49). Chicago: University of Chicago Press.

Cicchetti, D., Lynch, M., Shonk, S., & Manley, J. (1992). An organizational perspective on peer relations in maltreated children. In R. D. Parke & G. W. Ladd (Eds.), *Family–peer relationships: Modes of linkage* (pp. 345–383). Hillsdale, NJ: Erlbaum.

Cicchetti, D., & Olsen, K. (1990). The developmental psychopathology of child maltreatment. In M. Lewis & S. M. Miller (Eds.), *Handbook of developmental psychopathology* (pp. 261–279). New York: Plenum Press.

Cicchetti, D., & Rizley, R. (1981). Developmental perspectives on the etiology, intergenerational transmission, and sequelae of child maltreatment. *New Directions for Child Development, 11,* 31–55.

Cicchetti, D., & Rogosch, F. A. (1994). The toll of child maltreatment on the developing child. *Child and Adolescent Psychiatric Clinics of North America, 3,* 759–776.

Cicchetti, D., & Toth, S. L. (1995). A developmental psychopathology perspective on child abuse and neglect. *Journal of the American Academy of Child and Adolescent Psychiatry, 34,* 541–565.

Claussen, A. H., & Crittenden, P. M. (1991). Physical and psychological maltreatment: Relations among different types of maltreatment. *Child Abuse and Neglect, 15,* 5–18.

Cohen, H., & Weil, G. R. (1971). *Tasks of Emotional Development Test Manual.* Brookline, MA: T. E. D. Associates.

Cohen, J. A., & Mannarino, A. P. (1988). Psychological symptoms in sexually abused girls. *Child Abuse and Neglect, 12,* 571–577.

Cole, P. M., & Putnam, F. W. (1992). Effect of incest on self and social functioning: A developmental perspective. *Journal of Consulting and Clinical Psychology, 60,* 174–184.

Cole, P. M., Woolger, C., Power, T. G., & Smith, K. D. (1992). Parenting difficulties among adult survivors of father–daughter incest. *Child Abuse and Neglect, 16,* 239–249.

Conaway, L. P., & Hansen, D. J. (1989). Social behavior of physically abused and neglected children: A critical review. *Clinical Psychology Review, 9,* 627–652.

Conduct Problems Prevention Research Group. (1992). A developmental and clinical model for the prevention of conduct disorder: The FAST Track Program. *Development and Psychopathology, 4,* 509–527.

Conte, J. R., & Berliner, L. (1988). The impact of sexual abuse in children: Empirical findings. In L. E. Walker (Ed.), *Handbook on sexual abuse of children* (pp. 72–93). New York: Springer.

Conte, J. R., & Schuerman, J. R. (1987). Factors associated with an increased impact of child sexual abuse. *Child Abuse and Neglect, 11,* 201–211.

Conte, J. R., Wolf, S., & Smith, T. (1989). What sexual offenders tell us about prevention strategies. *Child Abuse and Neglect, 13,* 293–301.

Cosentino, C. E., Meyer-Bahlburg, H. F. I., Alpert, J. L., Weinberg, S. L., & Gaines, R. (1995). Sexual behavior problems and psychopathology symptoms in sexually abused girls. *Journal of the American Academy of Child and Adolescent Psychiatry, 34,* 1033–1042.

Coster, W., Gersten, M., Beeghly, M., & Cicchetti, D. (1989). Communicative functioning in maltreated toddlers. *Developmental Psychology, 25,* 1020–1029.

Crittenden, P. M. (1988). Relationships at risk. In J. Belsky & T. Nezworski (Eds.), *Clinical applications of attachment* (pp. 136–174). New York: Plenum Press.

Crittenden, P. M. (1992a). Children's strategies for coping with adverse home environments: An interpretation using attachment theory. *Child Abuse and Neglect, 16,* 329–343.

Crittenden, P. M. (1992b). Treatment of anxious attachment in infancy and early childhood. *Development and Psychopathology, 4,* 575–602.

Crittenden, P. M., & DiLalla, D. (1988). Compulsive compliance: The development of an inhibitory coping strategy in infancy. *Journal of Abnormal Child Psychology, 16,* 585–599.

Cummings, N. A. (1986). The dismantling of our health system. *American Psychologist, 41,* 426–431.

Cunningham, C., & MacFarlane, K. (1991). *When children molest other children: Group treatment strategies for young sexual abusers.* Orwell, VT: Safer Society Press.

Daro, D. (1991). Child sexual abuse prevention: Separating fact from fiction. *Child Abuse and Neglect, 5,* 1–4.

Daro, D., & McCurdy, K. (1991). *Current trends in child abuse reporting and fatalities: The results of the 1990 fifty state survey.* Chicago: National Committee for Prevention of Child Abuse.

Davis, N. (1990). *Once upon a time: Therapeutic stories to heal abused children.* New York: Institute for Rational Living.

Deblinger, E., McLeer, S. V., Atkins, M. S., Ralphe, D., & Foa, E. (1989). Posttraumatic stress in sexually abused, physically abused, and nonabused children. *Child Abuse and Neglect, 13,* 403–408.

Demb, J. M. (1991). Reported hyperphagia in foster children. *Child Abuse and Neglect, 15,* 77–88.

Denham, S. A., McKinley, M., Couchoud, E. A., & Holt, R. (1990). Emotional and behavioral predictors of preschool ratings. *Child Development, 61,* 1145–1152.

Derogatis, L. R. (1983). *Administration scoring and procedures manual—II for the revised version and other instruments of the psychopathology rating scale series.* Baltimore: Clinical Psychometrics Research.

Dodds, J. B. (1985). *A child psychotherapy primer.* New York: Human Services Press.

Dodge, K. A., Bates, J. E., & Pettit, G. S. (1990). Mechanisms in the cycle of violence. *Science, 250,* 1678–1683.

Dodge, K. A., Pettit, G. S., & Bates, J. E. (1994). Effects of physical maltreatment on the development of peer relations. *Development and Psychopathology, 6,* 43–55.

Dodge, K., & Richard, B. (1985). Peer perceptions, aggression, and the development of peer relations. In J. Pryor & J. Day (Eds.), *The development of social cognition* (pp. 35–58). New York: Springer Verlag.

Dubowitz, H., Black, M., Harrington, D., & Verschoore, A. (1993). A follow-up study of behavior problems associated with child sexual abuse. *Child Abuse and Neglect, 17,* 743–754.

Duncan, G. J., Brooks-Gunn, J., & Klebanov, P. K. (1994). Economic deprivation and early childhood development. *Child Development, 65,* 296–318.

Dunn, J., Bretherton, I., & Munn, P. (1987). Conversations about feeling states between mothers and their young children. *Developmental Psychology, 23,* 132–139.

Dunn, J., & Brown, J. (1991). Relationships, talk about feelings, and the development of affect regulation in early childhood. In J. Garber & K. A. Dodge (Eds.), *The development of emotion regulation and dysregulation* (pp. 89–108). New York: Cambridge University Press.

Eckenrode, J., Laird, M., & Doris, J. (1993). School performance and disciplinary problems among abused and neglected children. *Developmental Psychology, 29,* 53–62.

Edwards, R. (1995). American Indians rely on ancient healing techniques. *APA Monitor, 26*(8), 36.

Egeland, B. (1991). A longitudinal study of high-risk families: Issues and findings. In R. H. Starr, Jr., & D. A. Wolfe (Eds.), *The effects of child abuse and neglect: Issues and research* (pp. 33–56). New York: Guilford Press.

Egeland, B., Jacobvitz, D., & Sroufe, L. A. (1988). Breaking the cycle of abuse. *Child Development, 59,* 1080–1088.

Egeland, B., & Sroufe, L. A. (1981). Developmental sequelae of maltreatment in infancy. In R. Rizley & D. Cicchetti (Eds.), *Developmental perspectives in child maltreatment* (pp. 77–92). San Francisco: Jossey-Bass.

Einbender, A. J., & Friedrich, W. N. (1989). Psychological functioning and behavior of sexually abused girls. *Journal of Consulting and Clinical Psychology, 57,* 155–157.

Elmer, E., Gregg, G. S., & Ellison, P. (1969). Late results of the "Failure to Thrive" syndrome. *Clinical Pediatrics, 8,* 584–589.

Erickson, M., Egeland, B., & Pianta, R. (1989). The effects of maltreatment on the development of young children. In D. Cicchetti & V. Carlson (Eds.), *Child maltreatment: Theory and research on the causes and consequences of child abuse and neglect* (pp. 647–684). New York: Cambridge University Press.

Erickson, M. F., Korfmacher, J., & Egeland, B. R. (1992). Attachment past and present: Implications for therapeutic intervention with mother–infant dyads. *Development and Psychopathology, 4,* 495–507.

Everson, M. D., Hunter, W. M., Runyon, D. K., Edelsohn, G. A., & Coulter, M. L. (1989). Maternal support following disclosure of incest. *American Journal of Orthopsychiatry, 59,* 197–207.

Exner, J. (1993). *The Rorschach: A comprehensive system: Vol. 1. Basic foundations* (3rd ed.). New York: Wiley.

Eyberg, S., & Ross, A. (1978). Assessment of child behavior problems: The validation of a new inventory. *Journal of Clinical Child Psychology, 7,* 113–116.

Famularo, R., Fenton, T., Kinscherff, R., Ayoub, C., & Barnum, R. (1994). Maternal and child posttraumatic stress disorder among child victims of sexual abuse. *Child Abuse and Neglect, 18,* 27–36.

Feshbach, N. D., Feshbach, S., Fauvre, M., & Ballard-Campbell, M. (1983). *Learning to care.* Glenview, IL: Scott, Foresman.

Finkelhor, D. (1979). *Sexually victimized children*. New York: Free Press.

Finkelhor, D. (1995). The victimization of children: A developmental perspective. *American Journal of Orthopsychiatry, 65*, 177–193.

Finkelhor, D., & Berliner, L. (1995). Research on the treatment of sexually abused children: A review and recommendations. *Journal of the American Academy of Child and Adolescent Psychiatry, 34*, 1408–1423.

Finkelhor, D., & Browne, A. (1985). The traumatic impact of child sexual abuse: A conceptualization. *American Journal of Orthopsychiatry, 55*, 530–541.

Finkelhor, D., & Dziuba-Leatherman, J. (1994). Victimization of children. *American Psychologist, 49*, 173–183.

Finkelhor, D., Hotaling, G., Lewis, I. A., & Smith, C. (1989). Sexual abuse and its relationship to later sexual satisfaction, marital status, religion, and attitudes. *Journal of Interpersonal Violence, 4*, 279–399.

Flaherty, J. A., & Richman, J. A. (1986). Effects of childhood relationships on the adult's capacity to form social supports. *American Journal of Psychiatry, 143*, 851–855.

Foa, E. B., Steketee, G., & Rothbaum, B. (1989). Behavioral/cognitive conceptualizations of post-traumatic stress disorder. *Behavior Therapy, 20*, 155–176.

Fox, L., Long, S. H., & Langlois, A. (1988). Patterns of language comprehension deficits in abused and neglected children. *Journal of Speech and Hearing Disorders, 53*, 239–244.

Fraiberg, S., Adelson, E., & Shapiro, V. (1975). Ghosts in the nursery: A psychoanalytic approach to impaired infant–mother relationships. *Journal of the American Academy of Child Psychiatry, 14*, 387–421.

Frazier, D., & Levine, E. (1983). Reattachment therapy: Intervention with the very young physically abused child. *Psychotherapy: Theory, Research and Practice, 20*, 90–100.

Freud, A. (1966). *The ego and the mechanisms of defense* (Rev. ed.). New York: International Universities Press. (Original work published 1939)

Friedman, W. J. (1981). *The developmental psychology of time*. New York: Academic Press.

Friedrich, W. N. (1990). *Psychotherapy of sexually abused children and their families*. New York: W. W. Norton.

Friedrich, W. N. (1993). Sexual victimization and sexual behavior in children: A review of recent literature. *Child Abuse and Neglect, 17*, 59–66.

Friedrich, W. N., Beilke, R. L., & Urquiza, A. J. (1987). Children from sexually abusive families: A behavioral comparison. *Journal of Interpersonal Violence, 2*, 391–402.

Friedrich, W. N., Beilke, R. L., & Urquiza, A. J. (1988). Behavior problems in young sexually abused boys: A comparison study. *Journal of Interpersonal Violence, 3*, 21–28.

Friedrich, W. N., Grambsch, P., Broughton, D., Kuiper, J., & Beilke, R. L. (1991). Normative sexual behavior in children. *Pediatrics, 88*, 456–646.

Friedrich, W. N., Grambsch, P., Damon, L., Hewitt, S., Koverola, C., Lang, R., Wolfe, V., & Broughton, D. (1992). The child sexual behavior inventory: Normative and clinical findings. *Psychological Assessment, 4*, 303–311.

Gaensbauer, T. J., & Hiatt, S. (1984). Facial communication of emotion in early infancy. In N. A. Fox & R. J. Davidson (Eds.), *The Psychobiology of affective development* (pp. 207–230). Hillsdale, NJ: Erlbaum.

Gaensbauer, T., Mrazek, D., & Harmon, R. (1981). Emotional expression in abused and/or neglected infants. In N. Frude (Ed.), *Psychological approaches to child abuse* (pp. 120–135). Totowa, NJ: Roman and Littlefield.

Gaensbauer, T. J., & Sands, K. (1979). Distorted affective communication in abused/neglected infants and their potential impact on caregivers. *American Journal of Child Psychiatry, 18,* 236–250.

Garbarino, J., & Gilliam, G. (1980). *Understanding abusive families.* Lexington, MA: Lexington Press.

Garbarino, J., Guttman, E., & Seeley, J. (1986). *The psychologically battered child: Strategies for identification, assessment and intervention.* San Francisco: Jossey-Bass.

Garbarino, J., Stott, F. M., & Faculty of the Erikson Institute. (1989). *What children can tell us.* San Francisco: Jossey-Bass.

Gardner, L. I. (1972). Deprivation dwarfism. *Scientific American, 227,* 76–82.

Gardner, R. A. (1971). *Therapeutic communication with children: The mutual storytelling technique.* New York: Jason Aronson.

Garmezy, N., & Streitman, S. (1974). Children at risk: The search for antecedents to schizophrenia. Part I: Conceptual models and research methods. *Schizophrenia Bulletin, 8,* 14–90.

Gelles, R. J., & Straus, M. A. (1990). The medical and psychological costs of family violence. In M. A. Straus & R. J. Gelles (Eds.), *Physical violence in American families: Risk factors and adaptations to violence in 8,145 families* (pp. 425–430). New Brunswick, NJ: Transaction.

George, C., & Main, M. (1979). Social interactions of young abused children: Approach, avoidance, and aggression. *Child Development, 50,* 306–318.

Gersten, M., Coster, W., Schneider-Rosen, K., Carlson, V., & Cicchetti, D. (1986). The socio-emotional bases of communicative functioning: Quality of attachment, language development, and early maltreatment. In M. E. Lamb, A. L. Brown, & B. Rogoff (Eds.), *Advances in developmental psychology* (Vol. 4, pp. 105–151). Hillsdale, NJ: Erlbaum.

Gil, E. (1991). *The healing power of play: Working with abused children.* New York: Guilford Press.

Gil, E., & Johnson, T. C. (1993). *Sexualized children: Assessment and treatment of sexualized children and children who molest.* Rockville, MD: Launch Press.

Ginott, H. G. (1965). *Between parent and child.* New York: Avon Books.

Gittleman, R. (1980). The role of psychological tests for differential diagnosis in child psychiatry. *American Academy of Child Psychiatry, 19,* 413–438.

Glasser, H., Heagarty, M., Bullard, D. M., Jr., & Rivchik, E. C. (1968). Physical and psychological development of children with early failure to thrive. *Journal of Pediatrics, 73,* 690–698.

Goldberg, S. (1991). Recent developments in attachment theory and research. *Canadian Journal of Psychiatry, 36,* 393–400.

Goldenson, R. M. (Ed.). (1984). *Longman dictionary of psychology and psychiatry.* New York: Longman.

Gomes-Schwartz, B., Horowitz, J. M., Cardarelli, A. P., & Sauzier, M. (1990). The aftermath of child sexual abuse: 18 months later. In B. Gomes-Schwartz,

J. M. Horowitz, & A. P. Cardarelli (Eds.), *Child sexual abuse: The initial effects* (pp. 132–152). Newbury Park, CA: Sage.

Goodwin, J., McCarthy, T., & Divasto, P. (1981). Prior incest in mothers of sexually abused children. *Child Abuse and Neglect, 5,* 87–96.

Graziano, A. M., & Wells, J. R. (1992). Treatment for abused children: When is a partial solution acceptable? *Child Abuse and Neglect, 16,* 217–228.

Grizenko, N., & Pawliuk, N. (1994). Risk and protective factors for disruptive behavior disorders in children. *American Journal of Orthopsychiatry, 64,* 534–544.

Gutierrez, J. (1989). Using tests and other instruments. In J. Garbarino, F. M. Stott, & Faculty of the Erikson Institute, *What children can tell us* (pp. 203–225). San Francisco: Jossey-Bass.

Hagans, K. B., & Case, J. (1988). *When your child has been molested: A parent's guide to healing and recovery. Putting the pieces back together.* New York: Lexington Books.

Hall, D. K. (1993). *Assessing child trauma.* Toronto: Institute for the Prevention of Child Abuse.

Hansburg, H. G. (1972). *Adolescent separation anxiety: A method for the study of adolescent separation problems.* Springfield, IL: C. C. Thomas.

Hart, S. N., & Brassard, M. R. (1987). A major threat to children's mental health: Psychological maltreatment. *American Psychologist, 42,* 160–165.

Hart, S. N., Germain, R., & Brassard, M. R. (Eds.). (1983). *Proceedings Summary of the International Conference on Psychological Abuse of Children and Youth.* Bloomington: Indiana University, Office for the Study of the Psychological Rights of the Child.

Hart, S. N., Germain, R., & Brassard, M. R. (1987). The challenge: To better understand and combat the psychological maltreatment of children and youth. In M. R. Brassard, R. German, & S. N. Hart (Eds.), *Psychological maltreatment of children and youth* (pp. 3–24). New York: Pergamon Press.

Harter, S. (1977). A cognitive–developmental approach to children's expression of conflicting feelings and a technique to facilitate such expression in play therapy. *Journal of Consulting and Clinical Psychology, 45,* 417–432.

Harter, S. (1982). The Perceived Competence Scale for Children. *Child Development, 53,* 87–97.

Harter, S. (1983). Cognitive–developmental considerations in the conduct of play therapy. In C. E. Schaeffer & K. J. O'Connor (Eds.), *Handbook of play therapy* (pp. 95–127). New York: Wiley.

Haskett, M. E., & Kistner, J. A. (1991). Social interactions and peer perceptions of young physically abused children. *Child Development, 62,* 979–990.

Hathaway, S. R., & McKinley, J. C. (1989). *Manual for Minnesota Multiphasic Personality Inventory–2.* Minneapolis: University of Minnesota Press.

Hewitt, S. K., & Friedrich, W. N. (1991, January). *Preschool children's responses to alleged sexual abuse at intake and one-year follow up.* Paper presented at the meeting of the American Professional Society on the Abuse of Children, San Diego, CA.

Hibbard, R. A., & Hartman, G. L. (1992). Behavioral problems of alleged sexual abuse victims. *Child Abuse and Neglect, 16,* 755–762.

Hodges, J., & Tizard, B. (1989a). IQ and behavioral adjustment of ex-institutional adolescents. *Journal of Child Psychology and Psychiatry, 30,* 53–75.

Hodges, J., & Tizard, B. (1989b). Social and family relationships of ex-institutional adolescents. *Journal of Child Psychology and Psychiatry, 30,* 77–97.

Hoffman-Plotkin, D., & Twentyman, C. T. (1984). A multi-modal assessment of behavioral and cognitive deficits in abused and neglected preschoolers. *Child Development, 55,* 794–802.

Howes, C. (1984). Social interactions and patterns of friendships in normal and emotionally disturbed children. In T. Field, J. Roopnarine, & M. Segal (Eds.), *Friendships in normal and handicapped children* (pp. 163–185). Norwood, NJ: Ablex.

Howes, C., & Eldredge, R. (1985). Responses of abused, neglected, and nonmaltreated children to the behaviors of their peers. *Journal of Applied Developmental Psychology, 6,* 261–270.

Howes, C., & Espinosa, M. P. (1985). The consequences of child abuse for the formation of relationships with peers. *Child Abuse and Neglect, 9,* 397–404.

Hufton, I. W., & Oates, R. K. (1977). Nonorganic failure to thrive: A long term follow-up. *Pediatrics, 59,* 73–77.

James, B. (1989). *Treating traumatized children: New insights and creative interventions.* Lexington, MA: Lexington Books.

James, B. (1994). *Handbook for treatment of attachment–trauma problems in children.* Lexington, NY: Lexington Books.

Janoff-Bulman, R. (1979). Characterological versus behavioral self-blame: Inquiries into depression and rape. *Journal of Personality and Social Psychology, 37,* 1789–1809.

Johnstone, B. K., & Kenkel, M. B. (1991). Stress, coping, and adjustment in female adolescent incest victims. *Child Abuse and Neglect, 15,* 293–305.

Kagan, R. M. (1986). Game therapy for children in placement. In C. E. Schaefer & S. Reid (Eds.), *Game play: Therapeutic use of childhood games.* New York: Wiley.

Karen, R. (1994). *Becoming attached.* New York: Warner Books.

Katz, K. (1992). Communication problems in maltreated children: A tutorial. *Journal of Childhood Communication Disorders, 14,* 147–163.

Kaufman, A. S., & Kaufman, N. L. (1983). *Kaufman Assessment Battery for Children.* Circle Pines, MN: American Guidance Center.

Kaufman, J., & Cicchetti, D. (1989). Effects of maltreatment on school-age children's socio-emotional development: Assessments in a day camp setting. *Developmental Psychology, 25,* 516–524.

Kazdin, A. E., Moser, J., Colbus, D., & Bell, R. (1985). Depressive symptoms among physically abused and psychiatrically disturbed children. *Journal of Abnormal Psychology, 94,* 298–307.

Kendall, P. C., & Braswell, L. (1993). *Cognitive–behavioral therapy for impulsive children* (2nd ed.). New York: Guilford Press.

Kendall-Tackett, K. A., & Eckenrode, J. (1996). The effects of neglect on academic achievement and disciplinary problems: A developmental perspective. *Child Abuse and Neglect, 20,* 161–169.

Kendall-Tackett, K. A., Williams, L. M., & Finkelhor, D. (1993). Impact of sexual abuse on children: A review and synthesis of recent empirical studies. *Psychological Bulletin, 113,* 164–180.

Klagsbrun, M., & Bowlby, J. (1976). Responses to separation from parents: A clinical test for young children. *British Journal of Projective Psychology, 21,* 7–21.

Kluft, R. P. (1984). Multiple personality disorder in children. *Psychiatric Clinics of North America, 7,* 121–134.

Kluft, R. P. (1996). Outpatient treatment of Dissociative Identity Disorder and allied forms of Dissociative Disorder not otherwise specified in children and adolescents. *Child and Adolescent Psychiatric Clinics of North America, 5,* 471–494.

Kobak, R., & Sceery, A. (1988). Attachment in late adolescence: Working models, affect regulation, and representations of self and others. *Child Development, 59,* 135–146.

Kolko, D. J. (1992). Characteristics of child victims of physical violence: Research findings and clinical implications. *Journal of Interpersonal Violence, 7,* 244–276.

Kovacs, M. (1983). *The Children's Depression Inventory: A self-rated depression scale for school-aged youngsters.* Unpublished manuscript, University of Pittsburgh.

Koverola, C., Pound, J., Heger, A., & Lytle, C. (1993). Relationship of child sexual abuse to depression. *Child Abuse and Neglect, 17,* 393–400.

Kurtz, K. J., Gaudin, J. M., Wodarski, J. S., & Howing, P. T. (1993). Maltreatment and the school-aged child: School performance consequences. *Child Abuse and Neglect, 17,* 581–590.

Lamb, S. (1986). Treating sexually abused children: Issues of blame and responsibility. *American Journal of Orthopsychiatry, 56,* 303–307.

Lanktree, C. B., & Briere, J. (1995). Outcome of therapy for sexually abused children: A repeated measures study. *Child Abuse and Neglect, 19,* 1145–1155.

Lanktree, C. B., Briere, J., & Zaidi, L. Y. (1991). Incidence and impacts of sexual abuse in a child outpatient sample: The role of direct inquiry. *Child Abuse and Neglect, 15,* 447–453.

Leifer, M., Shapiro, J. P., & Kassem, L. (1993). The impact of maternal history and behavior upon foster placement and adjustment in sexually abused children. *Child Abuse and Neglect, 17,* 755–766.

Levine, M. D. (1985). *The ANSER System.* Cambridge, MA: Educators Publishing Service.

Levy, D. (1939). Release therapy. *American Journal of Orthopsychiatry, 9,* 713–736.

Lewandowdski, L. A., & Baranoski, M. V. (1994). Psychological aspects of acute trauma: Intervening with children and families in the inpatient setting. *Child and Adolescent Clinics of North America, 3,* 513–592.

Lewis, D. O. (1992). From abuse to violence: Psychophysiological consequences of maltreatment. *Journal of the American Academy of Child and Adolescent Psychiatry, 31,* 383–391.

Lewis, D. O. (1996). Diagnostic evaluation of the child with Dissociative Identity Disorder/Multiple Personality Disorder. *Child and Adolescent Psychiatric Clinics of North America, 5,* 303–331.

Lewis, D. O., Lovely, E., Yeager, C., & Della Femina, D. (1989). Toward a theory of the genesis of violence: A follow-up study of delinquents. *Journal of the American Academy of Child and Adolescent Psychiatry, 28,* 431–436.

Lewis, D. O., Lovely, E., Yeager, C., Ferguson, G., Friedman, M., Sloane, G., Friedman, H., & Pincus, J. H. (1988). Intrinsic and environmental characteristics of juvenile murderers. *Journal of the American Academy of Child and Adolescent Psychiatry, 27,* 582–587.

Lewis, D. O., & Yeager, C. A. (1994). Abuse, dissociative phenomena, and childhood multiple personality disorder. *Child and Adolescent Psychiatric Clinics of North America, 3,* 729–743.

Lewis, D. O., Yeager, C. A., Cobham-Portorreal, C. S., Klein, N., Showalter, C.,

& Anthony, A. (1991). A follow-up of female delinquents: Maternal contributions to the perpetuation of deviance. *Journal of the American Academy of Child and Adolescent Psychiatry, 30,* 197–201.

Lieberman, A. F. (1991). Attachment theory and infant–parent psychotherapy: Some conceptual, clinical, and research considerations. In D. Cicchetti & S. L. Toth (Eds.), *Rochester Symposium on Developmental Psychopathology: Vol. 3. Models and integrations* (pp. 375–398). Rochester, NY: University of Rochester Press.

Lieberman, A. F. (1992). Infant–parent psychotherapy with toddlers. *Development and Psychopathology, 4,* 559–574.

Lieberman, A. F., & Pawl, J. H. (1990). Disorders of attachment and secure base behavior in the second year of life: Conceptual issues and clinical intervention. In M. T. Greenberg, D. Cicchetti, & E. M. Cummings (Eds.), *Attachment in the preschool years* (pp. 375–398). Chicago: University of Chicago Press.

Lieberman, A. F., Weston, D., & Pawl, J. H. (1991). Preventive intervention and outcome with anxiously attached dyads. *Child Development, 62,* 199–209.

Lieberman, A. F., & Zeannah, C. H. (1995). Disorders of attachment in infancy. *Child and Adolescent Psychiatric Clinics of North America, 4,* 571–587.

Lipman, E. L., Offord, D. R., & Boyle, M. H. (1994). Relation between economic disadvantage and psychosocial morbidity in children. *Canadian Medical Association Journal, 151,* 431–437.

Littner, N. (1960). The child's need to repeat his past: Some implications for placement. *Social Services Review, 34,* 128–148.

Lochman, J. E., White, K. J., & Wayland, K. K. (1991). Cognitive–behavioral assessment and treatment with aggressive children. In P. C. Kendall (Ed.), *Child and adolescent therapy: Cognitive–behavioral procedures* (pp. 25–65). New York: Guilford Press.

Looney, J. G. (1984). Treatment planning in child psychiatry. *Journal of the American Academy of Child Psychiatry, 23,* 529–536.

Lyon, E. (1993). Hospital staff reactions to accounts by survivors of childhood abuse. *American Journal of Orthopsychiatry, 63,* 410–416.

Lyons-Ruth, K., Alpern, L., & Repacholi, B. (1993). Disorganized infant attachment classification and maternal psychosocial problems as predictors of hostile–aggressive behavior in the preschool classroom. *Child Development, 64,* 572–585.

Lyons-Ruth, K., Repacholi, B., McLeod, S., & Silva, E. (1991). Disorganized attachment behavior in infancy: Short-term stability, maternal and infant correlates, risk-related subtypes. *Development and Psychopathology, 3,* 377–396.

MacFarlane, K., & Cunningham, C. (1988). *Steps to healthy touching.* Mt. Dora, FL: Kidsrights.

Main, M. (1981). Avoidance in the service of attachment: A working paper. In K. Immelman, G. Barlow, L. Petrinovich, & M. Main (Eds.), *Behavioral development* (pp. 651–693). Cambridge, England: Cambridge University Press.

Main, M. (1990). Cross-cultural studies of attachment organization: Recent studies, changing methodologies, and the concept of conditional strategies. *Human Development, 33,* 48–61.

Main, M., & Cassidy, J. (1988). Categories of response to reunion with the parent at age 6: Predictable from infant classifications and stable over a 1-month period. *Developmental Psychology, 24,* 425–426.

Main, M., & George, C. (1985). Response of abused and disadvantaged toddlers to distress in agemates: A study in the day care setting. *Developmental Psychology, 21,* 407–412.

Main, M., & Goldwyn, R. (1984). Predicting rejection of her infant from other's representation of her own experience: Implications for the abused–abusing intergenerational cycle. *Child Abuse and Neglect, 8,* 203–217.

Main, M., & Hesse, E. (1990). Parents' unresolved traumatic experiences are related to infant disorganized attachment status: Is frightened and/or frightening parental behavior the linking mechanism? In M. Greenberg, D. Cicchetti, & E. M. Cummings (Eds.), *Attachment in the preschool years: Theory, research and intervention* (pp. 161–184). Chicago: The University of Chicago Press.

Main, M., Kaplan, N., & Cassidy, J. (1985). Security in infancy, childhood, and adulthood: A move to the level of representation. In I. Bretherton & E. Waters (Eds.), Growing points of attachment theory and research. *Monographs of the Society for Research in Child Development, 50*(1–2, Serial No. 209), 66–104.

Main, M., & Solomon, J. (1986). Discovery of an insecure disorganized/disoriented attachment pattern. In T. B. Brazelton & M. W. Yogman (Eds.), *Affective development in infancy* (pp. 95–124). Norwood, NJ: Ablex.

Main, M., & Solomon, J. (1990). Procedures for identifying infants as disorganized/disoriented during the Ainsworth strange situation. In M. Greenberg, D. Cicchetti, & M. Cummings (Eds.), *Attachment in the preschool years* (pp. 121–160). Chicago: University of Chicago Press.

Main, M., & Weston, D. (1982). Avoidance of the attachment figure in infancy: Descriptions and interpretations. In C. M. Parkes & J. Stevenson-Hinde (Eds.), *The place of attachment in human behavior* (Vol. 8, pp. 203–217). London: Tavistock.

Malinosky-Rummell, R., & Hansen, D. J. (1993). Long-term consequences of childhood physical abuse. *Psychological Bulletin, 114,* 68–79.

Malinosky-Rummell, R., & Hoeir, T. S. (1991). Validating measures of dissociation in sexually abused and nonabused children. *Behavioral Assessment, 13,* 341–357.

Mandell, J. G., & Damon, L. (1989). *Group treatment for sexually abused children.* New York: Guilford Press.

Manly, J. T., Cicchetti, D., & Barnett, D. (1994). The impact of maltreatment on child outcome: An exploration of dimensions within maltreatment. *Development and Psychopathology, 6,* 121–143.

Mann, E., & McDermott, J. F. (1983). Play therapy for victims of child abuse and neglect. In C. E. Schaefer & K. J. O'Connor (Eds.), *Handbook of play therapy* (pp. 283–307). New York: Wiley.

Mannarino, A. P., & Cohen, J. A. (1986). A clinical–demographic study of sexually abused children. *Child Abuse and Neglect, 10,* 17–23.

Mannarino, A. P., Cohen, J. A., & Berman, S. R. (1994). The Children's Attributions and Perceptions Scale: A new measure of sexual abuse-related factors. *Journal of Clinical Child Psychology, 23,* 204–211.

Mantzicopoulos, P. Y., & Morrison, D. (1994). A comparison of boys and girls with attention problems: Kindergarten through second grade. *American Journal of Orthopsychiatry, 64,* 522–533.

Martin, H. P., Beezley, P., Conway, E. F., & Kempe, C. H. (1974). The development of the abused child. *Advances in Pediatrics, 21,* 25–73.

Masten, A. S., Best, K. M., & Garmezy, N. (1990). Resilience and development: Contributions from the study of children who overcome adversity. *Development and Psychopathology, 2,* 425–444.

McArthur, D. S., & Roberts, G. E. (1982). *Roberts Apperception Test for Children manual.* Los Angeles: Western Psychological Services.

McCarthy, D. (1972). *McCarthy Scales of Children's Abilities manual.* New York: Psychological Corporation.

McCrone, E. R., Egeland, B., Kalkoske, M., & Carlson, E. A. (1994). Relations between early maltreatment and mental representations of relationships assessed with projective storytelling in middle childhood. *Development and Psychopathology, 6,* 99–120.

McGain, B., & McKinzey, R. K. (1995). The efficacy of group treatment in sexually abused girls. *Child Abuse and Neglect, 19,* 1157–1169.

McGee, R. A., & Wolfe, D. A. (1991). Psychological maltreatment: Toward an operational definition. *Development and Psychopathology, 3,* 3–18.

McLeer, S. V., Deblinger, E., Atkins, M. S., Foa, E. B., & Ralphe, D. L. (1988). Posttraumatic stress disorder in sexually abused children. *Journal of the American Academy of Child and Adolescent Psychiatry, 27,* 650–654.

Merry, S. N., & Andrews, L. K. (1994). Psychiatric status of sexually abused children 12 months after disclosure of abuse. *Journal of the American Academy of Child and Adolescent Psychiatry, 33,* 939–944.

Miller-Perrin, C. L., Wurtele, S. K., & Kondrick, P. A. (1990). Sexually abused and nonabused children's conceptions of personal body safety. *Child Abuse and Neglect, 14,* 99–112.

Mills, B., & Allan, J. (1992). Play therapy with the maltreated child: Impact upon aggressive and withdrawn patterns of interaction. *International Journal of Play Therapy, 1,* 1–20.

Mills, J. C., & Crowley, R. J. (1986). *Therapeutic metaphors for children and the child within.* New York: Brunner/Mazel.

Milner, J. S. (1986). *The Child Abuse Potential Inventory: Manual* (Rev. ed.). Webster, NC: Psytec Corporation.

Money, J. (1977). The syndrome of abuse dwarfism (psychosocial dwarfism or reversible hyposomatotropism). *American Journal of Diseases in Childhood, 131,* 508–513.

Money, J., & Annecillo, C. (1976). IQ change following change of domicile in the syndrome of reversible hyposomatotropism: Pilot investigation. *Psychoneuroendocrinology, 1,* 427–239.

Money, J., Annecillo, C., & Kelly, J. F. (1983). Abuse–dwarfism syndrome: After rescue, statural and intellectual catchup growth correlate. *Journal of Clinical Child Psychology, 12,* 279–283.

Mowrer, O. H. (1960). *Learning theory and behavior.* New York: Wiley.

Mrazek, P. B. (1981). Group psychotherapy with sexually abused children. In P. B. Mrazek & C. H. Kempe (Eds.), *Sexually abused children and their families* (pp. 199–210). New York: Pergamon Press.

Mueller, E., & Silverman, N. (1989). Peer relations in maltreated children. In D.

Cicchetti & V. Carlson (Eds.), *Child maltreatment: Theory and research on the causes and consequences of child abuse and neglect* (pp. 529–578). New York: Cambridge University Press.

Murray, H. (1938). *Explorations in personality.* New York: Oxford University Press.

Murray, H. (1943). *Thematic Apperception Test—manual.* Cambridge, MA: Harvard University Press.

National Center on Child Abuse and Neglect. (1981). *National incidence and prevalence of child abuse and neglect.* Washington, DC: U. S. Government Printing Office.

Nelson, K., & Gruendal, J. (1981). Generalized event representations: Basic building blocks of cognitive development. In M. Lamb & A. Brown (Eds.), *Advances in developmental psychology* (Vol. I, pp. 131–158). Hillsdale, NJ: Erlbaum.

Ney, P. G., Fung, T., & Wickett, A. R. (1994). The worst combinations of child abuse and neglect. *Child Abuse and Neglect, 18,* 705–714.

Oates, R. K., Peacock, A., & Forrest, D. (1985). Long-term effects of nonorganic failure to thrive. *Pediatrics, 75,* 36–40.

Ollendick, T. H. (1983). Reliability and validity of the Revised Fear Survey Schedule for Children (FSSCR-R). *Behavior Research and Therapy, 21,* 685–692.

Parker, G. B., Barrett, B. A., & Hickie, I. B. (1992). From nurture to network: Examining links between perceptions of parenting received in childhood and social bonds in adulthood. *American Journal of Psychiatry, 149,* 877–885.

Patterson, G. R. (1980). *Living with children: New methods for parents and teachers.* Champaign, IL: Research Press.

Patterson, G. R., Redi, J. B., Jones, R. R., & Conger, R. E. (1975). *A social learning approach to family intervention: Vol. 1. Families with aggressive children.* Eugene, OR: Castalia.

Pearce, J. W., & Pezzot-Pearce, T. D. (1994). Attachment theory and its implications for psychotherapy with maltreated children. *Child Abuse and Neglect, 18,* 425–438.

Petersen, C., & Seligman, M. E. P. (1983). Learned helplessness and victimization. *Journal of Social Issues, 39,* 103–116.

Peterson, G. (1991). Children coping with trauma: Diagnosis of "dissociation identity disorder." *Dissociation, 4,* 152–164.

Pezzot, T. D. (1978). *Battered and neglected children: Developmental characteristics and the familial–environmental factors involved in abuse.* Unpublished master's thesis, University of Manitoba, Winnipeg, Manitoba, Canada.

Piaget, J. (1952). *The origins of intelligence.* New York: Norton.

Piaget, J. (1967). *Six psychological studies.* New York: Random House.

Piers, E. V., & Harris, D. B. (1969). *The Piers–Harris Children's Self-Concept Scale.* Nashville, TN: Counselor Recordings and Tests.

Polansky, N. A., Chalmers, M. A., Buttenwieser, E., & Williams, D. P. (1981). *Damaged parents: An anatomy of child neglect.* Chicago: University of Chicago Press.

Powell, G. F., Brasel, J. A., & Blizzard, R. M. (1967). Emotional deprivation and growth retardation simulating idiopathic hypopituitarism: I. Clinical evaluation of the syndrome. *New England Journal of Medicine, 276,* 1271–1278.

Powell, G. F., Brasel, J. A., Raiti, S., & Blizzard, R. M. (1967). Emotional deprivation and growth retardation simulating idiopathic hypopituitarism: I. Endocrinologic evaluation of the syndrome. *New England Journal of Medicine, 276,* 1279–1283.

Province of Alberta. (1984). *Child Welfare Act, Chapter C-8.1.* Edmonton, Alberta, Canada: Queen's Printer.

Psychological Corporation. (1992). *Wechsler Individual Achievement Test manual.* San Antonio: Harcourt Brace Jovanovich.

Putnam, F. W. (1989). *Diagnosis and treatment of multiple personality disorder.* New York: Guilford Press.

Putnam, F. W. (1991). Dissociative disorders in children and adolescents: A developmental perspective. *Psychiatric Clinics of North America, 14,* 519–531.

Putnam, F. W. (1993). Dissociative disorders in children: Behavioral profiles and problems. *Child Abuse and Neglect, 17,* 39–45.

Putnam, F. W. (1995). Development of dissociative disorders. In D. Cicchetti & D. J. Cohen (Eds.), *Developmental psychopathology: Vol. 2. Risk, disorder, and adaptation* (pp. 581–608). New York: Wiley.

Putnam, F. W., Helmers, K., & Trickett, P. K. (1993). Development, reliability, and validity of a child dissociation scale. *Child Abuse and Neglect, 17,* 731–741.

Pynoos, R. S., & Eth, S. (1986). Witness to violence: The child interview. *Journal of the American Academy of Child Psychiatry, 25,* 306–319.

Rasmussen, L. A., & Cunningham, C. (1995). Focused play therapy and nondirective play therapy: Can they be integrated? *Journal of Child Sexual Abuse, 4,* 1–20.

Reagor, P. A., Kasten, J. D., & Morelli, N. (1992). A checklist for screening dissociative disorders in children and adolescents. *Dissociation, 5,* 4–19.

Regehr, C. (1990). Parental responses to extrafamilial child sexual assault. *Child Abuse and Neglect, 14,* 113–120.

Reynolds, C. R., & Richmond, B. O. (1978). What I think and feel: A revised measure of children's anxiety. *Journal of Abnormal Child Psychology, 6,* 271–280.

Rieder, C., & Cicchetti, D. (1989). An organizational perspective on cognitive control functioning and cognitive–affective balance in maltreated children. *Developmental Psychology, 25,* 382–393.

Ross, A. O. (1964). Interruptions and termination of treatment. In M. R. Haworth (Ed.), *Child psychotherapy: Practice and theory* (pp. 292–297). New York: Basic Books.

Ross, C. A., Anderson, G., Fleisher, W. P., & Norton, G. R. (1991). The frequency of multiple personality disorder among psychiatric inpatients. *American Journal of Psychiatry, 148,* 1717–1720.

Runyan, D. K., Everson, M. D., Edelsohn, G. A., Hunter, W. M., & Coulter, M. L. (1988). Impact of legal intervention on sexually abused children. *Journal of Pediatrics, 113,* 647–653.

Russell, D. E. H. (1983). The incidence and prevalence of intrafamilial and extrafamilial sexual abuse of female children. *Child Abuse and Neglect, 7,* 133–146.

Rutter, M. (1985). Resilience in the face of adversity: Protective factors and resistance to psychiatric disorder. *British Journal of Psychiatry, 147,* 598–611.

Rutter, M. (1987). Psychosocial resilience and protective mechanisms. *American Journal of Orthopsychiatry, 57,* 316–331.

Rutter, M. (1993). Resilience: Some conceptual considerations. *Journal of Adolescent Health, 14,* 626–631.

Rutter, M. (1995). Clinical implications of attachment concepts: Retrospect and prospect. *Journal of Child Psychology and Psychiatry, 36,* 549–571.

Ryan, G. (1989). Victim to victimizer: Rethinking victim treatment. *Journal of Interpersonal Violence, 4,* 325–341.

Salzinger, S., Kaplan, S., Pelcovitz, D., Samit, C., & Krieger, R. (1984). Parent and teacher assessment of children's behavior in child maltreating families. *Journal of the American Academy of Child Psychiatry, 23,* 458–464.

Sanders, B., & Giolas, M. H. (1991). Dissociation and childhood trauma in psychologically disturbed adolescents. *American Journal of Psychiatry, 148,* 50–54.

Sandler, J., Kennedy, H., & Tyson, R. L. (1980). *The technique of child psychoanalysis—Discussions with Anna Freud.* Cambridge, MA: Harvard University Press.

Scerbo, A. S., & Kolko, D. J. (1995). Child physical abuse and aggression: Preliminary findings on the role of internalizing problems. *Journal of the American Academy of Child and Adolescent Psychiatry, 34,* 1060–1066.

Schene, P. (1987). Is child abuse decreasing? *Journal of Interpersonal Violence, 2,* 225–227.

Scherer, M. W., & Nakamura, C. Y. (1968). A Fear Survey Schedule for Children (FSS-FC): A factor-analytic comparison with manifest anxiety. *Behaviour Research and Therapy, 6,* 173–182.

Schowalter, J. E. (1985). Countertransference in work with children: Review of a neglected concept. *Journal of the American Academy of Child Psychiatry, 25,* 40–45.

Schutz, B. M., Dixon, E. B., Lindenberger, N. J., & Ruther, N. J. (1989). *Solomon's sword.* San Francisco: Jossey-Bass.

Scully, L. (Writer/Director). (1992). *Good things can still happen* [Video]. Montreal: National Film Board of Canada.

Sedlack, A. J. (1991). *National incidence and prevalence of child abuse and neglect: 1988 revised report.* Rockville, MD: Westat.

Shields, A. M., Cicchetti, D., & Ryan, R. M. (1994). The development of emotional and behavioral self-regulation and social competence among maltreated school-age children. *Development and Psychopathology, 6,* 57–76.

Shirk, S. R. (1988). The interpersonal legacy of physical abuse of children. In M. B. Straus (Ed.), *Abuse and victimization across the life span* (pp. 57–81). Baltimore: John Hopkins University Press.

Shirk, S. R., & Saiz, C. C. (1992). Clinical, empirical, and developmental perspectives on the therapeutic relationship in child psychotherapy. *Development and Psychopathology, 4,* 713–728.

Shouldice, A., & Stevenson-Hinde, J. (1992). Coping with security distress: The Separation Anxiety Test and attachment classification at 4.5 years. *Journal of Child Psychology and Psychiatry, 33,* 331–348.

Smith, J. D., Walsh, R. T., & Richardson, M. A. (1985). The clown club: A structured fantasy approach to group therapy with the latency-age child. *International Journal of Group Psychotherapy, 35,* 49–64.

Solomon, J., George, C., & De Jong, A. (1995). Children classified as controlling at age six: Evidence of disorganized representational strategies and aggression at home and at school. *Development and Psychopathology, 7,* 447–463.

Spanier, G. B. (1976). Measuring dyadic adjustment: New scales for assessing the quality of marriage and similar dyads. *Journal of Marriage and the Family, 38,* 15–28.

Sparrow, S., Balla, D., & Cicchetti, D. (1984). *Vineland Adaptive Behavior Scales.* Circle Pines, MN: American Guidance Service.

Spielberger, C. D. (1973). *State–Trait Anxiety Inventory for Children*. Palo Alto, CA: Consulting Psychologists Press.

Spitz, R. (1945). Hospitalism: An inquiry into the genesis of psychiatric conditions in early childhood. *Psychoanalytic Study of the Child, 1,* 53–74.

Spitz, R. (1946). Anaclitic depression. *Psychoanalytic Study of the Child, 2,* 313–342.

Spivak, G., Platt, J. J., & Shure, M. B. (1976). *The problem-solving approach to adjustment.* San Francisco: Jossey-Bass.

Sroufe, L. A. (1979). The coherence of individual development: Early care, attachment, and subsequent developmental issues. *American Psychologist, 34,* 834–841.

Sroufe, L. A. (1988). The role of infant–caregiver attachment in development. In J. Belsky & T. Nezworski (Eds.), *Clinical implications of attachment* (pp. 18–38). Hillsdale, NJ: Erlbaum.

Sroufe, L. A., & Fleeson, J. (1986). Attachment and the construction of relationships. In W. Hartup and Z. Rubin (Eds.), *Relationships and development* (pp. 51–71). Hillsdale, NJ: Erlbaum.

Sroufe, L. A., & Rutter, M. (1984). The domain of developmental psychopathology. *Child Development, 55,* 17–29.

Stauffer, L. B., & Deblinger, E. (1996). Cognitive behavioral groups for nonoffending mothers and their young sexually abused children: A preliminary treatment outcome study. *Child Maltreatment, 1,* 65–76.

Steele, B. F., & Pollock, C. B. (1968). A psychiatric study of parents who abuse infants and small children. In C. H. Kempe & R. E. Helfer (Eds.), *The battered child* (pp. 103–147). Chicago: University of Chicago Press.

Steinberg, M. (1996). Diagnostic tools for assessing dissociation in children and adolescents. *Child and Adolescent Psychiatric Clinics of North America, 5,* 333–349.

Stern, J. B., & Fodor, I. G. (1989). Anger control in children: A review of social skills and cognitive behavioral approaches to dealing with aggressive children. *Child and Family Behavior Therapy, 11,* 1–20.

Steward, M. S., Bussey, K., Goodman, G. S., & Saywitz, K. J. (1993). Implications of developmental research for interviewing children. *Child Abuse and Neglect, 17,* 25–38.

Stovall, G., & Craig, R. J. (1990). Mental representations of physically and sexually abused latency-aged females. *Child Abuse and Neglect, 14,* 233–242.

Straker, G., & Jacobson, R. S. (1989). Aggression, emotional maladjustment, and empathy in the abused child. *Developmental Psychology, 17,* 762–765.

Straus, M. (1979). Measuring intrafamily conflicts and violence: The Conflicts Tactic (CT) Scales. *Journal of Marriage and the Family, 41,* 75–88.

Terr, L. C. (1990). *Too scared to cry.* New York: Harper and Row.

Terr, L. C. (1991). Childhood traumas: An outline and overview. *American Journal of Psychiatry, 148,* 10–20.

Thorndike, R. L., Hagen, E. P., & Sattler, J. M. (1986). *Stanford–Binet Intelligence Scale: Guide for administering and scoring the fourth edition.* Chicago: Riverside.

Tong, L., Oates, K., & McDowell, M. (1987). Personality development following sexual abuse. *Child Abuse and Neglect, 11,* 371–383.

Toth, S. L., Manly, J. T., & Cicchetti, D. (1992). Child maltreatment and vulnerability to depression. *Development and Psychopathology, 4,* 97–112.

Trickett, P. K., McBride-Chang, C., & Putnam, F. W. (1994). The classroom per-

formance and behavior of sexually abused females. *Development and Psychopathology,*
6, 183–194.

Troy, M., & Sroufe, L. A. (1987). Victimization among preschoolers: The role
of attachment relationship history. *Journal of the American Academy of Child and
Adolescent Psychiatry, 26,* 166–172.

Trupin, E., Tarico, V., Low, B., Jemelka, R., & McClellan, J. (1993). Children
on child protective service caseloads: Prevalence and nature of serious emotional disturbance. *Child Abuse and Neglect, 17,* 345–355.

Tuft's New England Medical Center, Division of Psychiatry. (1984). *Sexually ex-
ploited children: Service and research project: Final report for the Office of Juvenile Justice
and Delinquency Prevention.* Washington, DC: U.S. Department of Justice.

Tutty, L. (1994). Developmental issues in young children's learning of sexual abuse
prevention concepts. *Child Abuse and Neglect, 18,* 179–192.

Urquiza, A. J., & Winn, C. (1994). *Treatment for abused and neglected children: Infancy to age 18.* Washington, DC: U.S. Department of Health and Human Services Administration for Children and Families.

van den Boom, D. C. (1994). The influence of temperament and mothering on
attachment and exploration: An experimental manipulation of sensitive responsiveness among lower-class mothers with irritable infants. *Child Development, 65,*
1457–1477.

Van de Putte, S. J. (1995). A paradigm for working with child survivors of sexual
abuse who exhibit sexualized behaviors during play therapy. *International Journal of Play Therapy, 4,* 27–49.

van IJzendoorn, M. H., Goldberg, S., Kroonenberg, P. M., & Frenkel, O. J. (1992).
The relative effects of maternal and child problems on the quality of attachment:
A meta-analysis of attachment in clinical samples. *Child Development, 63,* 840–858.

van IJzendoorn, M. H., Juffer, F., & Duyvesteyn, M. G. C. (1995). Breaking the
intergenerational cycle of insecure attachment: A review of the effects of
attachment-based interventions on maternal sensitivity and infant security. *Journal
of Child Psychology and Psychiatry, 36,* 225–248.

Veronen, L. J., & Kilpatrick, D. G. (1986). *The Impact of Event Scale.* Unpublished
manuscript, Medical University of South Carolina.

Vincent, M., & Pickering, R. (1988). Multiple personality disorder in childhood.
Canadian Journal of Psychiatry, 33, 524–529.

Vissing, Y. M., Straus, M. A., Gelles, R. J., & Harrop, J. W. (1991). Verbal aggression by parents and psychosocial problems of children. *Child Abuse and
Neglect, 15,* 223–238.

Vondra, J., Barnett, D., & Cicchetti, D. (1989). Perceived and actual competence
among maltreated and comparison school children. *Development and Psychopathology, 1,* 237–255.

Vondra, J., Barnett, D., & Cicchetti, D. (1990). Self-concept, motivation, and competence among preschoolers from maltreating and comparison families. *Child
Abuse and Neglect, 14,* 525–540.

Wachtel, P. L. (1973). *Psychoanalysis and behavior therapy: Toward an integration.* New
York: Basic Books.

Waterman, J., & Lusk, R. (1993). Psychological testing in evaluation of child sexual abuse. *Child Abuse and Neglect, 17,* 145–160.

Weaver, T. L., & Clum, G. A. (1995). Psychological distress associated with inter-personal violence: A meta-analysis. *Clinical Psychology Review, 15,* 115–140.

Webb, N. B. (Ed.). (1991). *Play therapy with children in crisis: A casebook for practitioners.* New York: Guilford Press.

Wechsler, D. (1991). *WISC-III manual.* San Antonio: Psychological Corporation.

Werner, E. E. (1989). High risk children in young adulthood: A longitudinal study from birth to 32 years. *American Journal of Orthopsychiatry, 59,* 72–81.

Werner, E. E. (1993). Risk, resilience, and recovery: Perspectives from the Kauai Longitudinal Study. *Development and Psychopathology, 5,* 503–515.

West, M. L., & Sheldon-Keller, A. E. (1994). *Patterns of relating: An adult attachment perspective.* New York: Guilford Press.

Widom, C. S. (1989). The cycle of violence. *Science, 244,* 160–166.

Wilkinson, G. S. (1993). *The Wide Range Achievement Test: Administration manual.* Wilmington, DE: Wide Range.

Winnicott, D. (1965). *The family and individual development.* London: Tavistock.

Winton, M. A. (1990). An evaluation of a support group for parents who have a sexually abused child. *Child Abuse and Neglect, 14,* 397–405.

Wolfe, D. A. (1988). Child abuse and neglect. In E. J. Mash & L. G. Terdal (Eds.), *Behavioral assessment of childhood disorders* (2nd ed., pp. 627–669). New York: Guilford Press.

Wolfe, D. A., Sas, L., & Wekerle, C. (1994). Factors associated with the development of posttraumatic stress disorder among child victims of sexual abuse. *Child Abuse and Neglect, 18,* 37–50.

Wolfe, V. V., Gentile, C., & Wolfe, D. A. (1989). The impact of sexual abuse on children: A PTSD formulation. *Behavior Therapy, 20,* 215–228.

Wolfe, V. V., & Wolfe, D. A. (1988). The sexually abused child. In E. J. Mash & L. G. Terdal (Eds.), *Behavioral assessment of childhood disorders* (2nd ed., pp. 670–714). New York: Guilford Press.

Wozencraft, T., Wagner, W., & Pellegrin, A. (1991). Depression and suicidal ideation in sexually abused children. *Child Abuse and Neglect, 15,* 505–512.

Wright, J. D., Binney, V., & Smith, P. K. (1995). Security of attachment in 8-12 year-olds: A revised version of the Separation Anxiety Test, its psychometric properties and clinical interpretation. *Journal of Child Psychology and Psychiatry, 36,* 757–774.

Youngblade, L. M., & Belsky, J. (1990). The social and emotional consequences of child maltreatment. In R. Ammerman & M. Hersen (Eds.), *Children at risk: An evaluation of factors contributing to child abuse and neglect.* New York: Plenum Press.

Zeanah, C. H., & Zeanah, P. D. (1989). Intergenerational transmission of maltreatment: Insights from attachment theory and research. *Psychiatry, 52,* 177–196.

Index